Fe Deficiency, Dietary Bioavailability and Absorption

Fe Deficiency, Dietary Bioavailability and Absorption

Special Issue Editor

Elad Tako

MDPI • Basel • Beijing • Wuhan • Barcelona • Belgrade

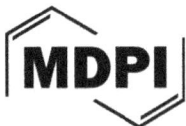

MDPI

Special Issue Editor
Elad Tako
Cornell University
USA

Editorial Office
MDPI
St. Alban-Anlage 66
Basel, Switzerland

This is a reprint of articles from the Special Issue published online in the open access journal *Nutrients* (ISSN 2072-6643) from 2017 to 2018 (available at: http://www.mdpi.com/journal/nutrients/special_issues/Fe_deficiency_bioavailbility_absorption)

For citation purposes, cite each article independently as indicated on the article page online and as indicated below:

LastName, A.A.; LastName, B.B.; LastName, C.C. Article Title. *Journal Name* **Year**, *Article Number*, Page Range.

ISBN 978-3-03897-230-3 (Pbk)
ISBN 978-3-03897-231-0 (PDF)

Contents

About the Special Issue Editor

Elad Tako holds degrees in animal science (B.S.), endocrinology (M.S.), and physiology/nutrigenomics (Ph.D.), with previous appointments at the Hebrew University of Jerusalem, North Carolina State University, and Cornell University. As a Research Physiologist with USDA/ARS, Dr. Tako's research focuses on various aspects of trace mineral deficiencies, emphasizing molecular, physiological and nutritional factors and practices that influence intestinal micronutrient absorption. With over 100 peer-reviewed publications and presentations, he leads a research team focused on understanding the interactions between dietary factors, physiological and molecular biomarkers, the microbiome, and intestinal functionality. His research accomplishments include the development of the Gallus gallus intra-amniotic administration procedure, and establishing recognized approaches for using animal models within mineral bioavailability and intestinal absorption screening processes. Specifically, he demonstrated that the broiler chicken (Gallus gallus) model exhibits appropriate responses to Fe deficiency and can serve as a model for Fe and Zn bioavailability and absorption. More recently, he also developed a zinc status physiological blood biomarker (red blood cell Linoleic Acid:Dihomo--Linolenic Acid Ratio), and molecular tissue biomarkers to assess the effect of dietary mineral deficiencies on intestinal functionality, and how micronutrients dietary deficiencies alter gut microbiota composition and function.

Preface to "Fe Deficiency, Dietary Bioavailability and Absorption"

Iron deficiency is widely observed worldwide, yet, paradoxically, iron (Fe) is the most plentiful heavy metal in the earth's crust. The World Health Organization (WHO) estimates that approximately one-third of worldwide infant deaths and one-half in developing countries can be attributed to malnutrition. More specifically, Fe deficiency is the most common nutritional deficiency worldwide and a major of infant mortality.

Although absorption of Fe from the gastrointestinal tract is strictly controlled, excretion is limited to Fe lost from exfoliation of skin and gastrointestinal cells, customary and abnormal blood loss, and menses. Individuals highly vulnerable to Fe deficiency have high iron needs, such as during growth or pregnancy; high Fe loss, such as during marked hemorrhage or excessive and/or frequent menstrual losses; or diets with low iron content or bioavailability. Food Fe is classified as heme or nonheme. Approximately half of the Fe in meat, fish, and poultry is heme Fe. Depending on an individual's Fe stores, 15% to 35% of heme Fe is absorbed. Food contains more nonheme Fe and, thus, it makes the larger contribution to the body's Fe pool despite its lower absorption rate of 2% to 20%. Absorption of nonheme Fe is markedly influenced by the levels of Fe stores and by concomitantly consumed dietary components. Enhancing factors, such as ascorbic acid and meat/fish/poultry, may increase nonheme iron bioavailability fourfold.

Fe deficiency is particularly widespread in low-income countries because of a general lack of consumption of animal products (which can promote non-heme Fe absorption and contain highly bioavailable heme Fe) coupled with a high consumption of a monotonous diet of cereal grains and legumes. Such diets are low in bioavailable Fe due to the presence of phytic acid and certain polyphenols that are inhibitors of Fe bioavailability. Further, recent research also suggests that cellular structures of legumes, such as the cotyledon cell walls, may also be a major factor limiting Fe absorption from legumes. Poor dietary quality is more often characterized by micronutrient deficiencies or reduced mineral bioavailability, than by insufficient energy intake. Diets with chronically poor Fe bioavailability which result in high prevalence of Fe deficiency and anemia, increase the risk of all-cause child mortalities and also may lead to many pathophysiological consequences, including stunted growth, low birth weight, delayed mental development and motor functioning, among others. Thus, a crucial step in alleviating Fe deficiency anemia is through understanding how specific dietary practices and components contribute to the Fe status in a particular region where Fe deficiency is prevalent.

In this context, one strategy to battle dietary Fe deficiency is biofortification (other strategies include, supplementation, fortification and diversification). Biofortification is the breeding of crops to increase their nutritional value, and has primarily focused on increased contents of Fe, Zn and pro-vitamin A. Biofortification aims to increase the nutrient density in crops during plant growth rather than during processing of the crops into foods. Developing staple food crops for enhanced nutritional quality often requires high throughput methods capable of examining hundreds and sometimes thousands of samples. In general, for zinc and pro vitamin A, the content of these micronutrients has been more positively correlated with enhanced nutritional quality; whereas for Fe, enhanced content does not always equate to improved nutritional quality. Understanding the factors related to the bioavailability of Fe may therefore be the key to developing sustainable Fe-biofortified crops, hence, the development of the appropriate screening tools is vital to properly guide the crop breeding process. For example, research has demonstrated that the Caco-2 cell bioassay is a fast and cost effective approach for screening hundreds of samples prior to the selection of the most promising lines to be assessed in vivo (Gallus gallus model) and, preferably, prior to human efficacy trials.

In the current manuscripts collection, we present a selection of recent advances and research developments related to improvements of dietary Fe bioavailability, metabolism and absorption in an effort to alleviate dietary Fe deficiency.

Elad Tako
Special Issue Editor

nutrients

MDPI

Article

Iron Fortified Complementary Foods Containing a Mixture of Sodium Iron EDTA with Either Ferrous Fumarate or Ferric Pyrophosphate Reduce Iron Deficiency Anemia in 12- to 36-Month-Old Children in a Malaria Endemic Setting: A Secondary Analysis of a Cluster-Randomized Controlled Trial

Dominik Glinz [1,2,3], **Rita Wegmüller** [1], **Mamadou Ouattara** [4,5], **Victorine G. Diakité** [5,6], **Grant J. Aaron** [7], **Lorenz Hofer** [8], **Michael B. Zimmermann** [1], **Lukas G. Adiossan** [9], **Jürg Utzinger** [3,8], **Eliézer K. N'Goran** [4,5] **and Richard F. Hurrell** [1,*]

[1] Laboratory of Human Nutrition, Institute of Food, Nutrition, and Health, ETH Zurich, CH-8092 Zurich, Switzerland; dominik.glinz@usb.ch (D.G.); rita@groundworkhealth.org (R.W.); michael.zimmermann@hest.ethz.ch (M.B.Z.)
[2] Basel Institute for Clinical Epidemiology and Biostatistics, University Hospital Basel, CH-4031 Basel, Switzerland
[3] University of Basel, P.O. Box, CH-4003 Basel, Switzerland; juerg.utzinger@swisstph.ch
[4] Université Félix Houphouët-Boigny, 01 BP V34, Abidjan 01, Côte d'Ivoire; mamadou_ouatt@yahoo.fr (M.O.); eliezerngoran@yahoo.fr (E.K.N.)
[5] Centre Suisse de Recherches Scientifiques en Côte d'Ivoire, 01 BP 1303, Abidjan 01, Côte d'Ivoire; sebagnoh@gmail.com
[6] Département de Sciologie, Université Alassane Ouattara, 01 BP V18 Bouaké, Côte d'Ivoire
[7] Global Alliance for Improved Nutrition, CH-1202 Geneva, Switzerland; gjaaron@masimo.com
[8] Swiss Tropical and Public Health Institute, P.O. Box, CH-4002 Basel, Switzerland; lhofer92@gmail.com
[9] Hôpital Général de Taabo, Taabo Cité, BP 700 Toumodi, Côte d'Ivoire; adiossanlukas@yahoo.fr
[*] Correspondence: richard.hurrell@hest.ethz.ch; Tel.: +41-44-632-8421

Received: 30 May 2017; Accepted: 11 July 2017; Published: 14 July 2017

Abstract: Iron deficiency anemia (IDA) is a major public health problem in sub-Saharan Africa. The efficacy of iron fortification against IDA is uncertain in malaria-endemic settings. The objective of this study was to evaluate the efficacy of a complementary food (CF) fortified with sodium iron EDTA (NaFeEDTA) plus either ferrous fumarate (FeFum) or ferric pyrophosphate (FePP) to combat IDA in preschool-age children in a highly malaria endemic region. This is a secondary analysis of a 9-month cluster-randomized controlled trial conducted in south-central Côte d'Ivoire. 378 children aged 12–36 months were randomly assigned to no food intervention (n = 125; control group), CF fortified with 2 mg NaFeEDTA plus 3.8 mg FeFum for six days/week (n = 126; FeFum group), and CF fortified with 2 mg NaFeEDTA and 3.8 mg FePP for six days/week (n = 127; FePP group). The outcome measures were hemoglobin (Hb), plasma ferritin (PF), iron deficiency (ID; PF < 30 μg/L), and anemia (Hb < 11.0 g/dL). Data were analyzed with random-effect models and PF was adjusted for inflammation. The prevalence of *Plasmodium falciparum* infection and inflammation during the study were 44–66%, and 57–76%, respectively. There was a significant time by treatment interaction on IDA (p = 0.028) and a borderline significant time by treatment interaction on ID with or without anemia (p = 0.068). IDA prevalence sharply decreased in the FeFum (32.8% to 1.2%, p < 0.001) and FePP group (23.6% to 3.4%, p < 0.001). However, there was no significant time by treatment interaction on Hb or total anemia. These data indicate that, despite the high endemicity of malaria and elevated inflammation biomarkers (C-reactive protein or α-1-acid-glycoprotein), IDA was markedly reduced by provision of iron fortified CF to preschool-age children for 9 months, with no significant differences between a combination of NaFeEDTA with FeFum or NaFeEDTA with FePP. However, there was no overall effect on anemia, suggesting most of the anemia in this setting is not due to ID. This trial is registered at clinicaltrials.gov (NCT01634945).

Keywords: anemia; cluster-randomized controlled trial; complementary food; Côte d'Ivoire; infant cereal; iron deficiency; iron deficiency anemia; iron fortification; *Plasmodium falciparum*; sodium iron EDTA

1. Introduction

Iron deficiency (ID) and anemia are considerable public health problems in sub-Saharan Africa [1]. For example, in Côte d'Ivoire, 25–75% of the preschool- and school-age children in rural areas are reported to be iron deficient, and about 80% are anemic [2], which can result in irreversible impairments in cognitive performance and motor development [3,4] unless additional iron is provided. One strategy to provide iron is through iron fortified complementary food (CF). However, this approach is not without challenges due to a large variation in the bioavailability of commonly used iron fortification compounds, frequent unacceptable sensory changes caused by the water soluble iron compounds of highest bioavailability, and the presence of phytic acid (PA), a potent inhibitor of iron absorption in CF containing cereals or legumes [5].

The iron compounds most commonly utilized to fortify CF are ferrous fumarate (FeFum), ferric pyrophosphate (FePP), and electrolytic iron. Ferrous sulfate is less commonly employed as it often causes unacceptable sensory changes in CF [6]. In order to overcome the inhibitory effect of PA on iron absorption, commercially manufactured infant cereals usually contain additional ascorbic acid (AA) at 2:1 molar ratio (AA:Fe), as recommended by the World Health Organization (WHO) [7]. Sodium iron ethylenediaminetetraacetate (NaFeEDTA) is an alternative iron compound that will overcome PA inhibition and is the iron compound of choice for fortifying high PA foods [5]. The Joint Food and Agriculture Organization (FAO)/WHO Expert Committee on Food Additives approved this compound, but proposed an acceptable daily intake of EDTA of 0.2 mg/kg body weight per day which restricts its use in young children [8].

Another potential barrier to the efficacy of iron fortified CF in Côte d'Ivoire is the widespread persistent low-grade inflammation caused by *Plasmodium* spp. (the causative agent of malaria) parasitemia that is reported to decrease iron absorption through increase in hepcidin [9,10]. Previous efficacy studies with iron fortified foods conducted in malaria-endemic settings revealed conflicting results. Iron status improved in young Kenyan children fed NaFeEDTA-fortified maize porridge [11] and in Ivorian school-age children who received meals containing salt fortified with micronized ground FePP [12], which was in line with findings obtained from children in non-malaria endemic areas [13]. In contrast, another trial conducted in Ivorian school-age children found that electrolytic iron fortified biscuits did not improve children's iron status [14]; the authors suggested this was due to malaria-induced inflammation and use of an iron fortificant with low bioavailability (electrolytic iron) [14].

The aim of this secondary analysis was to determine whether an iron fortified maize-soy CF is efficacious in improving iron status of 12- to 36-month-old Ivorian children in a setting that is hyper-endemic for *Plasmodium falciparum*. We used a locally produced, commercially available fortified CF containing NaFeEDTA and FePP. Additionally, we manufactured a second CF in which FePP was replaced by FeFum. In both CFs, we used the maximum acceptable level of iron as NaFeEDTA (i.e., 2 mg, assuming a mean body weight of 10 kg in our study population of children aged 12–36 months at baseline) [8]. The iron level was completed with 3.8 mg Fe as either FeFum or FePP. Hence, daily feeding of our maize-soy CF provided an extra 5.8 mg iron, equivalent to 100% of the reference nutrient intake (RNI) for one- to three-year-old children assuming an intermediate iron bioavailability of 10% [7]. Children were fed the CF fortified with iron once per day, six days per week, for nine months. Hemoglobin (Hb), iron status (plasma ferritin, PF), prevalence of *P. falciparum*, and inflammation were monitored and compared to a control group of children consuming their normal diet. The main (primary) analysis of the study was to investigate the interaction between iron fortified CF and intermittent preventive treatment (IPT) of malaria in improving Hb concentration. These results have been published elsewhere [15]. In short, no evidence was found for a treatment interaction between IPT and iron fortified CF to increase Hb concentration.

2. Subjects and Methods

2.1. Study Site and Participants

The study was carried out in the Taabo health and demographic surveillance system (HDSS) in south-central Côte d'Ivoire [16,17]. Located in the transition zone from rainforest (in the South) to savannah (in the North), the Taabo HDSS has ≈43,000 registered inhabitants and is hyper-endemic for malaria [18]. Depending on season and age of the inhabitants, the prevalence of *P. falciparum* ranges from 35–77% [2,19]. Cassava, plantain, and yam are mainly planted for local consumption, whereas coffee and cacao are cash crops. There is a limited amount of fish consumption from local rivers and lakes.

In April 2012, we selected 840 children from five villages (i.e., Ahouaty, Kokoti-Kouamekro, Kotiessou, N'Denou, and Taabo Village) in the designated age range (12–36 months) from the readily available Taabo HDSS database. Children were invited to participate in a baseline screening done from mid-April to mid-May 2012.

2.2. Study Design and Procedure

We present a secondary analysis of the larger study with key findings published elsewhere [15]. The primary analysis comprised five study groups (Figure 1) and focused on the interaction of iron fortified CF and IPT of malaria on Hb concentration (primary outcome). We selected 629 eligible children at the baseline screening and grouped them into 40 clusters based on proximity of their residence, with at least five clusters in each of the five study villages. Each cluster included between 13 and 18 children. Inclusion criteria were as follows: (i) Hb ≥ 7 g/dL; (ii) no major chronic illnesses, as determined by a study physician; (iii) anticipated residence in the study area for the 9-month intervention; and (iv) no known allergies to albendazole (treatment of choice against soil-transmitted helminthiasis). The clusters were randomly assigned to five study groups by drawing cluster numbers from a hat (urn randomization) together with village authorities. The study groups were: group 1, no nutritional intervention (continuation with the normal diet) and IPT-placebo; group 2, iron fortified CF containing FeFum + NaFeEDTA (FeFum) and IPT-placebo; group 3, no nutritional intervention and IPT of malaria (3-month intervals, using sulfadoxine-pyrimethamine and amodiaquine); group 4, iron fortified CF containing FeFum + NaFeEDTA (FeFum) and IPT of malaria (3-month intervals, using sulfadoxine-pyrimethamine and amodiaquine); and group 5, iron fortified CF containing FePP + NaFeEDTA (FePP) and IPT-placebo. In the current analysis, we focus solely on the iron status of children in the study groups receiving the iron fortified CF (groups 2 and 5) and compare changes in children's iron status biomarkers over the 9-month intervention with children in the control group (group 1). Hence, 251 children (groups 3 and 4; 16 clusters overall) were excluded from the current analysis.

Study approval was obtained from the institutional review board of ETH Zurich (reference No. EK 2009-N-19) and the national ethics committee of Côte d'Ivoire (reference No. 061 MSLS/CNER). Village authorities, health authorities, and parents/guardians of participating children were informed about the purpose, procedures, and potential risks and benefits of the study. Written informed consent from parents/guardians of the participating children was received. The study progress was assessed by an independent Data and Safety Monitoring Board that provided expertise and evaluated the safety of the study. We registered the trial at clinicaltrials.gov (NCT01634945).

2.3. CF Production, Preparation, and Child Feeding

Protein Kissèe-La (Abidjan, Côte d'Ivoire) manufactured the cereal-based, pre-cooked, instant CF. The composition of both study CFs was identical except for the iron compounds. The first study CF-FeFum contained 2.0 mg iron in form of NaFeEDTA and 3.8 mg iron in form of FeFum in a daily serving of 25 g dry weight porridge. The second study CF-FePP is the commercial product from Protein Kissèe-La, sold in Abidjan and contains 2.0 mg iron in form of NaFeEDTA and 3.8 mg iron in form of FePP in the same 25 g serving.

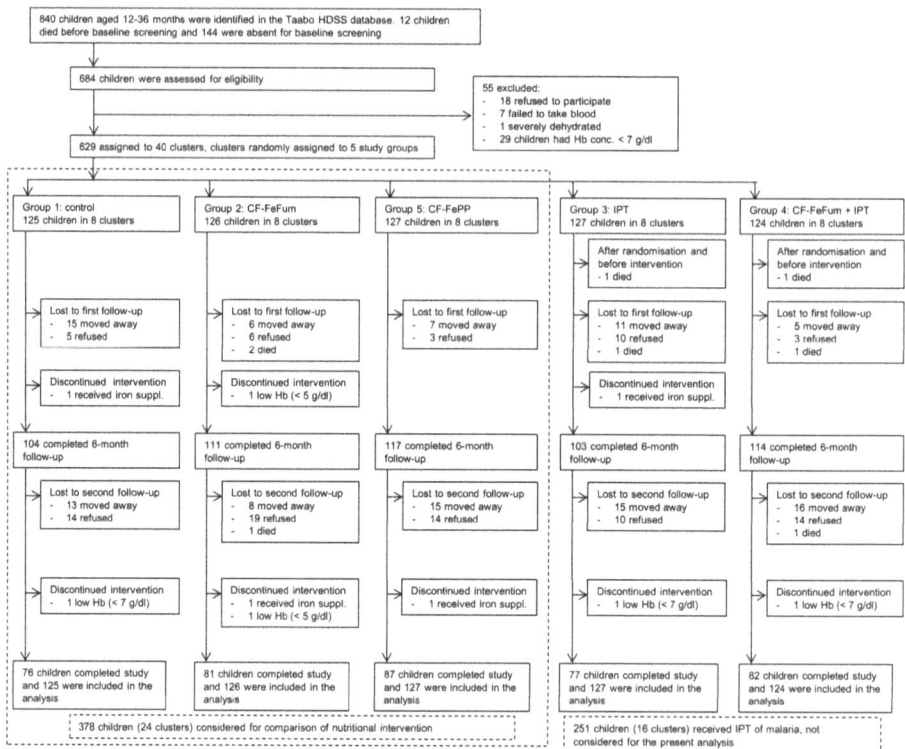

Figure 1. Flowchart. Study groups 1, 2, and 5 were considered for the current secondary analysis. Abbreviations: CF-FeFum, complementary food fortified with NaFeEDTA + ferrous fumarate; CF-FePP, complementary food fortified with NaFeEDTA + ferric pyrophosphate; Hb hemoglobin; HDSS, health and demographic surveillance system; IPT, intermittent preventive treatment of malaria.

The dried CF contained maize flour (49.9%), soy flour (21.4%), sucrose (20.0%), milk powder (7.0%), aroma (0.3%), salt (0.1%), and a vitamin/mineral premix (1.3%). The content of vitamins and minerals in a 25 g dry weight serving was 667 IU vitamin A, 100 IU vitamin D, 2.5 mg vitamin E, 0.25 mg vitamin B1, 0.25 mg vitamin B2, 0.25 mg vitamin B6, 0.45 µg vitamin B12, 15.0 mg ascorbic acid (AA), 0.075 mg folic acid, 3 mg niacin, 1 mg pantothenic acid, 0.045 mg iodine, 4.15 mg zinc, 0.28 mg copper, 0.6 mg manganese, 66.5 mg calcium, and 0.004 mg biotin. The AA:iron molar ratio was 0.8:1.

Each roller-dried CF was manufactured at three-month intervals during the 9-month study period to avoid losses in product quality during storage. All ingredients were weighed and mixed by Protein Kissèe-La under strict quality control. The manufacturing plant was thoroughly cleaned before CF manufacture. The homogenous mixing of the vitamin/mineral premix into the dry CF powder was assured by quantifying total iron content in three powder samples collected at the onset, in the middle, and toward the end of the mixing. The iron content was measured at ETH Zurich using graphite-furnace atomic absorption spectrophotometry (AA240Z, Agilent Technologies; Santa Clara, CA, USA). The dried CF was filled into 5 kg bags, and each CF was color-coded. The cleaning of the manufacturing plant, mixing, packaging, and labeling was rigorously supervised. After manufacture, Protein Kissèe-La transported the fortified CF to the study site and we stored the dried CFs under temperature-controlled conditions (between 20 °C and max 25 °C). The bags of 5 kg CF were distributed to the villages every other week.

Eight clusters of children (*n* = 125) received no intervention (group 1), eight clusters of children (*n* = 126) received FeFum fortified CF (group 2), and eight clusters of children (*n* = 127) received FePP fortified CF (group 5). These three groups of children received IPT-placebo. One cooking area was installed in each cluster, and women were trained in porridge preparation, including correct dosage (25 mg dry matter), hygiene, and completion of information forms related to food consumption. At each cooking location, the cooking woman prepared the porridge for 13 to 18 children. Children were brought to the cooking areas in the morning and fed by their mothers/guardians under direct supervision. The amount of porridge consumed by each child was recorded daily by the women cooks. Volunteers from the Taabo HDSS monitored cooking locations and cooks daily.

The women cooks used plastic beakers holding approximately 25 g CF powder for dosage. Each porridge serving was individually prepared by mixing 25 g of CF with approximately 100 mL boiled water. Each child consumed the porridge once per day 6 days each week, which provided approximately 34.8 mg added iron per week (5.8 mg added iron per serving). The maize and soy in the CF provided a further 0.6 mg intrinsic iron per serving. The fortificant iron alone provided 100% of the RNI for children aged 1–3 years assuming an intermediate iron bioavailability of 10% [7].

Children assigned to group 1 (control) received no nutritional intervention and continued with their normal dietary habits. Food intake in group 1 children was not monitored, however our previous studies in Côte d'Ivoire reported that young children (2–5 years) in rural areas consume mainly cassava and plantain with sauces based on okra or peanuts [20,21].

2.4. Blinding of Treatments

The control group was not blinded to either subjects or investigators. The two CFs were labeled with different colors (red or blue) and were single blinded, whereby the investigator was aware of the product difference. However, the study physician, parents/guardians of children, the cooking women, and the mothers/guardians who administered the porridge were not aware of group assignment.

2.5. Follow-Up

Mothers/guardians of participating children were encouraged to refer the child to the nearest health center as soon as the child presented a symptom of illness, especially fever, and to report the sick visit to the Taabo HDSS volunteer in each village. Each child had an individual study identity card. At the time of the study, all health consultations and treatments for children younger than 5 years were free of charge.

2.6. Laboratory Methods

Biomedical parameters were monitored at baseline, and after six months and nine months of intervention. We measured Hb, performed a malaria rapid diagnostic test, and prepared a thick and thin blood film from a venous blood sample. α-1-acid-glycoprotein (AGP), C-reactive protein (CRP), and PF were measured in plasma. Details of the laboratory procedures are available elsewhere [15]. We defined anemia as Hb concentration below 11.0 g/dL [22].

CRP above 5 mg/L or AGP concentrations above 1 g/L was considered as inflammation. Due to the high prevalence of inflammation, we defined ID as PF < 30 μg/L [23].

2.7. Statistical Analysis

The present report focuses on the impact of iron fortified CF on iron status and includes only three groups (1, 2, and 5) of a 5-arm intervention study. Hb concentration and anemia were our specified primary outcomes. PF concentration, the prevalence of ID, and *P. falciparum* prevalence were secondary outcomes. Results from all five study groups have been previously used to evaluate the interaction of IPT of malaria and iron fortified CF on Hb, anemia, and iron status [15]. The sample size calculation was based on Hb measurements from a 2010 study in preschool-age children in the same region of the Côte d'Ivoire [2]. In this previous study, the mean Hb concentration was 9.7 g/dL with a standard deviation of 2.0 g/dL. We estimated that 125 children per group were needed to detect an Hb difference of 0.8 g/dL at a 90% power level and a 5% level of significance, assuming 20% dropout.

Data were double entered into Microsoft Access 2010 (2010 Microsoft Corporation, Redmond, WA, USA). Double entries were compared using EpiInfo version 3.4.1 (Centers for Disease Control and Prevention, Atlanta, GA, USA) and differences were adjusted according to the original records. Data were analyzed with STATA version 13.1 (StataCorp LP; College Station, TX, USA). For the present analysis, we applied the same statistical approach as for the published paper presenting all five study groups, but restricted the analysis to the three groups receiving the nutritional intervention and corrected for multiple comparison. Briefly, all children randomized into study groups 1, 2, and 5 were analyzed (intention-to-treat). We analyzed the data with mixed (fixed and random) linear regression models to account for random effects due to repeated measures within clusters. The effectiveness was assessed by time-treatment interactions. For the between group comparison at follow-up, time was considered as categorical variable (0, 6, and 9 months). A Bonferroni correction was applied to multiple comparisons. Logistic regression models taking into account random effect were used for analysis of prevalence (i.e., binary) data. Treatment assignment was the fixed effect, and age and CRP concentration were the covariates in all models.

3. Results

3.1. Participant Characteristics and Compliance

We randomly assigned 378 children (mean age 29.8 ($\pm$8.4) months, 50.3% girls) to three study groups. Table 1 shows the biochemical measurements and anthropometry of the children at baseline, and after six months and nine months of intervention. The study period included almost the whole rainy season starting in April and was completed about one month after the onset of the dry season that begins in November. The only difference among the groups at baseline was a significantly higher CRP concentration in the CF-FePP group compared to the control group ($p = 0.009$) and the CF-FeFum group ($p = 0.013$), although the prevalence of inflammation (CRP > 5 mg/L and/or AGP > 1 g/L) did not differ between groups. At baseline, the overall prevalence of anemia, ID, and *P. falciparum* infection among all study children were 82.8%, 34.7%, and 62.0%, respectively. Nearly three-quarters (73%) of the children had elevated inflammation biomarkers (CRP and/or AGP). Helminth infections were rare, with only one child infected with *Ascaris lumbricoides* and another child with *Schistosoma haematobium* at baseline.

The daily amount of uneaten porridge was estimated for each child to the nearest one quarter of a serving. Overall, of the CF-FeFum and CF-FePP groups 92.5% and 94.8%, respectively, of the porridge was consumed.

Table 1. Between group comparison of anthropometric measures, *P. falciparum* infection prevalence, *P. falciparum* parasitemia, and inflammation biomarkers and prevalence at baseline, six months, and nine months in 12- to 36-month-old Ivorian children fed iron fortified complementary food (CF) containing NaFeEDTA combined with either ferrous fumarate (FeFum) or ferric pyrophosphate (FePP).

	Groups		
	Control	CF-FeFum	CF-FePP
	Participants N =		
Baseline	125	126	127
6 months	104	111	116
9 months	76	81	87
	Height (cm, mean, SD)		
Baseline	79.2 ± 9.8	78.5 ± 7.5	78.6 ± 6.8
6 months	86.2 ± 6.9	86.8 ± 6.9	85.8 ± 6.6
9 months	89.0 ± 6.6	89.3 ± 6.5	89.0 ± 6.3
	Body weight (kg, mean, SD)		
Baseline	10.7 ± 2.3	10.8 ± 2.9	10.7 ± 2.5
6 months	11.2 ± 2.0	11.1 ± 2.0	11.0 ± 1.8
9 months	11.7 ± 2.1	11.5 ± 1.9	11.4 ± 1.7
	P. falciparum prevalence		
Baseline	62.1%	57.7%	66.1%
6 months	62.5%	55.0%	64.7%
9 months	44.7%	46.9%	47.1%
	P. falciparum parasitemia (parasites/µL blood, geometric mean, 95% confidence interval)		
Baseline	1136 (729–1768)	896 (524–1534)	2182 (1409–3379)
6 months	3773 (2470–5762)	2268 (1427–3605)	2074 (1367–3146)
9 months	2820 (1460–5447)	2718 (1662–4445)	3130 (1913–5121)
	CRP (mg/L, median, interquartile range 25th 75th)		
Baseline	2.8 (1.0–11.1)	3.4 (1.4–8.7)	5.9 (1.9–21.3) *ᵟ
6 months	5.1 (1.8–18.6)	4.6 (1.2–20.4)	4.8 (1.5–14.6) **
9 months	2.6 (1.0–7.3)	4.3 (1.0–13.2)	3.2 (1.3–14.8) ᵟ
	AGP (g/L, median, 25th 75th)		
Baseline	1.12 (0.90–1.40)	1.27 (1.01–1.54)	1.26 (0.96–1.65)
6 months	1.13 (0.88–1.41)	1.25 (0.92–1.54)	1.10 (0.85–1.40)
9 months	1.07 (0.78–1.44)	1.13 (0.85–1.36)	1.06 (0.79–1.28) *
	Prevalence of inflammation (CRP > 5 mg/L and/or AGP > 1 g/L)		
Baseline	65.8%	76.8%	76.4%
6 months	72.1%	74.8%	65.5%
9 months	57.3%	64.2%	57.5%

Changes between baseline to six months and baseline to nine months were compared between groups with random effect models. Abbreviations: AGP, α-1-acid-glycoprotein; CRP, C-reactive protein; Hb, hemoglobin; SD, standard deviation. * $p < 0.05$ and ** $p < 0.01$ significant difference at baseline or increase/decrease in CF-FeFum or CF-FePP significantly different compared to increase/decrease in control. ᵟ $p < 0.05$ significant difference at baseline or increase/decrease in CF-FePP significantly different compared to CF-FeFum.

3.2. Hb Concentration and Anemia Prevalence

There were no significant time by treatment interactions on Hb concentrations or anemia (Table 2). There was, however, a significant time effect on Hb concentration and anemia. The increase in Hb of the control group from 9.8 g/dL at baseline to 10.3 g/dL at nine months was not significantly different compared to the increase from 9.9 g/dL to 10.4 g/dL in the CF-FeFum group ($p = 0.861$) and to the increase from 9.6 g/dL to 10.5 g/dL in the CF-FePP group ($p = 0.430$). The change in Hb from baseline to the 9-month follow-up was also not significantly different in both groups receiving iron fortified CF ($p = 0.535$). The decrease of anemia prevalence from baseline to nine months in the CF-FePP group was significantly greater than that in the control group (odds ratio (OR) = 0.42, 95% confidence interval (CI) 0.22–0.83, $p = 0.036$).

Table 2. Hemoglobin (Hb) concentration and iron status biomarkers at baseline, six months, and nine months in 12- to 36-month-old Ivorian children in the control group and in children consuming iron fortified complementary food (CF) containing NaFeEDTA combined with either ferrous fumarate (FeFum) or ferric pyrophosphate (FePP).

	Groups			Overall Effects			Between Group Comparisons		
	Control	CF-FeFum	CF-FePP	Time $p=$	Treatment $p=$	Time by Treatment Interaction $p=$	Control vs. CF-FeFum $p=$	Control vs. CF-FePP $p=$	CF-FeFum vs. CF-FePP $p=$
Participants N =									
Baseline	125	126	127						
6 months	104	111	116						
9 months	76	81	87						
Hb concentration (g/dL, mean, ±SD)									
Baseline	9.8 ± 1.3	9.9 ± 1.2	9.6 ± 1.2	<0.001	0.948	0.141			
6 months	9.9 ± 1.3	9.9 ± 1.3	10.0 ± 1.1				0.761	0.479	0.306
9 months	10.3 ± 1.3 *	10.4 ± 1.2 *	10.5 ± 1.2 **				0.871	0.226	0.161
Anemia (Hb < 11 g/dL)									
Baseline	81.6%	80.2%	86.6%	<0.001	0.475	0.237			
6 months	79.8%	77.5%	81.9%				0.216	0.953	0.746
9 months	71.1%	70.4%	65.5% *				0.083	0.036 [a]	0.069 [a]
PF (µg/L, median, interquartile range 25th 75th)									
Baseline	37.7 (18.3–72.4)	36.2 (21.6–66.0)	53.0 (28.4–115.7)	<0.001	0.068	0.458			
6 months	60.7 (35.1–114.0) ***	102.4 (48.3–159.5) ***	69.1 (41.8–139.7) ***				<0.003 [a]	0.048 [a]	0.214
9 months	49.6 (26.2–96.0) **	66.5 (45.4–117.4) ***	62.6 (41.1–107.2) ***				0.072 [a]	0.150	0.426
ID (PF < 30 µg/L)									
Baseline	37.4%	40.0%	26.7%	<0.001	0.004	0.068			
6 months	19.2% *	5.4% ***	8.6% ***				<0.003 [a]	0.006 [a]	0.368
9 months	29.3%	3.7% ***	10.3% ***				<0.003 [a]	0.003 [a]	0.171
IDA (PF < 30 µg/L and Hb < 11 g/dL)									
Baseline	33.3%	32.8%	23.6%	<0.001	0.003	0.028			
6 months	15.4% **	3.6% ***	4.3% ***				0.036 [a]	0.096 [a]	0.689
9 months	18.7%	1.2% ***	3.4% ***				0.027 [a]	0.018 [a]	0.388
ID and inflammation (PF < 30 µg/L and inflammation: CRP > 5 mg/L and/or AGP > 1 g/L)									
Baseline	21.1%	24.0%	14.2%	<0.001	0.001	0.080			
6 months	11.5% *	4.5% ***	4.3% ***				0.099 [a]	0.096 [a]	0.900
9 months	14.7%	2.5% **	2.3% **				0.033 [a]	0.021 [a]	0.919

Table 2. *Cont.*

	Groups			Overall Effects			Between Group Comparisons		
	Control	CF-FeFum	CF-FePP	Time p =	Treatment p =	Time by Treatment Interaction p =	Control vs. CF-FeFum p =	Control vs. CF-FePP p =	CF-FeFum vs. CF-FePP p =
Anemia, ID, and inflammation (Hb < 11 g/dL and PF < 30 µg/L and inflammation: CRP > 5 mg/L and/or AGP > 1 g/L)									
Baseline	18.7%	20.8%	13.4%	<0.001	0.003	0.040			
6 months	10.6%	2.7% **	3.4% ***				0.048 [a]	0.090 [a]	0.513
9 months	12.0%	1.2% **	1.1% **				0.063 [a]	0.048 [a]	0.944

[a] Changes between baseline to six months and baseline to nine months were compared between groups with random effect models. For the between group comparison at follow-up, time (0, 6, and 9 months) was considered as categorical variable. For group differences with significant *p*-values (<0.05) a Bonferroni correction was applied. Abbreviations: AGP, α-1-acid-glycoprotein; CRP, C-reactive protein; Hb, hemoglobin; PF, plasma ferritin; SD, standard deviation. * p < 0.05, ** p < 0.01, *** p < 0.001 significant difference within the same group from baseline to six months or baseline to nine months.

3.3. PF and Prevalence of ID

There were no differences between PF concentrations in the study groups at baseline. There was no significant time by treatment interaction on PF concentration, but a significant time effect ($p < 0.001$). PF concentrations within groups increased significantly at the two follow-up time points in all study groups. Although the overall time-treatment interaction was not significant, the increase in PF was significantly higher in children from the CF-FeFum group than in the control group at six months ($p < 0.003$), but was not any more significant at nine months of follow-up ($p = 0.072$). The increase of PF concentrations in the FePP group was significantly greater at six months ($p = 0.048$), but was not different from the control at nine months ($p = 0.150$) (Table 2).

There was a significant time by treatment interaction on IDA ($p = 0.028$) and a borderline significant time by treatment interaction on ID ($p = 0.068$) (Table 2). IDA prevalence sharply decreased in the FeFum (32.8% to 1.2%) and FePP groups (23.6% to 3.4%) (for both, $p < 0.001$). The prevalence of ID with or without anemia decreased significantly in the groups receiving the iron fortified CFs; from 40.0% to 3.7% in the group receiving CF-FeFum and from 26.7% to 10.3% in the group receiving CF-FePP (for both, $p < 0.001$). The decrease in ID prevalence observed in the children from CF-FeFum group was significantly greater than the decrease observed in the control group (OR = 0.06, 95% CI 0.02–0.25, $p < 0.003$). Similarly, the decrease in ID prevalence observed in the CF-FePP group was significantly greater than that observed in the control group (OR = 0.17, 95% CI 0.07–0.47, $p < 0.003$). The decreases in ID prevalence observed in the CF-FeFum and CF-FePP were not significantly different from each other (OR = 2.72, 95% CI 0.65–11.41, $p = 0.171$).

3.4. P. falciparum Prevalence and Inflammation

The prevalence of *P. falciparum* was around 60% in children from all groups at baseline and the 6-month follow-up (Table 1). *P. falciparum* prevalencedecreased slightly to around 45% at study completion during the dry season. Although there were some small differences in CRP and AGP values in children from different groups at different time points (Table 1), the prevalence of inflammation (CRP > 5 mg/L and/or AGP > 1 g/L) also remained high, ranging between 57.3% and 76.4% ($p > 0.05$), over the 9-month intervention period in children in all groups.

4. Discussion

The main finding of this study is that, despite the high *P. falciparum* prevalence and elevated inflammation biomarkers in 12- to 36-month-old children, consumption of iron fortified CF for nine months significantly decreased the prevalence of IDA. Our results indicate that, despite previous reports of decreased iron absorption from labelled single meal studies in adults and children infected with *P. falciparum* [9,24], iron absorption from the iron fortified CF in this study was sufficient to improve iron status and decrease IDA. Our findings suggest that, in the long term, the drive to increase iron absorption during ID can overcome the restriction in iron absorption from inflammation. This observation is consistent with previous studies showing that iron absorption is up-regulated in children with low iron status regardless of their inflammation status [25,26]. In addition, in a recent study in Gambian and Tanzanian children, hepcidin concentration was lower in iron deficient children infected with *P. falciparum* than in children of normal iron status infected with *P. falciparum* [27].

Although there was a significant reduction in IDA in this study, there was no significant overall reduction in anemia. This suggests that the major cause of anemia in this age group in this setting is not iron deficiency (ID). We have previously reported that anemia prevalence was high in our preschool-age children in rural Côte d'Ivoire and it was strongly linked to *P. falciparum* infection [2]. In our study, anemia prevalence was around 80% at baseline. Approximately 60% of our children were infected with *P. falciparum* at baseline and parasitemia remained approximately at the same level throughout the first six months during the rainy season. *Plasmodium falciparum* prevalence slightly declined to less than 50% at the end of the study in the dry season (Table 1). Between 57% and 77% of the children presented with elevated CRP and/or AGP at baseline, after six months, and after nine months. As inflammation, via its action on increasing hepcidin, would be expected to inhibit the recycling of red cell iron [28], much of the anemia in our study children would be expected to be anemia of inflammation, likely due to an infection with *P. falciparum* or other infectious agents. The lack of a substantial rise in overall Hb concentrations over the nine months of the study, despite an increase in iron stores, indicates that iron availability to the bone marrow for erythropoiesis was likely limited in many children by high rates of infection leading to hepcidin-mediated iron sequestration in macrophages of the reticulo-endothelial system. In addition, suppression of erythropoiesis and shortening of the red blood cell life span by malaria and infectious inflammation likely contributes to anemia in these children. High circulating hepcidin concentrations also decrease dietary iron absorption by inactivating the iron export protein ferroportin in duodenal enterocytes [29]. Previous absorption studies in women and children with *P. falciparum* parasitemia showed that iron absorption is only about half of the absorption measured after receiving antimalarial treatment [9,10]. Moreover, the malaria pigment hemozoin, a side product of the Hb digestion by *P. falciparum,* directly inhibits the erythropoiesis in the bone marrow [30]. It remains unclear whether an increase in iron stores in children in malaria-endemic settings, without an increase in Hb, will lead to an improvement in health. It is likely that a portion of this extra iron would be utilized by the iron requiring enzymes of the brain, energy metabolism, and immune system. Nevertheless, it appears that the children in our study were still able to absorb some iron from the iron fortified CF, despite the inhibitory effects of malaria and infectious inflammation.

At baseline, 24–33% of the children had ID in the presence of anemia. While ID could have been an additional cause of the observed anemia, it is conceivable that a considerable amount of the observed anemia is due to inflammation either separately or concurrent with IDA. Inherited hemoglobinopathies are unlikely to contribute to anemia, as a previous study in the Taabo HDSS reported 83% of subjects to have normal Hb genotype, and only 7%, 8%, and 1% carried the C allele, S allele, or had sickle cell anemia, respectively [2]. Vitamin A deficiency has been reported to be prevalent, but was not associated with anemia in young children [2] and infections with soil-transmitted helminths or *Schistosoma* spp. were rare in our study cohort, and thus unlikely to contribute to anemia in a substantial manner.

The inability of iron fortified foods to impact on anemia in malaria-endemic settings may be partly related to the relatively low amount of iron provided. The higher levels of iron used in iron supplements [31] and added to micronutrient powders [32] used for home fortification have been reported to decrease anemia prevalence in children in malaria-endemic areas. The lower levels of iron in fortified foods have two advantages. First, unlike with iron supplementation, there is no spike in iron absorption so there is little or no formation in plasma of non-transferrin bound iron, which is considered responsible for increasing the severity of *P. falciparum* infection [33,34]. Second, less unabsorbed iron reaches the colon, so there is a lower risk of changing the gut microbiome to a more pathogenic profile [35].

The fortified CF provided each child with its RNI for iron (5.8 mg added iron) for six days each week. Based mainly on adult absorption studies, the relative iron absorption from NaFeEDTA added to cereal foods would be expected to be 2–3 times greater than that from FeFum and 4–6 times greater than that from FePP [5]. It was somewhat surprising therefore that the CF fortified with FePP was as efficacious in improving iron status as the CF fortified with FeFum. One likely explanation is that the fortified CF provided considerably more iron than the gap between the child's iron intake from their regular diet and the child's daily iron requirement. Earlier studies from our group in Côte d'Ivoire reported that preschool-age children (2–5 years) consumed 5.5 mg Fe per day [20] which is close to the RNI of 5.8 mg recommended for one- to three-year-old children and to the 6.3 mg iron recommended for four- to six-year-old children assuming 10% iron absorption [7]. The iron bioavailability of the diet is not known but could approach 10% as the main staples of cassava and plantain are low in PA. It is possible therefore that the 2 mg of highly bioavailable iron from NaFeEDTA provided most or all of the iron lacking in the diet, and that any difference in iron absorption from CF-FeFum and CF-FePP had little or no effect. In Côte d'Ivoire, the commercial CF is identical to the CF (FePP) used in the present study. Our study confirms that this formulation will benefit the child's iron status.

Our study has several strengths. It was conducted in infants and young children in a rural region of West Africa where anemia and ID are very common and where *P. falciparum* is hyperendemic. We used iron compounds with highly bioavailable NaFeEDTA, and we maximized its content and completed with one of the two compounds, FeFum or FePP, which have relatively good bioavailability. It remains unclear whether most of the iron was absorbed from NaFeEDTA and whether by only using NaFeEDTA the effect would have been the same; this should be addressed in future research. Limitations of our study include possible confounding by seasonal variations in malaria transmission, the use of a single iron biomarker (PF) to define iron status, and the lack of plasma hepcidin measurements. A further limitation is that we did not consistently record potential adverse events in the different intervention groups because of limited financial and human resources and at times difficult access to some of the most remote communities.

In conclusion, our study confirms the high prevalence of anemia (> 80%) and ID (> 30%) in young children living in rural Côte d'Ivoire. This is a major public health concern that needs to be urgently addressed. Iron fortified, cereal-based CFs are highly efficacious in correcting IDA in young children living in malaria-endemic settings. Our study shows the usefulness of using the maximum amount of NaFeEDTA as permitted by its acceptable daily intake and completing the iron fortification level with other iron compounds. The current study, however, found that iron-fortified foods had no significant overall impact on anemia, presumably because the anemia is mainly attributable to malaria and infectious inflammation, and not ID. Our findings highlight the importance of assessing the etiology of anemia in order to design and implement appropriate intervention(s) [36]. Further research is needed to better understand the overlapping causes of anemia, and to develop methods to quantify ID in the presence of malaria-induced inflammation.

Acknowledgments: We express our gratitude to all participants and their mothers/caregivers, the village chiefs, and the communities supporting our study. The porridge was prepared during the nine months by volunteers, whose commitment was very much appreciated. We are thankful for all the support of the Centre Suisse de Recherches Scientifiques en Côte d'Ivoire (CSRS). Special thanks go to the Director-General of CSRS, Bassirou Bonfoh. We thank Jürgen Erhardt for measuring iron status and assuring the quality of the data. We are grateful to the members of the Data Safety and Monitoring Board, namely Thomas A. Smith, Sean Lynch, and Maria Andersson, who carefully assessed the study protocol and monitored outcomes. Supported by the Swiss National Science Foundation (Bern, Switzerland; project No. IZ70Z0_123900), Fairmed (Bern, Switzerland), Global Alliance for Improved Nutrition (grant agreement 30CI01-ML), and ETH Zurich (Zurich, Switzerland).

Author Contributions: The authors' responsibilities were as follows—D.G., R.F.H., R.W., G.J.A. and M.B.Z. designed research; D.G., M.O., V.G.D., L.H., L.G.A., J.U. and E.K.N. conducted research; D.G., R.F.H. and R.W. analyzed data or performed statistical analysis; D.G., R.F.H., R.W. and G.J.A. wrote paper; D.G., R.F.H. and R.W. had primary responsibility for final content. All authors read and approved the final manuscript.

Conflicts of Interest: The authors declare no conflict of interest.

Abbreviations

AA	ascorbic acid
AGP	α-1-acid glycoprotein
CF	complementary food
CRP	C-reactive protein
FAO	Food and Agriculture Organization
Fe	iron
FeFum	ferrous fumarate
FePP	ferric pyrophosphate
Hb	hemoglobin
HDSS	health and demographic surveillance system
ID	iron deficiency
IDA	iron deficiency anemia

IPT	intermittent preventive treatment
NaFeEDTA	sodium iron ethylenediaminetetraacetate
PA	phytic acid
PF	plasma ferritin
RNI	reference nutrient intake
WHO	World Health Organization

References

1. World Health Organization (WHO). *Worldwide Prevalence of Anaemia 1993–2005*; World Health Organization: Geneva, Switzerland, 2008.

2. Righetti, A.A.; Koua, A.Y.G.; Adiossan, L.G.; Glinz, D.; Hurrell, R.F.; N'Goran, E.K.; Niamké, S.; Wegmüller, R.; Utzinger, J. Etiology of anemia among infants, school-aged children, and young non-pregnant women in different settings of south-central Côte d'Ivoire. *Am. J. Trop. Med. Hyg.* **2012**, *87*, 425–434. [CrossRef] [PubMed]

3. Lozoff, B.; Georgieff, M.K. Iron deficiency and brain development. *Semin. Pediatr. Neurol.* **2006**, *13*, 158–165. [CrossRef] [PubMed]

4. Shafir, T.; Angulo-Barroso, R.; Jing, Y.; Angelilli, M.L.; Jacobson, S.W.; Lozoff, B. Iron deficiency and infant motor development. *Early Hum. Dev.* **2008**, *84*, 479–485. [CrossRef] [PubMed]

5. Hurrell, R.; Egli, I. Iron bioavailability and dietary reference values. *Am. J. Clin. Nutr.* **2010**, *91*, 1461S–1467S. [CrossRef] [PubMed]

6. Hurrell, R.F. Fortification: Overcoming technical and practical barriers. *J. Nutr.* **2002**, *132* (Suppl. 4), 806S–812S. [PubMed]

7. Food and Agriculture Organization (FAO)/World Health Organization (WHO). *Guidelines on Food Fortification with Micronutrients*; World Health Organization: Geneva, Switzerland, 2006.

8. World Health Organization (WHO). *Evaluation of Certain Food Additives and Contaminants*; WHO Technical Report Series Fifty-Third Report of the Joint FAO/WHO Expert Committee on Food Additives; World Health Organization: Geneva, Switzerland, 2000.

9. Cercamondi, C.I.; Egli, I.M.; Ahouandjinou, E.; Dossa, R.; Zeder, C.; Salami, L.; Tjalsma, H.; Wiegerinck, E.; Tanno, T.; Hurrell, R.F.; et al. Afebrile *Plasmodium falciparum* parasitemia decreases absorption of fortification iron but does not affect systemic iron utilization: A double stable-isotope study in young Beninese women. *Am. J. Clin. Nutr.* **2010**, *92*, 1385–1392. [CrossRef] [PubMed]

10. Glinz, D.; Hurrell, R.F.; Righetti, A.A.; Zeder, C.; Adiossan, L.G.; Tjalsma, H.; Utzinger, J.; Zimmermann, M.B.; N'Goran, E.K.; Wegmüller, R. In Ivorian school-age children, infection with hookworm does not reduce dietary iron absorption or systemic iron utilization, whereas afebrile *Plasmodium falciparum* infection reduces iron absorption by half. *Am. J. Clin. Nutr.* **2015**, *101*, 462–470. [CrossRef] [PubMed]

11. Andang'o, P.E.; Osendarp, S.J.; Ayah, R.; West, C.E.; Mwaniki, D.L.; De Wolf, C.A.; Kraaijenhagen, R.; Kok, F.J.; Verhoef, H. Efficacy of iron-fortified whole maize flour on iron status of schoolchildren in Kenya: A randomised controlled trial. *Lancet* **2007**, *369*, 1799–1806. [CrossRef]

12. Wegmüller, R.; Camara, F.; Zimmermann, M.B.; Adou, P.; Hurrell, R.F. Salt dual-fortified with iodine and micronized ground ferric pyrophosphate affects iron status but not hemoglobin in children in Côte d'Ivoire. *J. Nutr.* **2006**, *136*, 1814–1820. [PubMed]

13. Zimmermann, M.B.; Wegmueller, R.; Zeder, C.; Chaouki, N.; Rohner, F.; Saissi, M.; Torresani, T.; Hurrell, R.F. Dual fortification of salt with iodine and micronized ferric pyrophosphate: A randomized, double-blind, controlled trial. *Am. J. Clin. Nutr.* **2004**, *80*, 952–959. [PubMed]

14. Rohner, F.; Zimmermann, M.B.; Amon, R.J.; Vounatsou, P.; Tschannen, A.B.; N'Goran, E.K.; Nindjin, C.; Cacou, M.C.; Té-Bonlé, M.D.; Aka, H.; et al. In a randomized controlled trial of iron fortification, anthelmintic treatment, and intermittent preventive treatment of malaria for anemia control in Ivorian children, only anthelmintic treatment shows modest benefit. *J. Nutr.* **2010**, *140*, 635–641. [CrossRef] [PubMed]

15. Glinz, D.; Hurrell, R.F.; Ouattara, M.; Zimmermann, M.B.; Brittenham, G.M.; Adiossan, L.G.; Righetti, A.A.; Seifert, B.; Diakité, V.G.; Utzinger, J.; et al. The effect of iron-fortified complementary food and intermittent preventive treatment of malaria on anaemia in 12- to 36-month-old children: A cluster-randomised controlled trial. *Malar. J.* **2015**, *14*, 347. [CrossRef] [PubMed]

16. Fürst, T.; Silué, K.D.; Ouattara, M.; N'Goran, D.N.; Adiossan, L.G.; N'Guessan, Y.; Zouzou, F.; Koné, S.; N'Goran, E.K.; Utzinger, J. Schistosomiasis, soil-transmitted helminthiasis, and sociodemographic factors influence quality of life of adults in Côte d'Ivoire. *PLoS Negl. Trop. Dis.* **2012**, *6*, e1855. [CrossRef] [PubMed]

17. Koné, S.; Baikoro, N.; N'Guessan, Y.; Jaeger, F.N.; Silué, K.D.; Fürst, T.; Hürlimann, E.; Ouattara, M.; Séka, M.C.; N'Guessan, N.A.; et al. Health & Demographic Surveillance System Profile: The Taabo Health and Demographic Surveillance System, Côte d'Ivoire. *Int. J. Epidemiol.* **2015**, *44*, 87–97. [CrossRef] [PubMed]

18. Bassa, F.K.; Ouattara, M.; Silué, K.D.; Adiossan, L.G.; Baikoro, N.; Koné, S.; N'Cho, M.; Traoré, M.; Bonfoh, B.; Utzinger, J.; et al. Epidemiology of malaria in the Taabo health and demographic surveillance system, south-central Côte d'Ivoire. *Malar. J.* **2016**, *15*, 9. [CrossRef] [PubMed]

19. Righetti, A.A.; Wegmüller, R.; Glinz, D.; Ouattara, M.; Adiossan, L.G.; N'Goran, E.K.; Utzinger, J.; Hurrell, R.F. Effects of inflammation and *Plasmodium falciparum* infection on soluble transferrin receptor and plasma ferritin concentration in different age groups: A prospective longitudinal study in Côte d'Ivoire. *Am. J. Clin. Nutr.* **2013**, *97*, 1364–1374. [CrossRef] [PubMed]

20. Staubli Asobayire, F. *Development of a Food Fortification Strategy to Combat Iron Deficiency in the Ivory Coast*; ETH Zurich: Zürich, Switzerland, 2000; pp. 1–239.

21. Wegmüller, R. *Dual Fortification of Salt with Iodine and Iron in Africa*; ETH Zurich: Zürich, Switzerland, 2005; pp. 1–211.

22. World Health Organization (WHO). *Iron Deficiency Anaemia: Assessment, Prevention and Control: A Guide for Programme Managers*; World Health Organization: Geneva, Switzerland, 2001.

23. Word Health Organization (WHO). *Assessing the Iron Status of Populations*, 2nd ed.; Word Health Organization, Centers for Disease Control and Prevention: Geneva, Switzerland, 2007.

24. Glinz, D.; Kamiyango, M.; Phiri, K.S.; Munthali, F.; Zeder, C.; Zimmermann, M.B.; Hurrell, R.F.; Wegmüller, R. The effect of timing of iron supplementation on iron absorption and haemoglobin in post-malaria anaemia: A longitudinal stable isotope study in Malawian toddlers. *Malar. J.* **2014**, *13*, 397. [CrossRef] [PubMed]

25. Bezwoda, W.R.; Bothwell, T.H.; Torrance, J.D.; MacPhail, A.P.; Charlton, R.W.; Kay, G.; Levin, J. The relationship between marrow iron stores, plasma ferritin concentrations and iron absorption. *Scand. J. Haematol.* **1979**, *22*, 113–120. [CrossRef] [PubMed]

26. Collings, R.; Harvey, L.J.; Hooper, L.; Hurst, R.; Brown, T.J.; Ansett, J.; King, M.; Fairweather-Tait, S.J. The absorption of iron from whole diets: A systematic review. *Am. J. Clin. Nutr.* **2013**, *98*, 65–81. [CrossRef] [PubMed]

27. Pasricha, S.R.; Atkinson, S.H.; Armitage, A.E.; Khandwala, S.; Veenemans, J.; Cox, S.E.; Eddowes, L.A.; Hayes, T.; Doherty, C.P.; Demir, A.Y.; et al. Expression of the iron hormone hepcidin distinguishes different types of anemia in African children. *Sci. Transl. Med.* **2014**, *6*, 235re3. [CrossRef] [PubMed]

28. Ganz, T. Macrophages and systemic iron homeostasis. *J. Innate Immun.* **2012**, *4*, 446–453. [CrossRef] [PubMed]

29. Drakesmith, H.; Prentice, A.M. Hepcidin and the iron-infection axis. *Science* **2012**, *338*, 768–772. [CrossRef] [PubMed]

30. Skorokhod, O.A.; Caione, L.; Marrocco, T.; Migliardi, G.; Barrera, V.; Arese, P.; Piacibello, W.; Schwarzer, E. Inhibition of erythropoiesis in malaria anemia: Role of hemozoin and hemozoin-generated 4-hydroxynonenal. *Blood* **2010**, *116*, 4328–4337. [CrossRef] [PubMed]

31. Pasricha, S.R.; Hayes, E.; Kalumba, K.; Biggs, B.A. Effect of daily iron supplementation on health in children aged 4–23 months: A systematic review and meta-analysis of randomised controlled trials. *Lancet Glob. Health* **2013**, *1*, 77–86. [CrossRef]

32. De-Regil, L.M.; Suchdev, P.S.; Vist, G.E.; Walleser, S.; Pena-Rosas, J.P. Home fortification of foods with multiple micronutrient powders for health and nutrition in children under two years of age. *Evid. Based Child Health* **2013**, *8*, 112–201. [CrossRef] [PubMed]

33. Hurrell, R.F. Iron fortification: Its efficacy and safety in relation to infections. *Food Nutr. Bull.* **2007**, *28* (Suppl. 4), S585–S594. [CrossRef] [PubMed]

34. Brittenham, G.M.; Andersson, M.; Egli, I.; Foman, J.T.; Zeder, C.; Westerman, M.E.; Hurrell, R.F. Circulating non-transferrin-bound iron after oral administration of supplemental and fortification doses of iron to healthy women: A randomized study. *Am. J. Clin. Nutr.* **2014**, *100*, 813–820. [CrossRef] [PubMed]

35. Jaeggi, T.; Kortman, G.A.; Moretti, D.; Chassard, C.; Holding, P.; Dostal, A.; Boekhorst, J.; Timmerman, H.M.; Swinkels, D.W.; Tjalsma, H.; et al. Iron fortification adversely affects the gut microbiome, increases pathogen abundance and induces intestinal inflammation in Kenyan infants. *Gut* **2014**, *64*, 731–742. [CrossRef] [PubMed]

36. Suchdev, P.S.; Namaste, S.M.; Aaron, G.J.; Raiten, D.J.; Brown, K.H.; Flores-Ayala, R. Overview of the biomarkers reflecting inflammation and nutritional determinants of anemia (BRINDA) project. *Adv. Nutr.* **2016**, *7*, 349–356. [CrossRef] [PubMed]

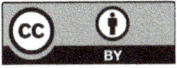

nutrients

MDPI

Article

Iron Bioavailability Studies of the First Generation of Iron-Biofortified Beans Released in Rwanda

Raymond Glahn [1,*], Elad Tako [1], Jonathan Hart [1], Jere Haas [2], Mercy Lung'aho [3] and Steve Beebe [4]

1   USDA-ARS Robert Holley Center for Agriculture and Health, Ithaca, NY 14853, USA;
     elad.tako@ars.usda.gov (E.T.); jon.hart@ars.usda.gov (J.H.)
2   Division of Nutritional Sciences, 220 Savage Hall, Cornell University, Ithaca, NY 14853, USA;
     jdh12@cornell.edu
3   International Center for Tropical Agriculture (CIAT), Regional Office for Africa, P.O. Box 823-00621,
     Nairobi 00100, Kenya; m.lungaho@cgiar.org
4   International Center for Tropical Agriculture (CIAT), Km 17, Recta Cali–Palmira CP 763537,
     Apartado Aéreo 6713, Cali, Colombia; s.beebe@cgiar.org
*   Correspondence: raymond.glahn@ars.usda.gov; Tel.: +1-607-255-2452

Received: 22 June 2017; Accepted: 17 July 2017; Published: 21 July 2017

Abstract: This paper represents a series of in vitro iron (Fe) bioavailability experiments, Fe content analysis and polyphenolic profile of the first generation of Fe biofortified beans (*Phaseolus vulgaris*) selected for human trials in Rwanda and released to farmers of that region. The objective of the present study was to demonstrate how the Caco-2 cell bioassay for Fe bioavailability can be utilized to assess the nutritional quality of Fe in such varieties and how they may interact with diets and meal plans of experimental studies. Furthermore, experiments were also conducted to directly compare this in vitro approach with specific human absorption studies of these Fe biofortified beans. The results show that other foods consumed with beans, such as rice, can negatively affect Fe bioavailability whereas potato may enhance the Fe absorption when consumed with beans. The results also suggest that the extrinsic labelling approach to measuring human Fe absorption can be flawed and thus provide misleading information. Overall, the results provide evidence that the Caco-2 cell bioassay represents an effective approach to evaluate the nutritional quality of Fe-biofortified beans, both separate from and within a targeted diet or meal plan.

Keywords: beans; *Phaseolus vulgaris*; iron; bioavailability; biofortification

1. Introduction

Studies on iron (Fe) biofortification of the common bean were published as early as 2000, approximately a year or two before the term "biofortification" was coined [1]. Prior to 2000, experiments were primarily conducted in rodent models using intrinsically labelled crops, or in humans with extrinsically labelled foods and meals [2]. The cost and limitations of such in vivo studies often prevented the experimental approach from addressing important aspects of bean Fe bioavailability, such as the effects of polyphenols, phytate, and the influence of other foods consumed with beans. Since then, advances have been achieved that allow for more extensive screening of foods and development of staple food crops and food products for improved nutritional quality of Fe. The coupling of the in vitro digestion techniques with Caco-2 cell monolayers was a significant advance that enabled direct in vitro examination of factors that influence Fe bioavailability [3]. This approach utilizes Caco-2 cell ferritin formation as a marker of Fe uptake, which enables scientists to avoid the cost and methodological issues associated with isotopic labelling. Moreover, the ferritin formation approach is a sensitive, cost-effective marker of Fe uptake that dramatically increased the throughput of the system. As a result, this in vitro model has demonstrated the potential to be a tool that can be effectively coupled with modern plant breeding approaches to identify regions of the genome that can influence Fe bioavailability and identify varieties and processing effects that warrant further pursuit to increase the nutritional quality of Fe [4–6]. When this in vitro approach is further coupled with an established animal model of Fe bioavailability it represents an effective approach to refine the experimental approach for human studies [7]. This combination of in vitro and in vivo animal studies can also be used to address issues not feasible to conduct in human trials.

The present study is an excellent example of how the established Caco-2 cell bioassay can be applied to evaluate key nutritional factors that could influence the effectiveness of Fe-biofortified beans. Studies were designed to reflect bean consumption in the context of typical meals of Rwanda, and more specifically to compare meals used in human absorption trials and efficacy studies which used the same exact varieties and harvests of beans [8,9]. The objective of this work was to demonstrate how the Caco-2 cell bioassay for Fe bioavailability can be applied to thoroughly and cost-effectively evaluate Fe-biofortified crops prior to a human study or release in the food system. Where appropriate, direct comparisons of the in vitro results to parallel or similar human studies are presented and critically evaluated.

2. Materials and Methods

2.1. Chemicals, Enzymes, and Hormones

All chemicals, enzymes, and hormones were purchased from Sigma Chemical Co. (St. Louis, MO, USA) unless stated otherwise.

2.2. Food Samples and Preparation

The normal and high Fe beans are the same varieties, and the same harvests were used for an animal feeding trial and from a parallel a human efficacy trial in Rwanda [8,10]. These bean lines are best described as "cream seeded carioca" varieties. Approximately 15 kg of the normal and high Fe varieties were available, and subsamples were taken from this stock for the various studies presented herein. For all studies, the bean samples were not pre-soaked, cooked by autoclave for 15 min in a 3:1 volume of water:bean, then freeze-dried and ground into powder with a common coffee grinder.

The menu items from the human efficacy study, reported in Experiment 1, were samples taken directly from the serving line used in the human study in Rwanda [8]. The samples were freeze dried for shipment to the lab of the first author for assay. For the in vitro Fe bioavailability assay, 0.5 g of the lyophilized sample were used for each replicate of the assay, as per the in vitro digestion procedure described below.

The potato sample used in the results presented in Experiment 2 was an organically grown Idaho white potato purchased at a local supermarket that was peeled and cooked by autoclave, then ground to a powder. It was deemed to be nutritionally similar to the white potato served in the parallel human trials. The rice sample used in this figure was polished, and of the Nishiki variety, and purchased at a local supermarket. These test meals were designed to match the relative combinations of beans and rice or beans and potato used in a similar human study. However, it is important to note that in the results presented in Experiment 2, the additional amount of Fe added as a stable isotope in the human study was not included in this in vitro study. This fact is important, as studies have shown, that the primary assumption of extrinsic labelling studies (i.e., complete isotopic exchange and equilibration of the extrinsic isotope) may not occur [11]. This point will be addressed in the discussion.

In the results presented in Experiments 3 and 4, extrinsic Fe the form of ^{58}Fe was added to the bean sample in the exact same relative ratio as done in similar human studies [9]. However, unlike the human study, potato or rice were not included. The ratio was 0.4 mg ^{58}Fe per 55 g of beans (dry weight). At the in vitro level, these amounts correspond to 0.5 g of dry ground bean sample plus 4 μg ^{58}Fe.

2.3. Iron Content of Food Samples, and Caco-2 Cells

Dried, ground food samples (0.5 g) were treated with 3.0 mL of 60:40 HNO_3 and $HClO_4$ mixture into a Pyrex glass tube and left for overnight to destroy organic matter. The mixture was then heated to 120 °C for two hours and 0.25 mL of 40 µg/g Yttrium added as an internal standard to compensate for any drift during the subsequent inductively coupled plasma atomic emission spectrometer (ICP-AES) analysis. The temperature of the heating block was then raised to 145 °C for 2 h. If necessary, more nitric acid (1–2 mL) was added to destroy the brownish color of the organic matter. Then, the temperature of the heating block raised to 190 °C for ten minutes and turned off. The cooled samples in the tubes were then diluted to 20 mL, vortexed and transferred onto auto sampler tubes to analyze via ICP-AES. The model of the ICP used was a Thermo iCAP 6500 series (Thermo Jarrell Ash Corp., Franklin, MA, USA). For the measurement of ^{58}Fe isotopes in Caco-2 cells, cell isolates were treated as described above, and ^{58}Fe was quantified using inductively coupled plasma mass spectrometry (Agilent Model 7500CS, Agilent Technologies, 5301 Stevens Creek Blvd, Santa Clara, CA 95051, USA).

2.4. Phytic acid Content of Food Samples

Phytic acid content was measured as phosphorous released by phytase and alkaline phosphatase via a colorimetric assay kit (K-PHYT 12/12, Megazyme International, Wicklow, Ireland).

Phytate degradation was conducted via the methods of Petry et al. [9]. The maximal effect achievable was a 66% decrease in total phytate phosphorous. To make the "68%" phytic acid samples, a non-treated sample was mixed 50:50 with sample treated for maximal phytate degradation (i.e., 34% phytate).

2.5. Polyphenol Analysis of Bean Samples

Seed coat extracts and polyphenol standards were analyzed with an Agilent 1220 Infinity UPLC coupled to an Advion Expression L compact mass spectrometer (CMS). Two (2) µL samples were injected and passed through an Acquity UPLC BEH Shield RP18 1.7 µm 2.1 × 100 mm column (Waters) at 0.35 mL/min. The column was temperature-controlled at 45 °C. The mobile phase consisted of water with 0.1% formic acid (solvent A) and acetonitrile with 0.1% formic acid (solvent B). Polyphenols were eluted using linear gradients of 86.7% to 77.0% A in 0.5 min, 77.0% to 46.0% A in 5.5 min, 46.0% to 0% A in 0.5 min, hold at 0% A for 3.5 min, 0% to 86.7% A in 0.5 min, and hold at 86.7% A for 3.5 min for a total 14 min run time. From the column, flow was directed into a variable wavelength UV detector set at 278 nm. Flow was then directed into the source of an Advion Expression LCMS (Advion Inc., Ithaca, NY, USA) and electrospray ionization (ESI) mass spectrometry was performed in negative ionization mode using selected ion monitoring with a scan time of 50 msec for each of eight polyphenol masses of interest. Capillary temperature and voltages were 300 C and 100 V, respectively. ESI source voltage and gas temperature were 2.6 kV and 240 C respectively. Desolvation gas flow was 240 L/h. Liquid chromatography (LC) and CMS instrumentation and data acquisition were controlled by Advion Mass Express software. Identities of polyphenols in bean samples were confirmed by comparison of m/z and LC retention times with authentic standards. No "internal" standards were used. External calibration standards were used for all polyphenolic compounds known to affect Fe bioavailability.

2.6. In Vitro Digestion

The in vitro digestion protocol was conducted as per an established in vitro digestion model [12]. Briefly, exactly 1 g of each sample was used for each sample digestion. To initiate the gastric phase of digestion, 10 mL of fresh saline solution (0.9% sodium chloride) was added to each sample and mixed. The pH was then adjusted to 2.0 with 1.0 mol/L HCl, and 0.5 mL of the pepsin solution (containing 1 g pepsin per 50 mL; certified > 250 U per mg protein; Sigma #P7000) was added to each mixture. The mixtures were under gastric digestion for 1 h at 37 °C on a rocking platform (model RP-50, Laboratory

Instrument, Rockville, MD, USA) located in an incubator. After 1 h of gastric digestion, the pH of the sample mixture was raised to 5.5–6.0 with 1.0 mol/L of NaHCO$_3$ solution. 2.5 mL of the pancreatin–bile extract solution was added to each mixture. The pancreatin–bile extract solution contained 0.35 g pancreatin (Sigma #P1750) and 2.1 g bile extract (Sigma #B8631) in a total volume of 245 mL. The pH of the mixture was then adjusted to approximately 7.0, and the final volume of each mixture was adjusted to 15.0 mL by weight using a salt solution of 140 mmol/L of NaCl and 5.0 mmol/L of KCl at pH 6.7. At this point, the mixture was referred to as a "digest". The samples were then incubated for an additional two hours at 37 °C, at which point the digests were centrifuged, and supernatants and pellet fractions collected and transferred to tubes for analysis. Three independent replications of the in vitro digestion procedure were carried out for all of the food samples. For some samples, as noted in the specific results section, Fe bioavailability was assessed in both the presence and absence of ascorbic acid (AA). The AA was added to the digests at the start of the gastric digestion phase at a concentration of 10 µmol/L. This treatment has been shown to expose some additional differences between samples and thus provides further information on the matrix of the digest.

2.7. Statistical Analysis

Data were analyzed using the software package GraphPad Prism (GraphPad Software, San Diego, CA, USA). Data were analyzed using analysis of variance incorporating normalization of variance, if needed, and Tukey's post test to determine significant differences ($p < 0.05$) between groups. Unless noted otherwise values are expressed as mean ± standard error of the mean (SEM); $n = 3$ independent replications.

3. Results

Compositional Analyses of Beans, Potato and Rice Samples

Iron and phytic acid levels for the ground bean, potato and rice samples used in experiments one and two are supplied in Table 1. It is important to note that measurement of the Fe content of the bean samples can vary substantially depending on the sub-sampling of the overall harvest. For example, as shown in Table 2, from the same harvests of these lines we measured the Fe level in a separate sub-sample to be 59.9 µg/g in the normal bean and 96.9 µg/g in the high Fe variety. A previously published animal trial using the same harvest of these two lines yielded values of 58 and 106 µg/g for the normal and high Fe varieties, respectively. From experience, we have found that such variation in Fe content is quite common among sub-samples of bean harvests and is simply due to variance in the individual bean Fe content. Thorough mixing of the harvest does not negate this variance; however, the grinding of the sample for analysis makes the sample homogenous for Fe content, with variance of less than 5% between replicates of the ground sample. The amount used for the sub-sampling of the bean harvests of the bean samples should therefore be substantial whenever practical to do so. Based on our observations, we recommend a sub-sample of 200–300 g from thoroughly mixed larger batches, such as 5–10 kg.

Table 1. Iron (Fe) and phytic acid (PA) content of beans for Experiments 1 and 2. The rice and potato samples were used in Experiments 3 and 4 [1].

Food Sample	Fe (µg/g)	Phytic Acid g/100 g	Molar Ratio PA:Fe
Normal Fe bean	47.5	1.21	22:1
High Fe bean	82.5	1.52	16:1
Potato	19.1	0.33	14:1
Rice	2.2	0.14	53:1

[1] Values represent the average of three replicate measurements. Range of variance in measurement was <5% for all samples.

Iron analysis of cotyledon, seed coat and embryo fractions demonstrated that the increase in Fe content was consistent across all of the major fractions.

Table 2. Iron content of cotyledon, embryo and seed coat of the normal and high Fe beans [1].

Bean Variety	Cotyledon Fe (µg/g)	Embryo Fe (µg/g)	Seed Coat Fe (µg/g)	Total Fe (µg/g)
Normal	51.5 (78.3%)	67.1 (1.2%)	156.4 (20.6%)	59.9
High Fe	81.6 (75.7%)	103.3 (1.5%)	255.9 (22.8%)	96.9

[1] Values in parentheses represent the percent of the total Fe present in this fraction of the whole bean. Values represent the average of three replicate measurements. Range of variance in measurement was <5% in all samples.

Polyphenolic compounds that are known to influence Fe uptake or that contrasted significantly between the normal and high Fe lines are summarized in Table 3. It is important to note that although other molecular weights were evident in the analyses, only compounds that could be identified are included. Based on previous studies, kaempferol and glycosides thereof are possible Fe uptake promoters, as are catechin and 3,4 di-hydroxybenzoic acid. Inhibitors of Fe uptake are quercetin and procyanidin B [12].

The results in Table 4 represent a summary of Fe bioavailability, Fe content, and Al and Ti levels, which are indicators of soil contamination. The green vegetables, cabbage and carrots, tomato sauce, and sombe (a dish with cassava leaves) all appear to have some level of soil contamination. All of these menu items were samples received directly from the cafeteria meal plan of the parallel human study.

Table 3. Polyphenolic profile of the seed coat of the normal and high Fe beans [1].

Compound	Molecular Weight (*m/z*)	Normal Bean	High Fe Bean
Kaempferol-3-glucoside	447.0926	281	475
Kaempferol derivative	489.1030	108	251
Catechin	289.0710	237	182
AzIV	1083.5415	135	32
Kaempferol	285.0393	50	101
Procyanidin B	577.1348	106	84
Querctin-3-glucoside	463.0874	ND	81
Kaempferol-3-sambubioside	579.1354	ND	25
3,4-dihydroxybenzoic acid	153.0180	19	24
Quercetin	301.0347	ND	19

[1] Values for compound levels represent ion intensity, and therefore represent only relative differences in concentration. "ND" = non-detected.

Table 4. Experiment 1. In vitro Fe bioavailability, and mineral (Fe, Al, Ti) content of menu items from human efficacy trial of normal and high Fe beans [8] [1].

Menu Item	Occurrence on Menu (%)	Fe Bioavailability (ng Ferritin/mg Cell Protein)	Fe (µg/g)	Al (µg/g)	Ti (µg/g)
Normal bean	100	5.01 ± 0.2	47.5	5.2	0.2
High Fe bean	100	5.9 ± 0.2	82.5	5.9	0.4
Tomato sauce	100	24.2 ± 1.1	120.8	76.8	0.5
Rice	85	0.9 ± 0.1	4.7	1.7	0.2
Cooked rice with curry	unknown	1.7 ± 0.3	6.5	14.5	0.2
Cabbage + carrots	43	9.5 ± 0.3	80.0	80.2	1.8
Green vegetables	43	1.5 ± 0.3	312.7	448.1	14.4
Potato chips	28	20.9 ± 1.1	25.4	8.0	1.2
Banana chips	unknown	1.8 ± 0.2	10.5	2.5	0.4
Fried sweet potatoes	14	7.3 ± 1.1	22.1	10.0	0.6
Cassava bread	14	5.69 ± 0.55	22.2	22.8	1.3
Macaroni	14	2.04 ± 0.26	34.3	5.8	0.3
Sombe	14	1.40 ± 0.21	81.0	168.1	0.8
Fried Irish potatoes	7	25.51 ± 1.33	30.4	8.6	1.3
Boiled Irish potatoes	7	41.77 ± 2.82	37.7	3.5	0.6
Banana with tomato sauce	14	1.91 ± 0.04	20.0	11.7	0.7

[1] Fe bioavailability values are mean ± standard error, *n* = 3. Mineral content values are the mean of three replicates.

The results of Experiment 2 show two significant effects. First, the addition of rice to beans lowers the Fe bioavailability, eliminating the increase in Fe uptake from the high Fe bean. The addition of potato increases the overall Fe uptake from the meal. In both combinations, the bean is the major source of Fe; however, the potato does contribute more Fe to the food matrix relative to rice. For each condition, and it is important to note that the amount of rice or potato is the same as that published in a human study where these lines of beans were evaluated. The second effect shown in Experiment 2 is that the reduction of phytate results in a decrease in Fe uptake. This occurs for both the normal and high Fe beans when evaluated alone or in combination with potato.

The results in Experiments 3 and 4 are from the same series of experiments. In these studies, efforts were made to replicate the conditions of a human absorption study where the normal and high Fe beans were treated with phytase, and the labelled extrinsically with [58]Fe [9]. Similar to the results shown in Figure 1, the high Fe bean resulted in significantly more ferritin formation (Fe uptake) than the normal bean, regardless of the phytate content. The addition of the [58]Fe resulted in significantly higher ferritin formation (iron uptake) from the normal beans but not from the high Fe beans (Experiment 3; Figure 2). Direct measurement of [58]Fe in the Caco-2 cells showed significantly more [58]Fe uptake from the normal Fe beans vs the high Fe beans (Experiment 4; Figure 3). Decreased phytate content was associated with decreased [58]Fe uptake, exhibiting similar pattern of response in Fe uptake as measured via Caco-2 cell ferritin formation.

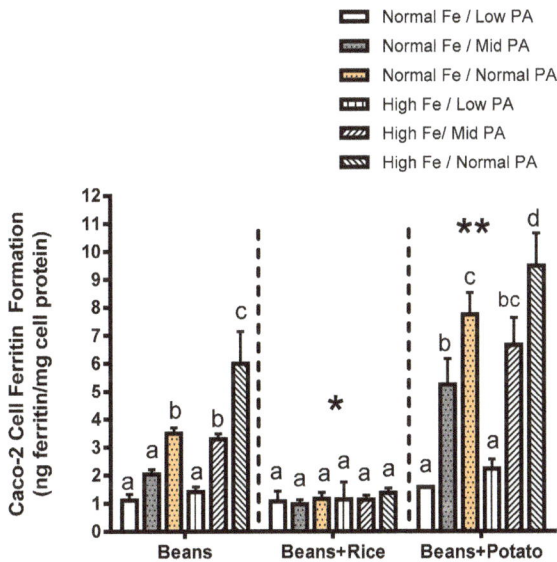

Figure 1. Experiment 2. Iron uptake as measured by Caco-2 cell ferritin formation from beans pre-treated with phytase. Values represent Fe uptake from normal or high Fe beans with normal phytate (PA; 100%) levels, or PA levels reduced to low (34%) or mid (68%) of the normal PA content. Bar values within food combination groups with no letters in common are significantly different ($p < 0.05$). A single asterisk indicates significant inhibitory effect ($p < 0.05$) of the addition of rice, whereas the double asterisk indicates significant promotional effect of the addition of potato.

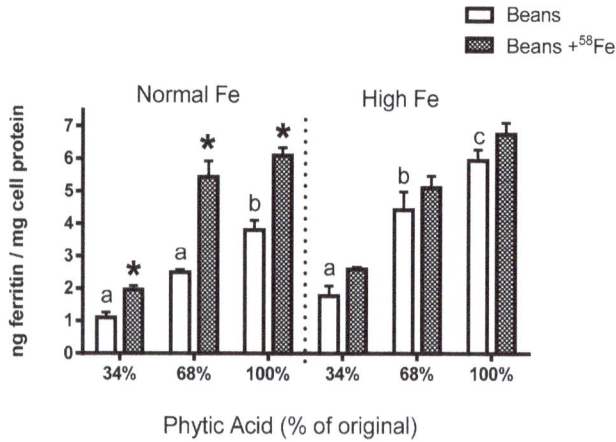

Figure 2. Experiment 3. Caco-2 cell Fe uptake as measured by ferritin formation from normal and high Fe beans that were extrinsically labelled with [58]Fe as per a published human study using the same harvest of these bean varieties [9]. Values are mean ± SEM, *n* = 3. Bars with no letters in common indicate significant difference (*p* < 0.05). Asterisks indicate significantly more ferritin formation relative to samples without the [58]Fe label.

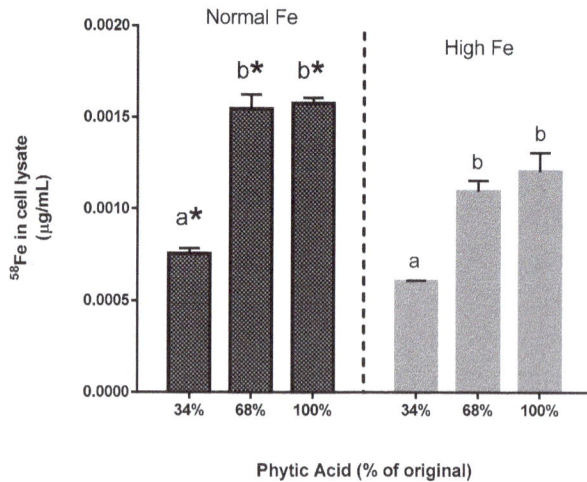

Figure 3. Experiment 4. Caco-2 cell [58]Fe content following exposure to in vitro digests of normal and high Fe beans extrinsically labelled with [58]Fe. Values are mean ± SEM, *n* = 3. Bars with no letters in common indicate significant difference (*p* < 0.05). Asterisks indicate significantly more [58]Fe (*p* < 0.05) relative to the same phytate content in the high Fe beans.

4. Discussion

The in vitro methodology for measuring Fe bioavailability utilized in the present study was first published in 1998 [3]. Since then it has been applied to estimate Fe bioavailability from many food products [13], forms of Fe [14], diet plans [15] and staple food crops [16]. It has been shown to be a robust model, capable not only of diverse application, but also able to handle high throughput [4,6]. Over the past few years, it has been shown to predict the overall outcome of two published human efficacy studies of Fe biofortification and the parallel animal studies [7,8,10,17,18]. A recent review article demonstrates that when coupled with a poultry feeding model, it can now be seen as an established and well-validated approach for the development of Fe-biofortified crops and food products [7].

The observations of the present study clearly suggest that several factors should be considered when evaluating and advancing Fe-biofortified beans for either human study or release to farmers. First, it is important to consider how other foods commonly consumed with beans can affect the Fe bioavailability. For example, Experiment 2 indicates that the consumption of beans with rice negates the nutritional benefits of the higher Fe content, whereas the consumption of beans with potato appears to enhance the Fe uptake from the meal. Consumption of beans with rice or potato has been documented as common throughout countries such as Rwanda and other African nations. These combinations were used as test meals in human absorption studies of these same lines of beans, yet it appears that potential differences in these meal combinations were not considered by the investigators [9].

In the above-mentioned human studies, ^{58}Fe was added extrinsically to the meal, at levels equalling 11.9% of the total Fe for the normal Fe beans, and at 7.6% of the total Fe for the high Fe variety [9]. Also, in this human study the investigators modified the levels of phytic acid in the bean samples by pre-treating the beans with phytase, claiming to achieve >95% reduction of phytate content. The present study mimicked these treatments using the exact same lines of beans, and used what should be a very effective phytase treatment, but only achieved a maximum decrease in phytate content of 66%. We also explored additional conditions such as increased enzyme concentration and duration of exposure to phytase, but no additional decrease in phytate was observed. Thus, we do not know how the other group was able to achieve almost complete removal of the phytate. This would be of concern as more prolonged treatment could also be more likely to alter other factors in the bean samples, such as polyphenolic profiles that would confound the results relative to the native phytate and polyphenol profiles of these lines.

The present study yields some key observations on Fe bioavailability with the reduction of phytate content. First, the decrease in phytic acid resulted in a surprising decrease in Fe uptake by the Caco-2 cells (Experiments 2–4), an observation which is in contrast to the claim from the human study that dephytinization increased Fe uptake. One possible explanation for the in vitro decrease in Fe uptake could be that the decrease in phytate facilitated greater opportunity for the seed coat polyphenols to complex the Fe and inhibit Fe bioavailability. However, with the addition of ^{58}Fe to the bean samples, there is an interesting observation that could explain the apparent difference between the human study results and this in vitro study when phytate content is decreased. Consider the following: the addition of the extrinsic ^{58}Fe was clearly associated with an increased ferritin formation effect (i.e., Fe uptake) in the normal beans but not in the high Fe beans (Experiment 3). Indeed, for the normal bean samples, where phytate values were reduced to 34% and 68% of the natural content, the addition of the ^{58}Fe approximately doubled the Caco-2 cell Fe uptake. A similar trend was evident in the high Fe beans although the difference was not statistically significant. The lesser effect in the high Fe bean samples is probably due to the increased intrinsic Fe content or possibly to other factors such as the differences in polyphenol content (Table 3). Direct measurement of the ^{58}Fe in the Caco-2 cells also indicates that the increased ferritin formation is due to the extrinsic ^{58}Fe (Experiment 4). Indeed, the addition of an extrinsic Fe source at an amount equal to 11.9% of the total Fe approximately doubles the Caco-2 cell ferritin formation. Taken together, these observations indicate that the uptake of the extrinsic Fe was much greater than that of the intrinsic Fe of the bean. In other words, the extrinsic ^{58}Fe has a different bioavailability relative to the intrinsic Fe of the bean and is clear evidence of incomplete isotopic exchange and equilibration of the extrinsic label. It should be noted that previous studies have shown that the cotyledon cell walls of beans are a potential barrier to Fe uptake from a bean meal, and could also be a barrier that prevents equilibration of the extrinsic Fe with the intrinsic Fe [19].

As noted in studies decades ago, extrinsic labelling of food Fe is dependent upon the assumption of complete isotopic exchange and equilibration [20]. Hence, the above observation indicates that extrinsic labelling of the bean samples as conducted in the human study would yield inaccurate measurement of Fe bioavailability from the beans under these feeding conditions. It is therefore entirely possible that in the human study, the decrease in phytate did indeed result in less overall Fe uptake, an effect that would have been masked due a flawed assumption of complete extrinsic label equilibration. The human study depends entirely upon this assumption, whereas the in vitro model does not.

In consideration of the above, it is also important to note that the human study [9] did not separate out the effects of rice versus potatoes on Fe uptake from the meals; thus, the Fe uptake in the human study represents the combined effects of rice and potato on isotopic Fe uptake. This combined food effect, plus the fact that the human study did not simply measure Fe uptake from just the beans, limits further useful comparison of the in vitro and human results. Certainly, future studies should follow up on the individual effects of rice and potatoes on bean Fe bioavailability as it negates the benefit of a crop in a given food system. In regards to comparing the human absorption study with the in vitro model, the question that remains is which approach is more accurate and effective at evaluating the Fe bioavailability of beans? The human model is based on an assumption that has seen a fair share of criticism and doubt by other scientists [11,20,21]; whereas, the in vitro approach bears the caveat of simply being an in vitro model, albeit one that is now validated by direct comparison to human efficacy and animal feeding trials [7].

The present study also demonstrates that the high Fe beans also contained higher levels of uptake-inhibiting polyphenols in the seed coats (Table 2). For these bean varieties, the inhibitory compounds of most significance are quercetin and quercetin-3-glucoside. These compounds have been shown to be inhibitory of Fe uptake, even when potential promoting polyphenols, such as kaempferol (and glycosides thereof) are present in greater amounts [12]. Increased inhibitory polyphenols were also demonstrated in high Fe black beans and high Fe pearl millet [22,23]. This consistent association of enhanced Fe content with greater polyphenol levels reinforces the need to perform bioavailability assessments of lines targeted for biofortification. Moreover, the finding of increased inhibitory polyphenols with increased Fe content is an example of how breeding solely for enhanced Fe content could result in a misdirection of breeding. Such a misdirection could result in an end product with no nutritional benefit, despite enhanced content, or one that achieves a less than maximal benefit. It is important to note that the compounds listed in the present study represent the ones that are currently known to be among the list of polyphenols found in bean seed coats and are known to influence Fe bioavailability. There may be others, but this list is simply based upon what has been identified and characterized from previous work that utilized the Caco-2 cell bioassay and LC-MS technology [12].

Evaluation of the results presented on the menu items of the Rwandan human trial (Experiment 1) must consider that these results are based on the dry weight of the menu items. We do not have data for the water content of these menu items. In general, it could be expected that for items such as tomato sauce the water content could be 90–95%, perhaps slightly less for items such as green vegetables, cabbage, carrots, and banana. The potato items could be of key nutritional interest, depending on their water content, as the Caco-2 cell ferritin formation and Fe content values were relatively high. The green vegetables appear to be contaminated with soil Fe as Fe, Al and Ti values were very high and ferritin values were low, measurements that are clear indicators of the presence of soil Fe. The occurrence of the items on the menu are also potentially important; and although it was beyond the scope of the present study, it should be noted that the experimental approach outlined in this manuscript could certainly be applied to evaluate the meal plan in greater detail, provided that information such as water content and consumption rate are available.

5. Conclusions

The present study clearly shows that the high Fe bean variety delivers more absorbable Fe relative to the normal bean variety. Such observations agree with previous in vitro, animal and human studies of these particular varieties and harvests [8,10]. Indeed, the level of validation of this in vitro approach is now quite extensive; hence, observations generated from its proper application should be confidently applied to direct nutritional studies and bean breeding. In addition, the results from the present study provide more evidence that the assessment of the Fe bioavailability of beans via extrinsic labelling yields potentially inaccurate information.

Acknowledgments: Research funded by the United States Department of Agriculture, Agricultural Research Service. The authors thank Yongpei Chang and Mary Bodis for their excellent technical support.

Author Contributions: For research articles with several authors, a short paragraph specifying their individual contributions must be provided. R.G. conceived and designed the experiments, analyzed the results and wrote the manuscript. E.T. consulted on project and contributed to manuscript content. J.H. (Hart) analyzed bean samples for polyphenolic profile and contributed to manuscript editing. J.H. (Haas) contributed to experimental design and manuscript content. M.L. provided bean and meal samples for analyses and contributed to manuscript content. S.B. provided bean samples and contributed to manuscript content.

Conflicts of Interest: The authors declare no conflict of interest.

References

1. Welch, R.M.; House, W.A.; Beebe, S.; Cheng, Z. Genetic selection for enhanced bioavailable levels of iron in bean (*Phaseolus vulgaris* L.) seeds. *J. Agric. Food Chem.* **2000**, *48*, 3576–3580. [CrossRef] [PubMed]

2. Van Campen, D.R.; Glahn, R.P. Micronutrient bioavailability techniques: Accuracy, problems and limitations. *Field Crops Res.* **1999**, *60*, 93–113. [CrossRef]

3. Glahn, R.P.; Lee, O.A.; Yeung, A.; Goldman, M.I.; Miller, D.D. Caco-2 Cell Ferritin Formation Predicts Nonradiolabeled Food Iron Availability in an In Vitro Digestion/Caco-2 Cell Culture Model. *J. Nutr.* **1998**, *128*, 1555–1561. [PubMed]

4. Lung'aho, M.G.; Mwaniki, A.M.; Szalma, S.J.; Hart, J.J.; Rutzke, M.A.; Kochian, L.V.; Glahn, R.P.; Hoekenga, O.A. Genetic and physiological analysis of iron biofortification in maize kernels. *PLoS ONE* **2011**, *6*, 20429. [CrossRef] [PubMed]

5. Dellavalle, D.M.; Vandenberg, A.; Glahn, R.P. Seed coat removal improves iron bioavailability in cooked lentils: Studies using an in vitro digestion/Caco-2 cell culture model. *J. Agric. Food Chem.* **2013**, *61*, 8084–8489. [CrossRef] [PubMed]

6. Wiesinger, J.A.; Cichy, K.A.; Glahn, R.P.; Grusak, M.A.; Brick, M.A.; Thompson, H.J.; Tako, E. Demonstrating a nutritional advantage to the fast-cooking dry bean (*Phaseolus vulgaris* L.). *J. Agric. Food Chem.* **2016**. [CrossRef] [PubMed]

7. Tako, E.; Bar, H.; Glahn, R.P. The Combined Application of the Caco-2 Cell Bioassay Coupled with In Vivo (*Gallus gallus*) Feeding Trial Represents an Effective Approach to Predicting Fe Bioavailability in Humans. *Nutrients* **2016**, *8*, 732. [CrossRef] [PubMed]

8. Haas, J.D.; Luna, S.V.; Lung'aho, M.G.; Wenger, M.J.; Murray-Kolb, L.E.; Beebe, S.; Gahutu, J.B.; Egli, I.M. Consuming Iron Biofortified Beans Increases Iron Status in Rwandan Women after 128 Days in a Randomized Controlled Feeding Trial. *J. Nutr.* **2016**, *146*, 1586–1592. [CrossRef] [PubMed]

9. Petry, N.; Egli, I.; Gahutu, J.; Tugirimana, P.; Boy, E.; Hurrell, R. Phytic acid concentration influences iron bioavailability from biofortified beans in Rwandese women with low iron status. *J. Nutr.* **2014**, *144*, 1681–1687. [CrossRef] [PubMed]

10. Tako, E.; Reed, S.; Anandaraman, A.; Beebe, S.E.; Hart, J.J.; Glahn, R.P. Studies of Cream Seeded Carioca Beans (*Phaseolus vulgaris* L.) from a Rwandan Efficacy Trial: In Vitro and In Vivo Screening Tools Reflect Human Studies and Predict Beneficial Results from Iron Biofortified Beans. *PLoS ONE* **2015**, *10*, 0138479. [CrossRef] [PubMed]

11. Glahn, R.P.; Cheng, Z.; Giri, S. Extrinsic labeling of staple food crops with isotopic iron does not consistently result in full equilibration: Revisiting the methodology. *J. Agric. Food Chem.* **2015**, *6*, 9621–9628. [CrossRef] [PubMed]

12. Hart, J.; Tako, E.; Raymond, P.; Glahn, R.P. Characterization of Polyphenol Effects on Inhibition and Promotion of Iron Uptake by Caco-2 Cells Jonathan. *J. Agric. Food Chem.* **2017**, *65*, 3285–3294. [CrossRef] [PubMed]

13. Etcheverry, P.; Wallingford, J.; Miller, D.D.; Glahn, R.P. Calcium, zinc and iron bioavailabilities from a commercial human milk fortifier: A comparison study. *J. Dairy Sci.* **2004**, *87*, 3629–3637. [CrossRef]

14. Yun, S.; Habicht, J.P.; Miller, D.D.; Glahn, R.P. An in vitro digestion/Caco-2 cell culture system accurately predicts the effects of ascorbic acid and polyphenolic compounds on iron bioavailability in humans. *J. Nutr.* **2004**, *134*, 2717–2721. [PubMed]

15. Pachón, H.; Stoltzfus, R.J.; Glahn, R.P. Homogenization, lyophilization or acid-extraction of meat products improves iron uptake from cereal-meat product combinations in an in vitro digestion/Caco-2 cell model. *Br. J. Nutr.* **2009**, *101*, 816–821. [CrossRef] [PubMed]

16. Dellavalle, D.M.; Thavarajah, D.; Thavarajah, P.; Vandenberg, A.; Glahn, R.P. Lentil (*Lens culinaris* L.) as a candidate crop for iron biofortification: Is there genetic potential for iron bioavailability? *Field Crops Res.* **2013**, *144*, 119–125. [CrossRef]

17. Finkelstein, J.L.; Mehta, S.; Udipi, S.A.; Ghugre, P.S.; Luna, S.V.; Wenger, M.J.; Murray-Kolb, L.E.; Przybyszewski, E.M.; Haas, J.D. A Randomized Trial of Iron-Biofortified Pearl Millet in School Children in India. *J. Nutr.* **2015**, *145*, 1576–1581. [CrossRef] [PubMed]

18. Tako, E.; Blair, M.W.; Glahn, R.P. Biofortified red mottled beans (*Phaseolus vulgaris* L.) in a maize and bean diet provide more bioavailable iron than standard red mottled beans: Studies in poultry (*Gallus gallus*) and an in vitro digestion/Caco-2 model. *Nutr. J.* **2011**, *10*, 113. [CrossRef] [PubMed]

19. Glahn, R.P.; Tako, E.; Cichy, K.A.; Wiesinger, J. The Cotyledon Cell Wall of the Common Bean (*Phaseolus vulgaris*) Resists Digestion in the Upper Intestine and Thus May Limit Iron Bioavailability. *Food Funct.* **2016**, *7*, 3193. [CrossRef] [PubMed]

20. Consaul, J.R.; Lee, K. Extrinsic tagging in iron bioavailability research. *J. Agric. Food Chem.* **1983**, *31*, 684–689. [CrossRef] [PubMed]

21. Jin, F.; Cheng, Z.; Rutzke, M.A.; Welch, R.M.; Glahn, R.P. Extrinsic labeling method may not accurately measure Fe absorption from cooked pinto beans (*Phaseolus vulgaris*): Comparison of extrinsic and intrinsic labeling of beans. *J. Agric. Food Chem.* **2008**, *56*, 6881–6885. [CrossRef] [PubMed]

22. Tako, E.; Beebe, S.E.; Reed, S.; Hart, J.J.; Glahn, R.P. Polyphenolic compounds appear to limit the nutritional benefit of biofortified higher iron black bean (*Phaseolus vulgaris* L.). *Nutr. J.* **2014**, *13*, 28. [CrossRef] [PubMed]

23. Tako, E.; Reed, S.M.; Budiman, J.; Hart, J.J.; Glahn, R.P. Higher iron pearl millet (*Pennisetum glaucum* L.) provides more absorbable iron that is limited by increased polyphenolic content. *Nutr. J.* **2015**, *14*, 11. [CrossRef] [PubMed]

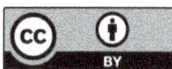

MDPI

Article

Iron Supplementation during Three Consecutive Days of Endurance Training Augmented Hepcidin Levels

Aya Ishibashi [1,2], Naho Maeda [2], Akiko Kamei [1] and Kazushige Goto [2,*]

[1] Department of Sports Science, Japan Institute of Sports Science, Nishigaoka, Kitaku, Tokyo 115-0056, Japan; aya.ishibashi@jpnsport.go.jp (A.I.); akiko.kamei@jpnsport.go.jp (A.K.)
[2] Graduate School of Sport and Health Science, Ritsumeikan University, Kusatsu, Shiga 525-8577, Japan; maeda.nh0709@gmail.com
* Correspondence: kagoto@fc.ritsumei.ac.jp; Tel./Fax: +81-77-599-4127

Received: 15 June 2017; Accepted: 28 July 2017; Published: 30 July 2017

Abstract: Iron supplementation contributes an effort to improving iron status among athletes, but it does not always prevent iron deficiency. In the present study, we explored the effect of three consecutive days of endurance training (twice daily) on the hepcidin-25 (hepcidin) level. The effect of iron supplementation during this period was also determined. Fourteen male endurance athletes were enrolled and randomly assigned to either an iron-treated condition (Fe condition, $n = 7$) or a placebo condition (Control condition; CON, $n = 7$). They engaged in two 75-min sessions of treadmill running at 75% of maximal oxygen uptake on three consecutive days (days 1–3). The Fe condition took 12 mg of iron twice daily (24 mg/day), and the CON condition did not. On day 1, both conditions exhibited significant increases in serum hepcidin and plasma interleukin-6 levels after exercise ($p < 0.05$). In the CON condition, the hepcidin level did not change significantly throughout the training period. However, in the Fe condition, the serum hepcidin level on day 4 was significantly higher than that of the CON condition ($p < 0.05$). In conclusion, the hepcidin level was significantly elevated following three consecutive days of endurance training when moderate doses of iron were taken.

Keywords: iron related-hormone; endurance training; iron supplementation

---

1. Introduction

Iron deficiency (ferritin <20 ng/mL) is frequently observed among endurance athletes [1], as it is more common than iron-deficient anemia and affects 13–22% of elite athletes [2,3]. Several physiological mechanisms have been proposed to explain this phenomenon, including gastrointestinal bleeding [4], hemolysis [5], lack of dietary iron [6], and iron loss in sweat [7]. Additionally, the regulatory hormone hepcidin may be involved [8]. Hepcidin, a 25-amino acid peptide, is a crucial mediator of iron homeostasis and may be associated with iron deficiency in response to exercise training. Iron is taken up by enterocytes and is either bound to transferrin or stored as intracellular ferritin [9]. Hepcidin internalizes (degrades) the ferroportin export channels of the small intestine and macrophage surface, inhibiting gut absorption of dietary iron and preventing iron release by macrophages [10]. Hepcidin expression is upregulated by increased iron intake and/or storage [10,11] and inflammation [12,13]. In contrast, it is downregulated by iron deficiency anemia and hypoxia [14].

A low ferritin level with iron supplementation did not affect endurance performance (e.g., running economy, time to exhaustion) in iron-deficient non-anemic athletes [15,16]. In contrast, iron treatments may improve the iron status and endurance performance even in iron-deficient non-anemic athletes [17], although these findings are not consistent. Therefore, the question of whether iron supplementation during intense training might improve endurance performance has not been fully explored [18]. A high dose of iron supplementation can be applied among some competitive athletes [19,20], but high doses of iron supplementation may stimulate hepcidin production to maintain iron homeostasis [10,11]. Such high-level supplementation (60–240 mg daily) increased the serum hepcidin level after 24 h, and the fractional iron absorption fell by 35–45% [21]. However, the influence of moderate iron supplementation during strenuous training on the hepcidin level remains unclear. This is an important issue because iron supplementation is a widespread practice among endurance athletes.

Previous studies exploring the influence of acute exercise on iron metabolism found that the hepcidin level was transiently elevated about 3 h after exercise [8,22–24] and that this was associated with increases in exercise-induced inflammation and hemolysis [24]. Strenuous exercise promotes inflammation, as reflected by a marked increase in the interleukin-6 (IL-6) level [25]. Pro-inflammatory cytokines (e.g., IL-6) stimulate hepcidin production [10,26,27], and sustained inflammation caused by cumulative exercise may promote hepcidin production and iron deficiency. Peeling et al. [28] recently reported that resting iron status, in addition to post-exercise IL-6 level and exercise intensity, accounted for ~77% of the variance in post-exercise hepcidin elevation in elite athletes.

Two recent studies found that seven days of running and/or military training, followed by a 54-km skiing event, significantly increased the basal hepcidin level [29,30]. Furthermore, we previously observed that augmented monthly training significantly increased the hepcidin level in long-distance runner [31]. In contrast, other studies found that exercise did not significantly influence the hepcidin level [23,32]. However, the effects of several consecutive days of strenuous endurance training have not yet been determined.

In the present study, we investigated the impact of three consecutive days of endurance training on the hepcidin level. Training was performed twice daily, because the typical training programs among endurance athletes involve two daily sessions (with several hours of rest between). The influence of iron supplementation during training was also determined. We hypothesized that three consecutive days of endurance training would elevate the hepcidin level and that iron supplementation during training would further augment this level.

2. Materials and Methods

2.1. Subjects

Fourteen male endurance athletes (long-distance runners and triathletes) participated (means ± standard errors (SE): age: 19–22 years; height: 1.68 ± 0.01 m; weight: 55.9 ± 1.1 kg; maximal oxygen uptake ($\dot{V}O_{2max}$): 59.6 ± 0.8 mL/kg/min). All subjects were healthy and trained regularly on ≥4 days a week. The exclusion criteria were smoking and the use of herbs or medications. All subjects were informed about the study protocol, the possible benefits and risks, and they provided written informed consent. The study was approved by the Ethics Committee for Human Experiments of Ritsumeikan University, Japan (BKC-IRB-2015-023).

2.2. Experimental Design

This was a single-blinded placebo-controlled study. The 14 subjects were randomly assigned to either an iron-treatment (Fe condition; $n = 7$) or a placebo (CON condition; $n = 7$) condition; $\dot{V}O_{2max}$ level were evaluated prior to the experiment. All subjects completed three consecutive days of twice-daily endurance exercises (75 min bouts of treadmill running at 75% of $\dot{V}O_{2max}$ in the morning (Ex 1; 8:30–10:45) and afternoon (Ex 2; 13:00–14:15). The Fe condition received 12 mg of iron in a flavored drink (100 mL) before and immediately after Ex 1 (24 mg/day); CON subjects received the drink only. Iron supplementation among athletes often features 24 mg Fe/day [33].

Blood samples were collected from the antecubital vein at 08:00 during the training period (days 1–3) and on the next day (day 4).

During the three days of training, all subjects arrived at the laboratory at 08:00 following an overnight fast. Body weight, fatigue score, and muscle soreness were evaluated using a visual analog scale. All subjects completed the six exercise sessions at 75% of the $\dot{V}O_{2max}$. However, the running velocity was reduced when a subject could not maintain the prescribed velocity because of accumulated fatigue. Water was given ad libitum throughout all sessions, and standard meals were provided at 11:00, 13:30, and 19:00.

2.3. Measurements

2.3.1. Determination of Running Velocity

About two weeks prior to the training period, an incremental treadmill exercise test (Life Fitness 95T, Chicago, IL, USA) was used to assess $\dot{V}O_{2max}$. The initial running velocity was 6 km/h and was increased progressively by 2 km/h every minute. When the velocity attained 14.6 km/h, it was further increased by 0.6 km/h every minute to exhaustion. The treadmill gradient was 0% (flat) [34]. Respiratory gases were collected using a breath-by-breath methods; we evaluated oxygen uptake ($\dot{V}O_2$), carbon dioxide output ($\dot{V}CO_2$), ventilation volume ($\dot{V}E$), and the respiratory exchange ratio (RER) using a metabolic cart (AE300S, Minato Medical Science Co., Osaka, Japan). The oxygen, carbon dioxide, and flow sensors were calibrated before each test according to the manufacturer's instructions. The exercise test was terminated when the subject could not maintain the prescribed running speed or when the $\dot{V}O_2$ plateau was attained. The running velocity and $\dot{V}O_2$ were used to calculate the running speed associated with 75% of the $\dot{V}O_{2max}$.

2.3.2. Blood Sampling and Analyses

Resting blood samples from the antecubital vein were collected after an overnight fast (at least 12 h) during the experimental period (days 1–4) and 3 h after Ex 2 on day 1. Serum and plasma samples were stored at −80 °C after centrifugation for 10 min (3000 rpm, 4 °C). Two-milliliter samples were transferred to ethylenediaminetetraacetic acid (EDTA) containing tubes immediately after sampling for determination of hematological parameters; blood hemoglobin (Hb) levels were measured in a clinical laboratory (Falco Holdings Co., Kyoto, Japan). Serum total iron binding capacity (TIBC) and ferritin, iron, transferrin, creatine kinase (CK), high-sensitivity C reactive protein (hsCRP), and myoglobin levels were measured in another clinical laboratory (SRL Co., Tokyo, Japan). Transferrin saturation (TSAT) was calculated as the serum iron level/serum TIBC level × 100. Plasma IL-6 levels were determined using a commercial enzyme-linked immunosorbent assay (ELISA) kit (R and D Systems Inc., Minneapolis, MN, USA). Serum hepcidin levels were measured by cation-exchange chromatography followed by liquid chromatography-tandem mass spectrometry (LC-MS/MS).

The intra-assay coefficients of variation (CVs) were as follows: 0.6% for Hb, 3.8% for ferritin, 1.4% for iron, 1.6% for the TIBC, 2.3% for CK, 3.2% for hsCRP, 3.4% for myoglobin, and 5.2% for IL-6.

2.3.3. Scores of Fatigue and Muscle Soreness

Subjective fatigue and muscle soreness levels were evaluated using a visual analog scale (VAS). The subjects were instructed to draw lines on 100 mm scales that were marked with "not tired" or "no pain" on the left and with "extremely tired" or "the worst pain ever" on the right [35].

2.3.4. Nutritional Assessment and Standard Meal

All subjects were asked to maintain their usual dietary intake during the month before commencement of training. Regular food and nutrient consumption were calculated using dedicated software (Excel Eiyo-kun FFQg version 4.0; Kenpaku-sha, Tokyo, Japan). The FFQg yields average intake/week of 29 food groups and 10 forms of cookery in conventional units or portion sizes. No subject took an iron supplement. The standard meals were individually adjusted to reflect the usual food and nutrient consumptions.

2.3.5. Statistical Analyses

All data are presented as means ± SE. Changes over time in blood variables were evaluated using two-way analysis of variance (ANOVA) with repeated measures (condition (Fe, CON) × time (days 1–4)). When the ANOVA revealed a significant interaction or a main effect, Tukey's post-hoc analysis was performed to explore where the difference was located. In addition to p-values, we calculated Cohen's d-values (on independent t-test) or the partial η^2 values (when a two-way ANOVA with repeated measures was performed) to determine effect size (ES). All analyses were performed with the aid of SPSS version 22.0 software (SPSS Inc, Chicago, IL, USA). A p-value < 0.05 was considered to reflect statistical significance.

3. Results

3.1. General Information during Training Sessions

The running distance and the mean heart rate during exercise are shown in Table 1. There was no significant difference between the Fe and CON conditions for any variables. The total running distance over the three days of training (six exercise sessions) was 101.9 ± 2.6 km in the Fe condition and 98.0 ± 3.3 km in the CON condition; this difference did not reach statistical significance (p > 0.05).

Table 1. Running distances and HR during training period.

Condition		Day 1	Day 2	Day 3
Running distance	Fe	34.5 ± 0.9	34.5 ± 0.9	34.5 ± 0.9
(km)	CON	33.3 ± 0.7	33.3 ± 0.7	33.3 ± 0.7
Heart rate (bpm)				
Ex1	Fe	158 ± 4	157 ± 4	154 ± 3
	CON	156 ± 5	156 ± 4	154 ± 2
Ex2	Fe	158 ± 4	154 ± 4	156 ± 4
	CON	159 ± 5	158 ± 3	153 ± 3

The values are means ± SE.

3.2. Blood Parameters

3.2.1. Iron Parameter

The Hb level on day 1 did not differ significantly between the conditions (Fe: 15.4 ± 0.3 g/dL, CON: 15.4 ± 0.5 g/dL, p > 0.05). Table 2 presents the serum ferritin, iron, and TSAT levels.

Table 2. Resting serum ferritin, iron, TSAT during training period (days 1–3) and on the following day after training period.

Condition		Day 1	Day 2	Day 3	Day 4
Ferritin	Fe	47.9 ± 9.3	52.2 ± 9.3	56.9 ± 9.0	61.4 ± 10.0
(ng/mL)	CON	38.0 ± 9.5	39.8 ± 10.8	44.9 ± 11.2	47.6 ± 11.1
Iron	Fe	89.1 ± 11.5	115.6 ± 10.0	120.1 ± 9.3	91.3 ± 13.5
(μg/dL)	CON	73.3 ± 15.8	143.1 ± 23.3	120.1 ± 13.9	129.7 ± 7.5
TSAT	Fe	31.4 ± 5.0	40.9 ± 3.5	44.9 ± 5.6	34.1 ± 6.0
(%)	CON	24.4 ± 4.7	50.2 ± 10.1	42.4 ± 6.2	46.5 ± 3.7

The values are means ± SE. Serum ferritin: interaction (condition × time): p = 0.504 (ES = 0.005), main effect for condition: p = 0.445 (ES = 0.05), main effect for time: p = 0.008 (ES = 0.47). Serum iron: interaction (condition × time): p = 0.069 (ES = 0.19), main effect for condition (p = 0.321, ES = 0.08), main effect for time: p = 0.001 (ES = 0.36). Serum TSAT: interaction: p = 0.056 (ES = 0.19), main effect for condition: p = 0.598 (ES = 0.02), main effect for time: p = 0.001 (ES = 0.38).

3.2.2. Muscle Damage and Inflammatory Parameters

Figure 1 shows the serum myoglobin, CK and hsCRP levels over time. The myoglobin level exhibited no significant interaction or main effect for condition, and there was a significant main effect for time. The serum CK and hsCRP levels did not show significant interaction or main effect for condition, with a main effect for time.

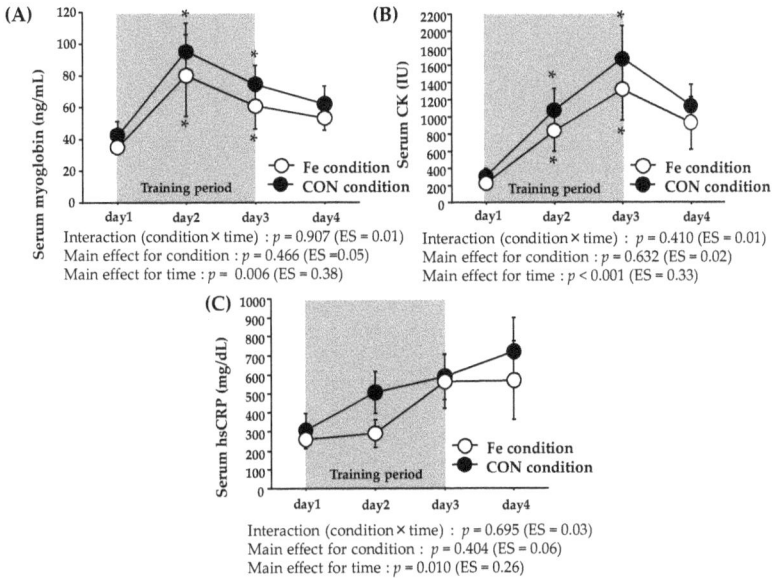

(A)
Interaction (condition × time) : $p = 0.907$ (ES = 0.01)
Main effect for condition : $p = 0.466$ (ES = 0.05)
Main effect for time : $p = 0.006$ (ES = 0.38)

(B)
Interaction (condition × time) : $p = 0.410$ (ES = 0.01)
Main effect for condition : $p = 0.632$ (ES = 0.02)
Main effect for time : $p < 0.001$ (ES = 0.33)

(C)
Interaction (condition × time) : $p = 0.695$ (ES = 0.03)
Main effect for condition : $p = 0.404$ (ES = 0.06)
Main effect for time : $p = 0.010$ (ES = 0.26)

Figure 1. Serum myoglobin (**A**); CK (**B**); and hsCRP (**C**) levels on days 1–4. The values are means ± SE. * Significant difference from day 1.

Figure 2 shows the plasma IL-6 levels. The plasma IL-6 level did not show significant interaction or main effect for condition, with only a significant main effect for time.

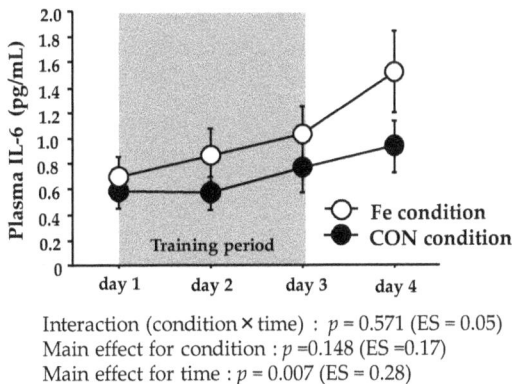

Interaction (condition × time) : $p = 0.571$ (ES = 0.05)
Main effect for condition : $p = 0.148$ (ES = 0.17)
Main effect for time : $p = 0.007$ (ES = 0.28)

Figure 2. Plasma IL-6 levels during days 1–4. The values are means ± SE.

3.2.3. Serum Hepcidin Level

Figure 3 shows the serum hepcidin levels. The serum hepcidin level exhibited significant interaction (condition × time) over days 1–4. On day 4, the serum hepcidin level was significantly higher in the Fe condition (12.6 ± 1.9 (range: 3.2–20.5) ng/mL) than the CON condition (6.9 ± 1.9 (range: 2.5–14.5) ng/mL).

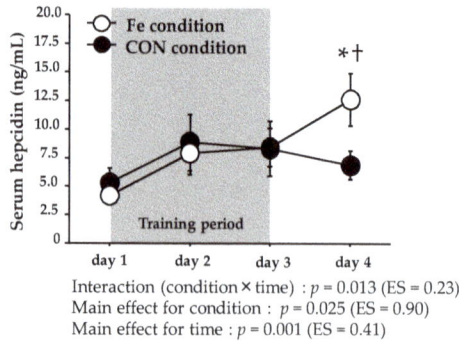

Interaction (condition × time) : $p = 0.013$ (ES = 0.23)
Main effect for condition : $p = 0.025$ (ES = 0.90)
Main effect for time : $p = 0.001$ (ES = 0.41)

Figure 3. Serum hepcidin levels during days 1–4. The values are means ± SE. * Significant difference from day 1. † Significant difference between conditions.

3.3. *Score of Fatigue and Muscle Soreness*

Table 3 presents the fatigue and muscle soreness scores. The score of fatigue and muscle soreness exhibited no significant interaction or main effect for condition, and there was a significant main effect for time.

Table 3. Scores of fatigue and muscle soreness during training period.

Condition		Day 1	Day 2	Day 3	Day 4
Fatigue	Fe	25 ± 7	30 ± 7	41 ± 10	42 ± 6
(mm)	CON	26 ± 4	39 ± 9	43 ± 7	42 ± 7
Muscle Soreness	Fe	16 ± 5	36 ± 6	57 ± 9	55 ± 7
(mm)	CON	23 ± 4	43 ± 9	59 ± 5	53 ± 7

The values are means ± SE. Fatigue: interaction (condition × time): $p = 0.889$ (ES = 0.02), main effect for condition: $p = 0.690$ (ES = 0.01), main effect for time: $p = 0.020$ (ES = 0.61). Muscle soreness; interaction (condition × time): $p = 0.881$ (ES = 0.02), main effect for condition: $p = 0.498$ (ES = 0.04), main effect for time: $p < 0.001$ (ES = 0.55).

3.4. *Dietary Intake during the Training Periods*

Table 4 presents the data on dietary intake. We found no significant differences in energy, carbohydrate, protein, or fat intake during training between the conditions. The average carbohydrate intake over the three days were 7.0 ± 0.2 g/kg (Fe condition) and 6.9 ± 0.3 g/kg (CON condition). Due to iron supplementation during training period, the Fe condition exhibited a significantly higher Fe intake than the CON condition ($p < 0.001$, ES = 2400).

Table 4. Total energy and macronutrient intakes during training period.

Condition		Day 1			Day 2			Day 3		
Total energy	Fe	10,850	±	130	11,005	±	110	10,761	±	136
(KJ)	CON	10,560	±	65	10,621	±	74	10,661	±	71
CHO	Fe	395.3	±	7.8	402.5	±	7.7	388.2	±	6.8
(g)	CON	378.4	±	3.4	381.0	±	3.7	383.7	±	3.7
Protein	Fe	87.0	±	0.2	87.9	±	0.8	88.9	±	1.4
(g)	CON	86.8	±	0.2	88.0	±	0.7	87.2	±	0.2
Fat	Fe	65.2	±	0.04	65.9	±	0.47	65.3	±	0.04
(g)	CON	65.2	±	0.04	65.2	±	0.04	65.3	±	0.04
Iron	Fe	30.5	±	0.01	30.5	±	0.01	30.5	±	0.01
(mg)	CON	6.5	±	0.01	6.5	±	0.01	6.5	±	0.01

The values are means ± SE.

4. Discussion

This is the first study to explore the effect of iron supplementation on the hepcidin level during three consecutive days of endurance training. Our principal finding is that three days of training (twice daily) did not significantly change the hepcidin level in the CON condition without iron supplementation. However, in the Fe condition, hepcidin levels were significantly elevated after training accompanied by moderate iron supplementation (24 mg/day). Contrary to our hypothesis, no change in the serum hepcidin level was observed throughout training in the CON condition. Although the hepcidin level is commonly elevated after a single bout of exercise [21,22], the cumulative effect of daily endurance training on the hepcidin level has not previously been fully evaluated. Sim et al. [29] found that that seven consecutive days of running training significantly increased the resting urine hepcidin level. McClung et al. [30] reported that seveb days of winter training (four days of military training followed by three days of cross-country skiing) significantly elevated the serum hepcidin level. Moreover, increases in training intensity and duration elevated the serum hepcidin level in athletes [31,36,37]. In contrast, eight weeks of endurance training (continuous or interval running) did not increase the hepcidin level [32]. Similarly, the serum hepcidin level was not affected by nine weeks of basic combat training in female soldiers [38]. Thus, the cumulative effects of endurance training on the hepcidin level remain unclear. In consequence, our present findings suggest that three consecutive days of such training (75 min of running twice daily) did not strongly impact the serum hepcidin level. Erythropoiesis is one of the stimulating factors of hepcidin expression [39], and hypoxia augments erythropoiesis [40]. However, because all exercises were conducted under normoxic conditions, it is unlikely that erythropoiesis was augmented in the Fe condition.

The exercise-induced increase in the IL-6 level has been suggested to stimulate hepcidin production [41,42]. Although we did not measure IL-6 levels immediately after exercise, several studies have found that the levels become markedly elevated at this time [43–45]. The exercise-induced IL-6 elevation was followed by an increase in the hepcidin level, peaking about 3 h later [8,21,22,41,42,45]. On day 1, we observed a significant increase in the hepcidin level 3 h after Ex 2, which was consistent with previous findings (data not shown). We also measured the serum myoglobin and CK levels (indirect markers of muscle damage) because sustained muscle damage and/or inflammation have been suggested to increase the hepcidin level [46]. Both the myoglobin and CK levels were significantly elevated on days 2 and 3 in both conditions and did not differ significantly between the conditions. Furthermore, the myoglobin level peaked on day 2, and the CK level peaked on day 3; it tended to return to normal on day 4. It is, thus, possible that the duration of augmented muscle damage/inflammation was too short to alter the hepcidin level in the CON condition.

Hepcidin production is affected by the energy balance; a lower energy balance and/or depletion of muscle glycogen may increase the hepcidin level, which is attributable to an increase in IL-6 production [47,48]. In a previous study by Badenhorst et al. [49], subjects performed intensive running to deplete muscle glycogen, and they were then given either a low (3 g kg^{-1}) or a high (8 g kg^{-1}) CHO diet during the next 24 h. On the following day, both the pre- and post-exercise hepcidin levels were significantly elevated in those who had consumed the lower CHO diet. Therefore, high CHO intake may inhibit hepcidin elevation, although any benefit thus afforded was not fully evident in recent studies [49–52]. In the present study, all subjects consumed prescribed diets during training; the CHO intake was about 7 g kg^{-1}/day. However, as training was conducted twice daily (150 min of running per day),the negative CHO balance during training would be equal in the two conditions. Therefore, the elevated hepcidin level on day 4 in the Fe condition cannot be associated with a lower energy balance and/or a decreased muscle glycogen level compared to the CON condition.

Running transiently increases the serum iron level, and this is attributable to hemolysis [53]. Furthermore, an elevated iron level, per se, upregulates hepcidin production [54]. Thus, the post-exercise hepcidin elevation may reflect the iron homeostasis. Exercise-induced IL-6 elevation is the most significant factor for increasing the post-exercise hepcidin level. However, Peeling et al. [28] recently reported that iron status plays a more important role in the post-exercise hepcidin elevation seen in elite athletes; lower serum ferritin and iron levels attenuate the exercise-induced rise in hepcidin. Therefore, an elevated iron level due to iron supplementation in the Fe condition may explain the observed increase in the hepcidin level. However, the serum iron levels were elevated in both conditions during days 2–4. Moreover, the serum ferritin levels did not differ significantly between the conditions, suggesting that the altered iron status caused by iron supplementation did not affect the hepcidin level in the Fe condition.

We performed a unique exploration of the impact of iron supplementation during training on hepcidin level. During the three consecutive days of training, subjects in the Fe condition received a moderate dose (24 mg) of iron supplementation. The daily absorption of iron supplements ranges from 2.3% to 8.5% when the supplement is taken with and without food, respectively [55]. Thus, only small proportions of the iron are absorbed. Higher iron doses may be toxic, as iron catalyzes the production of reactive oxygen products. Hence, iron supplementation theoretically increases the hepcidin level [56]. An earlier study found that higher-dose iron (>40 mg) augmented the hepcidin level in females [23]. Moreover, Deli et al. [57] indicated that a moderate dose of iron supplementation over three weeks promoted pro-oxidant action, and augmented inflammation. Although the detailed mechanism still remains unclear, the findings in the Fe condition on day 4 suggests that even a moderate dose of iron supplementation during short-term endurance training may augment the hepcidin level.

One limitation of our present study is the relatively small sample size. However, we confirmed that the hepcidin level was significantly elevated in the Fe condition; the ES for reflecting condition difference was sufficient ($p = 0.025$, ES = 0.90). Another limitation is the short-term (three consecutive days) nature of the training; further work is needed to explore whether our findings are relevant to long-term training. We used short-term endurance training in an effort to mimic a realistic situation featuring a rapid increase in training stress. Moreover, since we strictly controlled daily energy and iron intake, it was not easy to prepare a long–term training period. Additionally, long-term iron supplementation may be associated with a risk of gastrointestinal disease.

5. Conclusions

The hepcidin level was significantly elevated after three consecutive days of endurance training in subjects taking moderate (24 mg/day) iron supplementation. The results suggest that moderate doses of iron supplementation during consecutive days of endurance training may increase resting hepcidin levels. The present findings would also provide an important message that even a moderate dose of iron supplementation during endurance training may not be a recommendable treatment to improve physical condition in athletes. Future work should explore effect of long-term iron supplementation during training on hepcidin. Moreover, whether other nutritional interventions (e.g., increased CHO intake, antioxidant supplementation) during training attenuate the rise of hepcidin level in endurance athletes would be a valuable topic to explore.

Acknowledgments: We thank all subjects for cooperation with the research. We are also grateful to the laboratory members for technical support during the experiment.

Author Contributions: The present study was designed by A.I. and K.G.; data were collected and analyzed by A.I., N.M., and K.G.; data interpretation and manuscript preparation were undertaken by A.I. and K.G. All authors approved the final version of the paper. The present study was supported by a research grant from Ritsumeikan University.

Conflicts of Interest: The authors declare no conflict of interest.

Abbreviations

IL-6	interleukin-6
Hb	hemoglobin
TIBC	total iron-binding capacity
CK	creatine kinase
TSAT	transferrin saturation
CV	coefficients of variation
ES	effect size

References

1. Beard, J.; Tobin, B. Iron status and exercise. *Am. J. Clin. Nutr.* **2000**, *72*, 594S–597S. [PubMed]
2. Dubnov, G.; Constantini, N.W. Prevalence of iron depletion and anemia in top-level basketball players. *Int. J. Sport Nutr. Exerc. Metab.* **2004**, *14*, 30–37. [CrossRef]
3. Eliakim, A.; Nemet, D.; Constantini, N. Screening blood tests in members of the Israeli National Olympic team. *J. Sports Med. Phys. Fit.* **2002**, *42*, 250–255.
4. Stewart, J.G.; Ahlquist, D.A.; McGill, D.B.; Ilstrup, D.M.; Schwartz, S.; Owen, R.A. Gastrointestinal blood loss and anemia in runners. *Ann. Int. Med.* **1984**, *100*, 843–845. [CrossRef] [PubMed]
5. Miller, B.; Pate, R.; Burgess, W. Foot impact force and intravascular hemolysis during distance running. *Int. J. Sport* **1988**, *9*, 56–60. [CrossRef] [PubMed]
6. King, N.; Fridlund, K.E.; Askew, E.W. Nutrition issues of military women. *J. Am. Coll. Nutr.* **1993**, *12*, 344–348. [CrossRef] [PubMed]
7. Brune, M.; Magnusson, B.; Persson, H.; Hallberg, L. Iron losses in sweat. *Am. J. Clin. Nutr.* **1986**, *43*, 438–443. [PubMed]
8. Peeling, P.; Dawson, B.; Goodman, C.; Landers, G.; Wiegerinck, E.T.; Swinkels, D.W.; Trinder, D. Training surface and intensity: Inflammation, hemolysis, and hepcidin expression. *Med. Sci. Sports Exerc.* **2009**, *41*, 1138–1145. [CrossRef] [PubMed]
9. Ganz, T.; Nemeth, E. Iron imports IV. Hepcidin and regulation of body iron metabolism. *Am. J. Physiol.* **2006**, *290*, 199–203. [CrossRef] [PubMed]
10. Nemeth, E.; Rivera, S.; Gabayan, V.; Keller, C.; Taudorf, S.; Pedersen, B.K.; Ganz, T. IL-6 mediates hypoferremia of inflammation by inducing the synthesis of the iron regulatory hormone hepcidin. *J. Clin. Investig.* **2004**, *113*, 1271–1276. [CrossRef] [PubMed]
11. Zimmermann, M.B.; Troesch, B.; Biebinger, R.; Egli, I.; Zeder, C.; Hurrell, R.F. Plasma hepcidin is a modest predictor of dietary iron bioavailability in humans, whereas oral iron loading, measured by stable-isotope appearance curves, increases plasma hepcidin. *Am. J. Clin. Nutr.* **2009**, *90*, 1280–1287. [CrossRef] [PubMed]
12. Wrighting, D.M.; Andrews, N.C. Interleukin-6 induces hepcidin expression through STAT3. *Blood* **2006**, *108*, 3204–3209. [CrossRef] [PubMed]
13. Song, S.-N.J.; Tomosugi, N.; Kawabata, H.; Ishikawa, T.; Nishikawa, T.; Yoshizaki, K. Down-regulation of hepcidin resulting from long-term treatment with an anti–IL-6 receptor antibody (tocilizumab) improves anemia of inflammation in multicentric Castleman disease. *Blood* **2010**, *116*, 3627–3634. [CrossRef] [PubMed]
14. Nicolas, G.; Chauvet, C.; Viatte, L.; Danan, J.L.; Bigard, X.; Devaux, I.; Beaumont, C.; Kahn, A.; Vaulont, S. The gene encoding the iron regulatory peptide hepcidin is regulated by anemia, hypoxia, and inflammation. *J. Clin. Investig.* **2002**, *110*, 1037–1044. [CrossRef] [PubMed]
15. Pedlar, C.R.; Whyte, G.P.; Burden, R.; Moore, B.; Horgan, G.; Pollock, N. A case study of an iron-deficient female Olympic 1500-m runner. *Int. J. Sports. Physiol. Perform.* **2013**, *8*, 695–698. [CrossRef] [PubMed]

16. Burden, R.J.; Pollock, N.; Whyte, G.P.; Richards, T.; Moore, B.; Busbridge, M.; Srai, S.K.; Pedlar, C.R. Impact of intravenous iron on aerobic capacity and iron metabolism in elite athletes. *Med. Sci. Sports Exerc.* **2014**, *47*, 1399–1407. [CrossRef] [PubMed]
17. Hinton, P.S.; Giordano, C.; Brownlie, T.; Haas, J.D. Iron supplementation improves endurance after training in iron-depleted, nonanemic women. *J. Appl. Physiol.* **2000**, *88*, 1103–1111. [PubMed]
18. Nielsen, P.; Nachtigall, D. Iron supplementation in athletes. Current recommendations. *Sports Med.* **1998**, *26*, 207–216. [CrossRef] [PubMed]
19. Zotter, H.; Robinson, N.; Zorzoli, M.; Schattenberg, L.; Saugy, M.; Mangin, P. Abnormally high serum ferritin levels among professional road cyclists. *Br. J. Sports Med.* **2004**, *38*, 704–708. [CrossRef] [PubMed]
20. Deugnier, Y.; Loréal, O.; Carré, F.; Duvallet, A.; Zoulim, F.; Vinel, J.P.; Paris, J.C.; Blaison, D.; Moirand, R.; Turlin, B.; et al. Increased body iron stores in elite road cyclists. *Med. Sci. Sports Exerc.* **2002**, *34*, 876–880. [CrossRef] [PubMed]
21. Peeling, P.; Dawson, B.; Goodman, C.; Landers, G.; Wiegerinck, E.T.; Swinkels, D.W.; Trinder, D. Effects of exercise on hepcidin response and iron metabolism during recovery. *Int. J. Sport Nutr. Exerc. Metab.* **2009**, *19*, 583–597. [CrossRef]
22. Newlin, M.K.; Williams, S.; McNamara, T.; Tjalsma, H.; Swinkels, D.W.; Haymes, E.M. The effects of acute exercise bouts on hepcidin in women. *Int. J. Sport Nutr. Exerc. Metab.* **2012**, *22*, 79–88. [CrossRef]
23. Moretti, D.; Goede, J.S.; Zeder, C.; Jiskra, M.; Chatzinakou, V.; Tjalsma, H.; Melse-Boonstra, A.; Brittenham, G.; Swinkels, D.W.; Zimmermann, M.B. Oral iron supplements increase hepcidin and decrease iron absorption from daily or twice-daily doses in iron-depleted young women. *Blood* **2015**, *126*, 1981–1989. [CrossRef] [PubMed]
24. Roecker, L.; Meier-Buttermilch, R.; Brechtel, L.; Nemeth, E.; Ganz, T. Iron-regulatory protein hepcidin is increased in female athletes after a marathon. *Eur. J. Appl. Physiol.* **2005**, *95*, 569–571. [CrossRef] [PubMed]
25. Ronsen, O.; Lea, T.; Bahr, R.; Pedersen, B.K. Enhanced plasma IL-6 and IL-1ra responses to repeated vs. single bouts of prolonged cycling in elite athletes. *J. Appl. Physiol.* **2002**, *92*, 2547–2553. [CrossRef] [PubMed]
26. Ganz, T. Hepcidin, a key regulator of iron metabolism and mediator of anemia of inflammation. *Blood* **2003**, *102*, 783–788. [CrossRef] [PubMed]
27. Ganz, T.; Nemeth, E. Iron sequestration and anemia of inflammation. *Semin. Hematol.* **2009**, *46*, 387–393. [CrossRef] [PubMed]
28. Peeling, P.; McKay, A.K.A.; Pyne, D.B.; Guelfi, K.J.; McCormick, R.H.; Laarakkers, C.M.; Swinkels, D.W.; Garvican-Lewis, L.A.; Ross, M.L.R.; Sharma, A.P.; et al. Factors influencing the post-exercise hepcidin-25 response in elite athletes. *Eur. J. Appl. Physiol.* **2017**, *117*, 1233–1239. [CrossRef] [PubMed]
29. Sim, M.; Dawson, B.; Landers, G.J.; Swinkels, D.W.; Tjalsma, H.; Wiegerinck, E.T.; Trinder, D.; Peeling, P. A seven day running training period increases basal urinary hepcidin levels as compared to cycling. *J. Int. Soc. Sports Nutr.* **2014**, *11*, 14. [CrossRef] [PubMed]
30. McClung, J.P.; Martini, S.; Murphy, N.E.; Montain, S.J.; Margolis, L.M.; Thrane, I.; Spitz, M.G.; Blatny, J.-M.; Young, A.J.; Gundersen, Y.; et al. Effects of a 7-day military training exercise on inflammatory biomarkers, serum hepcidin, and iron status. *Nutr. J.* **2013**, *12*, 141. [CrossRef] [PubMed]
31. Ishibashi, A.; Maeda, N.; Sumi, D.; Goto, K. Elevated Serum Hepcidin Levels during an Intensified Training Period in Well-Trained Female Long-Distance Runners. *Nutrients* **2017**, *9*, 277. [CrossRef] [PubMed]
32. Auersperger, I.; Knap, B.; Jerin, A.; Blagus, R.; Lainscak, M.; Skitek, M.; Skof, B. The effects of 8 weeks of endurance running on hepcidin concentrations, inflammatory parameters, and iron status in female runners. *Int. J. Sport Nutr. Exerc. Metab.* **2012**, *22*, 55–63. [CrossRef]
33. Rietjens, G.J.; Kuipers, H.; Hartgens, F.; Keizer, H.A. Red blood cell profile of elite olympic distance triathletes. A three-year follow-up. *Int. J. Sports Med.* **2002**, *23*, 391–396. [CrossRef] [PubMed]
34. Sumi, D.; Kojima, C.; Goto, K. Impact of Endurance Exercise in Hypoxia on Muscle Damage, Inflammatory and Performance Responses. *J. Strength Cond. Res.* **2017**. [CrossRef] [PubMed]
35. McCormack, H.M.; Horne, D.J.; Sheather, S. Clinical applications of visual analogue scales: A critical review. *Psychol. Med.* **1988**, *18*, 1007–1019. [CrossRef] [PubMed]
36. Dzedzej, A.; Ignatiuk, W.; Jaworska, J.; Grzywacz, T.; Lipińska, P.; Antosiewicz, J.; Korek, A.; Ziemann, E. The effect of the competitive season in professional basketball on inflammation and iron metabolism. *Biol. Sport* **2016**, *33*, 223–229. [CrossRef] [PubMed]

37. Ziemann, E.; Kasprowicz, K.; Kasperska, A.; Zembro, A. Do High Blood Hepcidin Concentrations Contribute to Low Ferritin Levels in Young Tennis Players at the End of Tournament Season? *J. Sports Sci. Med.* **2013**, *12*, 249–258. [PubMed]

38. Karl, J.P.; Lieberman, H.R.; Cable, S.J.; Williams, K.W.; Young, A.J.; McClung, J.P. Randomized, double-blind, placebo-controlled trial of an iron-fortified food product in female soldiers during military training: Relations between iron status, serum hepcidin, and inflammation. *Am. J. Clin. Nutr.* **2010**, *92*, 93–100. [CrossRef] [PubMed]

39. Pak, M.; Lopez, M.; Gabayan, V.; Ganz, T.; Rivera, S. Suppression of hepcidin during anemia requires erythropoietic activity. *Blood* **2006**, *108*, 3073–3075. [CrossRef] [PubMed]

40. Shah, Y.; Xie, L. Hypoxia-inducible factors link iron homeostasis and erythropoiesis. *Gastroenterology* **2014**, *146*, 630–642. [CrossRef] [PubMed]

41. Sim, M.; Dawson, B.; Landers, G.; Swinkels, D.W.; Tjalsma, H.; Trinder, D.; Peeling, P. Effect of exercise modality and intensity on post-exercise interleukin-6 and hepcidin levels. *Int. J. Sport Nutr. Exerc. Metab.* **2013**, *23*, 178–186. [CrossRef]

42. Peeling, P.; Sim, M.; Badenhorst, C.E.; Dawson, B.; Govus, A.D.; Abbiss, C.R.; Swinkels, D.W.; Trinder, D. Iron Status and the Acute Post-Exercise Hepcidin Response in Athletes. *PLoS ONE* **2014**, *9*, e93002. [CrossRef] [PubMed]

43. Steensberg, A.; Febbraio, M.A.; Osada, T.; Schjerling, P.; van Hall, G.; Saltin, B.; Pedersen, B.K. Interleukin-6 production in contracting human skeletal muscle is influenced by pre-exercise muscle glycogen content. *J. Physiol.* **2001**, *537*, 633–639. [CrossRef] [PubMed]

44. Pedersen, B.K.; Steensberg, A.; Schjerling, P. Exercise and interleukin-6. *Curr. Opin. Hematol.* **2001**, *8*, 137–141. [CrossRef] [PubMed]

45. Peeling, P.; Dawson, B.; Goodman, C.; Landers, G.; Wiegerinck, E.T.; Swinkels, D.W.; Trinder, D. Cumulative effects of consecutive running sessions on hemolysis, inflammation and hepcidin activity. *Eur. J. Appl. Physiol.* **2009**, *106*, 51–59. [CrossRef] [PubMed]

46. Zhang, A.-S.; Enns, C.A. Iron homeostasis: Recently identified proteins provide insight into novel control mechanisms. *J. Biol. Chem.* **2009**, *284*, 711–715. [CrossRef] [PubMed]

47. Keller, C.; Steensberg, A.; Pilegaard, H.; Osada, T.; Saltin, B.; Pedersen, B.K.; Neufer, P.D. Transcriptional activation of the IL-6 gene in human contracting skeletal muscle: Influence of muscle glycogen content. *FASEB J.* **2001**, *15*, 2748–2750. [CrossRef] [PubMed]

48. Badenhorst, C.E.; Dawson, B.; Cox, G.R.; Laarakkers, C.M.; Swinkels, D.W.; Peeling, P. Acute dietary carbohydrate manipulation and the subsequent inflammatory and hepcidin responses to exercise. *Eur. J. Appl. Physiol.* **2015**, *115*, 2521–2530. [CrossRef] [PubMed]

49. Badenhorst, C.E.; Dawson, B.; Cox, G.R.; Laarakkers, C.M.; Swinkels, D.W.; Peeling, P. Timing of post-exercise carbohydrate ingestion: Influence on IL-6 and hepcidin responses. *Eur. J. Appl. Physiol.* **2015**, *115*, 2215–2222. [CrossRef] [PubMed]

50. Sim, M.; Dawson, B.; Landers, G.; Wiegerinck, E.T.; Swinkels, D.W.; Townsend, M.-A.; Trinder, D.; Peeling, P. The effects of carbohydrate ingestion during endurance running on post-exercise inflammation and hepcidin levels. *Eur. J. Appl. Physiol.* **2012**, *112*, 1889–1898. [CrossRef] [PubMed]

51. Robson-Ansley, P.; Walshe, I.; Ward, D. The effect of carbohydrate ingestion on plasma interleukin-6, hepcidin and iron concentrations following prolonged exercise. *Cytokine* **2011**, *53*, 196–200. [CrossRef] [PubMed]

52. Badenhorst, C.E.; Dawson, B.; Cox, G.R.; Sim, M.; Laarakkers, C.M.; Swinkels, D.W.; Peeling, P. Seven days of high carbohydrate ingestion does not attenuate post-exercise IL-6 and hepcidin levels. *Eur. J. Appl. Physiol.* **2016**, *116*, 1715–1724. [CrossRef] [PubMed]

53. Buchman, A.L.; Keen, C.; Commisso, J.; Killip, D.; Ou, C.N.; Rognerud, C.L.; Dennis, K.; Dunn, J.K. The effect of a marathon run on plasma and urine mineral and metal concentrations. *J. Am. Coll. Nutr.* **1998**, *17*, 124–127. [CrossRef] [PubMed]

54. Nemeth, E.; Tuttle, M.S.; Powelson, J.; Vaughn, M.B.; Donovan, A.; Ward, D.M.; Ganz, T.; Kaplan, J. Hepcidin regulates cellular iron efflux by binding to ferroportin and inducing its internalization. *Science* **2004**, *306*, 2090–2093. [CrossRef] [PubMed]

55. Asobayire, F.S.; Adou, P.; Davidsson, L.; Cook, J.D.; Hurrell, R.F. Prevalence of iron deficiency with and without concurrent anemia in population groups with high prevalences of malaria and other infections: A study in Côte d'Ivoire. *Am. J. Clin. Nutr.* **2001**, *74*, 776–782. [PubMed]

56. Papanikolaou, G.; Tzilianos, M.; Christakis, J.I.; Bogdanos, D.; Tsimirika, K.; MacFarlane, J.; Goldberg, Y.P.; Sakellaropoulos, N.; Ganz, T.; Nemeth, E. Hepcidin in iron overload disorders. *Blood* **2005**, *105*, 4103–4105. [CrossRef] [PubMed]

57. Deli, C.K.; Fatouros, I.G.; Paschalis, V.; Tsiokanos, A.; Georgakouli, K.; Zalavras, A.; Avloniti, A.; Koutedakis, Y.; Jamurtas, A.Z. Iron supplementation effects on redox status following septic skeletal muscle trauma in adults and children. *Oxid. Med. Cell. Longev.* **2017**, *2017*, 4120421. [CrossRef] [PubMed]

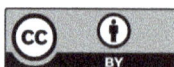

nutrients

MDPI

Article

Iron Fortification of Lentil (*Lens culinaris* Medik.) to Address Iron Deficiency

Rajib Podder [1], Bunyamin Tar'an [1], Robert T. Tyler [2], Carol J. Henry [3], Diane M. DellaValle [4] and Albert Vandenberg [1,*]

[1] Department of Plant Sciences, University of Saskatchewan, Saskatoon, SK S7N 5A8, Canada; rap039@mail.usask.ca (R.P.); bunyamin.taran@usask.ca (B.T.)
[2] Department of Food and Bioproduct Sciences, University of Saskatchewan, Saskatoon, SK S7N 5A8, Canada; bob.tyler@usask.ca
[3] College of Pharmacy and Nutrition, University of Saskatchewan, Saskatoon, SK S7N 5C9, Canada; carol.henry@usask.ca
[4] Department of Nutrition and Dietetics, Marywood University, 2300, Adams Avenue, Scranton, PA 18509, USA; ddellavalle@maryu.marywood.edu
* Correspondence: bert.vandenberg@usask.ca; Tel.: +1-306-221-2039

Received: 28 June 2017; Accepted: 7 August 2017; Published: 11 August 2017

Abstract: Iron (Fe) deficiency is a major human health concern in areas of the world in which diets are often Fe deficient. In the current study, we aimed to identify appropriate methods and optimal dosage for Fe fortification of lentil (*Lens culinaris* Medik.) dal with $FeSO_4 \cdot 7H_2O$ (ferrous sulphate hepta-hydrate), NaFeEDTA (ethylenediaminetetraacetic acid iron (III) sodium salt) and $FeSO_4 \cdot H_2O$ (ferrous sulphate mono-hydrate). We used a colorimetric method to determine the appearance of the dal fortified with fortificants at different Fe concentrations and under different storage conditions. Relative Fe bioavailability was assessed using an in vitro cell culture bioassay. We found that NaFeEDTA was the most suitable fortificant for red lentil dal, and at 1600 ppm, NaFeEDTA provides 13–14 mg of additional Fe per 100 g of dal. Lentil dal sprayed with fortificant solutions, followed by shaking and drying at 75 °C, performed best with respect to drying time and color change. Total Fe and phytic acid concentrations differed significantly between cooked unfortified and fortified lentil, ranging from 68.7 to 238.5 ppm and 7.2 to 8.0 mg g^{-1}, respectively. The relative Fe bioavailability of cooked fortified lentil was increased by 32.2–36.6% compared to unfortified cooked lentil. We conclude that fortification of lentil dal is effective and could provide significant health benefits to dal-consuming populations vulnerable to Fe deficiency.

Keywords: lentil; iron; fortification; NaFeEDTA; $FeSO_4 \cdot 7H_2O$; $FeSO_4 \cdot H_2O$

1. Introduction

Lentil (*Lens culinaris* Medikus) is an important legume crop, cultivated for food and feed since prehistoric times. As a source of dietary protein, lentil can be combined with cereals to prepare human diets and animal feeds that provide a balance of essential amino acids and essential micronutrients such as iron, zinc and selenium [1,2]. Lentil is a good source of non-heme iron, ranging from 73 to 90 mg kg^{-1} [3]. The crude protein content ($N \times 6.25$) of Western Canadian lentil is reported to range from 25.8 to 27.1% [4]. Lentil also is considered to be a starchy legume as it contains 27.4–47.1% starch, with a significant level of amylose (23.5–32.2)% [5,6]. Although lentil is a good source of intrinsic Fe, the bioavailability/absorption is low [7]. These authors reported that the mean Fe absorption from lentil dal was 2.2%, which was significantly lower than the 23.6% observed for a similar amount of Fe given as ferrous sulphate to women with poor Fe status. Low bioavailability may be due to the presence of phytic acid and polyphenols in the lentil dal [7,8].

Iron (Fe) is the most abundant element in the earth's crust and is an essential micronutrient for both plants and animals. In plants, Fe deficiency affects key metabolic processes such as the electron transfer system for photosynthesis and respiration [9]. Iron deficiency in humans refers to a condition in which an insufficient amount of bioavailable Fe results in Fe deficiency anemia [10]. This deficiency has become a major nutritional disorder, widespread in both developing and developed countries [11]. The major consequences of Fe deficiency are reduction of physical activity, fitness and work capability, a reduced ability to maintain body temperature, a lowered resistance to infection, and an increase in mortality during pregnancy and in newborns [12]. According to Food and Agriculture Organization (FAO) and World Health Organization (WHO) recommendations, the estimated daily average Fe requirements for females and males 19–50 years of age are 29.4 mg and 10.8 mg, respectively, based on 10% bioavailability [13].

Several strategies are used around the world to address micronutrient malnutrition. Micronutrient supplementation, dietary diversification, biofortification, food fortification, nutrition education, public health interventions and food safety measures are approaches that can solely or in combination be applied to address micronutrient deficiency in a target population [14]. Supplementation is an effective means of providing immediate benefits to "at risk groups" but not for other household or community members [15] since it requires supplemental Fe consumption on a long-term basis, in tablet form for example. Dietary improvement through supplementation requires a change in dietary behavior, and this process also requires changes in food supply and availability that may require a long time to achieve success [14]. Also, public health intervention can help prevent micronutrient malnutrition, but micronutrient malnutrition can also be associated with a high prevalence of microbial infection that causes a variety of different diseases. Food fortification can overcome this limitation due to its sustainability in improving the dietary quality of a targeted group or population without changing dietary habits. Food fortification is a potentially cost-effective way to add micronutrients to processed foods in a way that can rapidly mitigate micronutrient malnutrition [13].

A successful Fe fortification program was first reported in Canada in 1944, when the government began fortifying wheat flour with Fe along with thiamine, riboflavin and niacin [14]. A remarkable reduction in child mortality was observed from 102/1000 live births in 1944 (first year) to 61/1000 in 1947 in Canada [16]. During the twentieth century, Fe fortification became mandatory in several developing countries, including Bolivia, Chile, Colombia, Costa Rica, Ecuador, Guatemala, Indonesia and others [17]. In every country, either wheat or maize flour was chosen as the food vehicle. The requirements for selecting an appropriate food vehicle for fortification were established by FAO in 1995 [17]. In 1980, the FDA (U.S. Food and Drug Administration) established a "Food Fortification Policy" that was guided by six basic principles [18]. The WHO has recommended Fe compounds and concentration for fortification of wheat flour in 13 countries [19]. To optimize iron bioavailability and maintain the organoleptic attributes that influence consumer acceptability of fortified foods, selected food vehicles and Fe fortificants need to be well matched. The food vehicle should be safe, widely accepted by the target consumers, have good storage capability after fortification, and the added Fe should be stable with high bioavailability [20].

Fortifying lentil with suitable Fe fortificants is a research area with potential application to reduce Fe deficiency. We hypothesized that it would be possible to increase the amount of bioavailable Fe in dehulled (decorticated) pulses (dal) such as lentil, in a biologically and culturally meaningful way, to a level that could prevent Fe deficiency in humans. Our experimental approach had two main objectives, first, to determine the most suitable iron fortificant and the appropriate dose of Fe for dehulled lentil based on ease of fortification, and second, to determine the optimal processing technology to fortify iron in dehulled lentil based on current processing practices. To fulfill the first objective, research was focused on selection of the appropriate genotype and product type of dehulled lentil, and identifying the best form of Fe solution with which to fortify dehulled lentil products. The Fe fortificants, ferrous sulphate heptahydrate ($FeSO_4 \cdot 7H_2O$), NaFeEDTA (ethylenediaminetetraacetic acid iron (III) sodium salt) and ferrous sulphate monohydrate ($FeSO_4 \cdot H_2O$), are acceptable fortificants that have potential for fortifying dehulled lentil seed [13]. The second objective was fulfilled by conducting studies to help standardize the protocol for lentil fortification. These included assessments of the appropriate dose of Fe solution, selection of the most appropriate fortification method in the context of changes in organoleptic properties and storage capability, assessment of the best temperature for drying lentil after the addition of fortificants, and the effect of fortification on boiling time.

2. Materials and Methods

The procedure followed for development of a lentil fortification protocol is shown in Figure 1, and is discussed below.

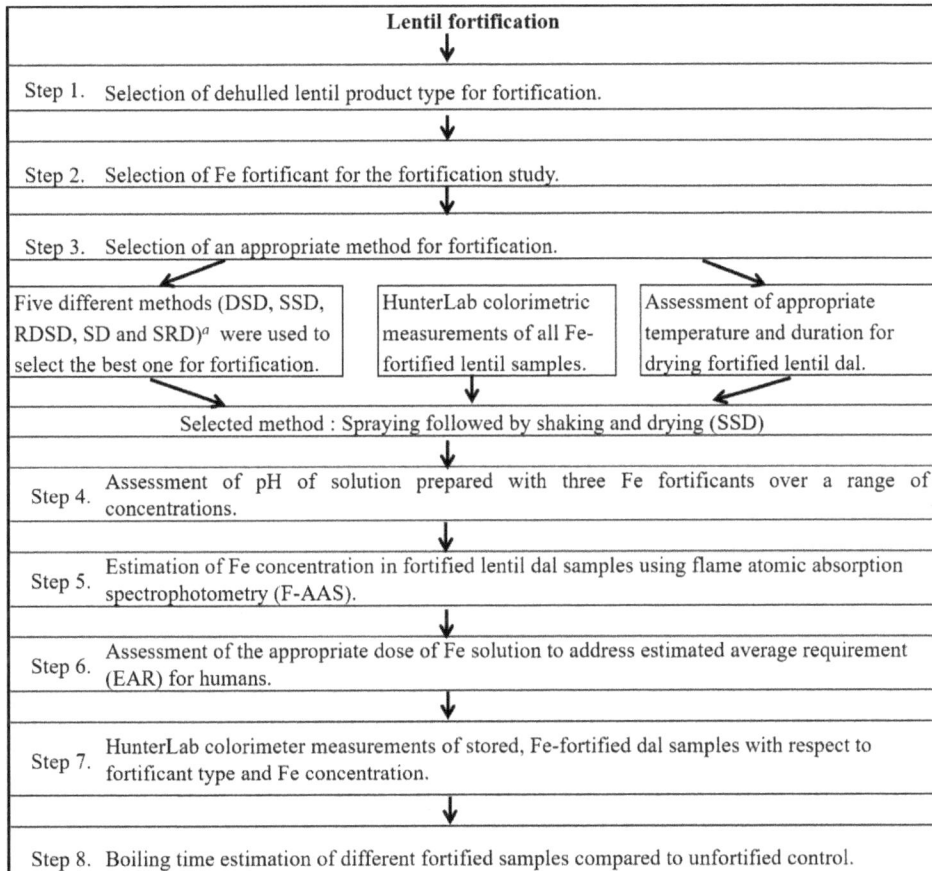

Lentil fortification ↓
Step 1. Selection of dehulled lentil product type for fortification. ↓
Step 2. Selection of Fe fortificant for the fortification study. ↓
Step 3. Selection of an appropriate method for fortification.

Five different methods (DSD, SSD, RDSD, SD and SRD)[a] were used to select the best one for fortification.	HunterLab colorimetric measurements of all Fe-fortified lentil samples.	Assessment of appropriate temperature and duration for drying fortified lentil dal.

Selected method : Spraying followed by shaking and drying (SSD) ↓
Step 4. Assessment of pH of solution prepared with three Fe fortificants over a range of concentrations. ↓
Step 5. Estimation of Fe concentration in fortified lentil dal samples using flame atomic absorption spectrophotometry (F-AAS). ↓
Step 6. Assessment of the appropriate dose of Fe solution to address estimated average requirement (EAR) for humans. ↓
Step 7. HunterLab colorimeter measurements of stored, Fe-fortified dal samples with respect to fortificant type and Fe concentration. ↓
Step 8. Boiling time estimation of different fortified samples compared to unfortified control.

Figure 1. Flow chart for development of a lentil fortification protocol. [a] Oven dried, soaked and oven dried (DSD); sprayed followed by shaking and drying (SSD); rinsed, oven dried, soaked, and oven dried (RDSD); directly soaked in Fe solution (SD) and rinsed, soaked, and oven dried (SRD).

2.1. Selection of Lentil Genotype and Dehulled Lentil Product Type

Fifteen red cotyledon lentil cultivars/genotypes were analyzed to estimate the concentration (ppm) of Fe in seeds (data not shown). One widely grown and popular cultivated red lentil cultivar, CDC (Crop Development Centre) Maxim, developed at the Crop Development Centre, University of

Saskatchewan, Saskatoon, SK, Canada, was selected for fortification studies due to its having a high Fe concentration (75–90 ppm) compared to other red lentil cultivars grown in Saskatchewan [21].

Four different types of dehulled lentil products are usually available in the red lentil market: polished football (dehulled, unsplit), polished splits, unpolished football and unpolished splits (Figure 2a). The Fe concentration in each product type was measured to determine the range of variability in Fe concentration. The product types then were used in a fortification study and samples of 200 g of each product type were mixed with 20 mL of NaFeEDTA solution (1600 ppm Fe) with four replications. The best product type in relation to uniformity of absorption of Fe solution, drying time and concentration of Fe in the fortified product was selected. The statistical analysis was conducted using SAS version 9.4 (SAS Inc., Cary, NC, USA). One-way analysis of variance (ANOVA) was used to compare the Fe concentration of unfortified and fortified red lentil product types. The least significant difference (LSD) was calculated and the level of significance set at $p < 0.05$.

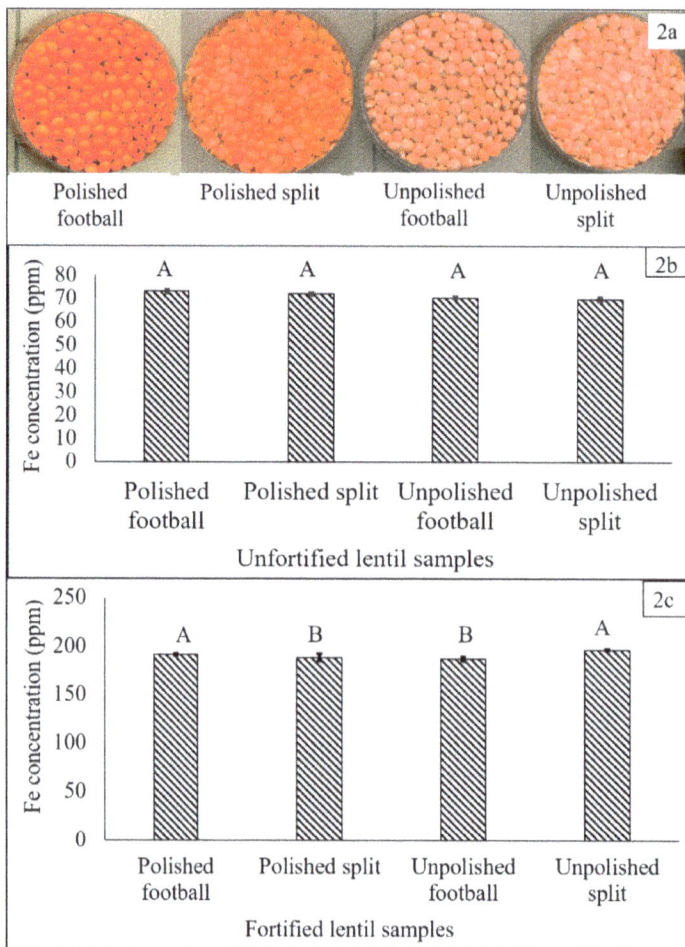

Figure 2. (**a**) Four dehulled, red lentil product types; (**b**) Fe concentration (ppm) in four dehulled, unfortified, red lentil product types; and (**c**) Fe concentration (ppm) in red lentil product types fortified with $FeSO_4 \cdot 7H_2O$ solution (400 ppm Fe). Different letters within each figure represent significant differences ($p < 0.05$).

2.2. Selection and Evaluation of the Most Suitable Fe Fortificant for Lentil

The selection of the most appropriate Fe fortificant is challenging due to possible interactions between the food product and the Fe compound. Three water-soluble Fe compounds, $FeSO_4 \cdot 7H_2O$, NaFeEDTA and $FeSO_4 \cdot H_2O$ were selected from a list of iron fortificants published in the WHO and FAO document "Guidelines on Food Fortification with Micronutrients" [13]. The $FeSO_4 \cdot 7H_2O$ and $FeSO_4 \cdot H_2O$ were supplied by Crown Technology, Inc., Indianapolis, IN, USA, and NaFeEDTA by Akzo Nobel Functional Chemicals, LLC, Chicago, IL, USA. The three fortificants were food grade and were selected on the basis of their relative bioavailability, interaction with the food vehicle and cost of fortification [14].

2.3. Selection of an Appropriate Method of Fortification

2.3.1. Techniques Used for Lentil Fortification

An experiment was designed to determine the most appropriate method for fortifying dehulled, polished, football lentil dal with an Fe solution prepared with $FeSO_4 \cdot 7H_2O$, one of the three Fe fortificants studied. Five methods were used to fortify lentil dal with $FeSO_4 \cdot 7H_2O$ solution (1600 ppm Fe) at 10 mL fortificant solution/100g dal. The 1600 ppm Fe concentration was selected with the aim that this concentration may provide a major part of the recommended daily allowances (RDAs) for humans. However, each method to fortify lentil dal is described below.

Method 1 (Dry-Soak-Dry). Lentil dal was oven dried at 80 °C for 10 min, soaked in 10 mL of fortificant solution for 2 min, and then dried again at 80 °C to obtain a moisture content of 14%.

Method 2 (Spray-Shake-Dry). Lentil dal was sprayed with fortificant solution using a 473 mL clear, fine-mist spray bottle (SOFT 'N STYLE, Product Code VO-302564, SKS Bottle and Packaging, INC., Watervliet, NY, USA), shaken using a Barnstead Thermolyne M49235 Bigger Bill Orbital Shaker (Sigma-Aldrich Corp., St. Louis, MO, USA) at 400 rpm for 10 min to mix the solution with the dal sample, and subsequently dried to 14% moisture under a 250-watt electric heat lamp (NOMA incandescent, clear, 130 V heat lamp, Trileaf Distributors, Toronto, ON, Canada) which produced a temperature of approximately 70 °C at the surface of the fortified dal.

Method 3 (Rinse-Dry-Soak-Dry). The third method consisted of rinsing 100 g dal samples under a continuous flow of deionized water for 30 s followed by oven drying at 80 °C for 10 min. The dried sample then was soaked in the fortificant solution (10 mL fortificant solution/100 g lentil) for 2 min and then placed in the oven again for 15 min at 80 °C to reduce the moisture level to 14%.

Method 4 (Soak-Dry). Lentil dal was soaked in fortificant solution followed by oven drying at 80 °C to 14% moisture.

Method 5 (Soak-Rinse-Dry). Lentil dal was soaked in fortificant solution and then rinsed with deionized water for 30 s, followed by oven drying at 80 °C to 14% moisture.

2.3.2. HunterLab Colorimetric Measurements of Fe-Fortified Lentil Samples

The color of the Fe-fortified lentil sample from each of the five fortification methods was measured using a HunterLab instrument (Hunter Associates Laboratory Inc., Reston, VA, USA) to allow comparison with unfortified control samples. For each method, four samples were assessed. The dimensions L*, a* and b* were compared with those of the control sample, where L* indicates lightness (ranging from 0 to 100), a* indicates red (+) and green (−) and b* indicates yellow (+) and blue (−) with a range of +80 to −80 [22]. The L*, a* and b* values were analyzed using ANOVA in SAS 9.4.

2.3.3. Assessment of Appropriate Temperature and Duration for Drying Fortified Lentil Dal

Electric heat lamps of three power levels (100, 200 and 250 watts) (Trileaf Distributor) were used to dry fortified football dal after spraying with fortificant solution. The distance between the bulb and the lentil dal surface was 15 cm. Samples of 100 g of dal were fortified with 10 mL of $FeSO_4 \cdot 7H_2O$ solution

(1600 ppm Fe concentration). The maximum temperature (°C) in the middle of the fortified dal sample during drying with the three bulb types and shaking using a Barnstead Thermolyne M49235 Bigger Bill Orbital Shaker (Sigma-Aldrich Corp.) was assessed using a thermometer (VWR Scientific, Chicago, IL, USA). The time to achieve 14% moisture for each sample was recorded for each treatment method. Both temperature and drying time were assessed three times and the mean temperature and drying time were calculated.

2.4. Estimation of Fe Concentration in Fortified Lentil Dal Samples by Flame Atomic Absorption Spectrophotometry (F-AAS)

The iron concentration in the fortified lentil dal was analyzed by flame atomic absorption spectrophotometry (F-AAS, Nova 300, Analytic Jena AG, Konrad-Zuse-Strasse, Neu-Ulm, Germany). Each sample was sub-sampled and 0.5 g was digested in a 30-mL digestion tube with HNO_3-H_2O_2 using an automatic digester (Vulcan 84, Questron Technology, Ontario, CA, USA). All chemicals (nitric acid (70%), hydrogen peroxide (30%) and hydrochloric acid (37%)) used for digestion were of analytical grade. The digestion was repeated twice, with three technical replications per repeat. In the digestion chamber, a total of 72 samples were digested in each run, along with eight standards (yellow lentil laboratory check) and four blanks. Samples were first digested with HNO_3 at 90 °C for 45 min, followed by addition of 5 mL of 30% H_2O_2 and then further digested for another 65 min. The solutions were then reduced with 3 mL of 6 M HCl, followed by heating at 90 °C for 5 min prior to cooling to room temperature. All sample solutions were then diluted with deionized water to a volume of 25 mL. Six mL of each of the digested samples was then used to determine the Fe concentration as described previously [23]. The Fe concentration values were analyzed using ANOVA in SAS 9.4 to determine differences for Fe concentration among the fortified lentil samples within each of the three fortificants at concentrations ranging from 100 to 3200 ppm. The LSD was calculated and the level of significance set at $p < 0.001$.

2.5. Assessment of the Appropriate Dose of Fe Solution

A total of 51 different solutions of the three fortificants (17 solutions of each fortificant with Fe concentrations of 100, 200, 400, 600, 800, 1000, 1200, 1400, 1600, 1800, 2000, 2200, 2400, 2600, 2800, 3000 and 3200 ppm) were prepared to fortify dehulled lentil dal samples. Ten mL of each fortificant solution at each Fe concentration was added to a 100-g dal sample and processed using the SSD (Spray–Shake–Dry) method described earlier. Twenty-five Fe solutions were prepared using the three Fe fortificants at eight concentrations (200, 400, 800, 1200, 1600, 2000, 2800 and 3200 ppm of Fe plus deionized water as the control) to assess the effect of increasing fortificant concentration on the pH of the solutions, which was measured three times for each solution using a pH meter (Oakton H_2O proof BNC pH tester, Cole-Parmer Scientific Experts, Montreal, QC, Canada). Data were analyzed using SAS 9.4.

2.6. HunterLab Colorimeter Measurements of Stored Fe-Fortified Dal Samples

The initial color of Fe-fortified lentil dal samples was measured using a HunterLab (Hunter Associates Laboratory Inc., Reston, VA, USA) instrument. Twenty-seven samples (nine concentrations of each of the three Fe fortificants) and one control (unfortified lentil dal) with four replications were scored for their L*, a* and b* values. Samples of each treatment were stored individually at room temperature (25 °C) for one year in clear plastic bags (Ronco, Toronto, ON, Canada), similar to methods traditionally used to store dal products. After six months and one year of storage, the L*, a* and b* values of the lentil dal again were measured to determine if any color change had occurred. The one-year storage period was considered an approximate maximum storage period from processing to consumption by dal consumers. The L*, a* and b* values were analyzed using ANOVA in SAS 9.4.

2.7. Boiling Time Estimation of Fortified Lentil Dal Samples

Three fortified dal samples (FeSO$_4$·7H$_2$0, NaFeEDTA and FeSO$_4$·H$_2$O at 1600 ppm Fe concentration) and one unfortified control were used to determine if differences existed in boiling time between fortified samples and the control. Two hundred fifty grams of each of the lentil dal samples were cooked in 1L of deionized water containing 5 g of NaCl on a single burner gas stove at 104 °C. The boiling time was recorded as the point when >90% of the dehulled lentils were softened to the point that the mixture with water produced a thickened soup, a method of preparation like that commonly used in the South Asian Region [24]. This study was replicated three times and data were analyzed using SAS 9.4.

2.8. Relative Fe Bioavailability and Phytic Acid Content of Fortified Lentils

Lentil dishes were prepared for four different samples, including Fe-fortified lentil and the control (unfortified lentil). Both fortified and control samples were rinsed with 18 MΩ deionized water. A traditional Bangladeshi lentil dish (dal) was prepared in stainless steel cookware using a traditional Bangladeshi recipe [24] where salt, turmeric powder, onion, canola oil and deionized water were used as ingredients at a 15:75:5:3:2 ratio. The prepared dish was cooled to room temperature for 2 h, frozen at −80 °C for 24 h, freeze dried using a FreeZone 12 Liter Console Freeze Dry System with Stoppering Trays (Labconco, model 7759040, Kansas City, MO, USA) for 72 hand stored at room temperature [25]. Ten grams of freeze-dried dal from each dish was finely grounded and sent to the USDA-ARS Robert Holley Center for Agriculture and Health (Ithaca, New York, NY, USA) to assess iron concentration and bioavailability using an in vitro digestion/Caco-2 cell culture bioassay [26]. Total Fe concentration from the cooked lentil samples was measured using a standard HNO$_3$-HClO$_4$ method and atomic absorption spectrophotometry [23]. The phytic acid (total phosphorus) test kit (Megazyme International, County Wicklow, Ireland), a simple, quantitative, colorimetric and high throughput method [25,27], was used for the measurement and analysis of phytic acid in the four cooked lentil samples used for the bioavailability assessment. The ANOVA was conducted using SAS 9.4 to determine differences in iron concentration, relative iron bioavailability and phytic acid concentration among the cooked fortified lentil dishes. The LSD was calculated and the level of significance set at $p < 0.001$.

3. Results and Discussion

3.1. Selection of Dehulled Lentil Product Type for Fortification

Prior to fortification, no significant differences in Fe concentration existed among product types (70–73 ppm Fe) (Figure 2b). After fortification with 200 ppm of Fe, significant differences in Fe concentration were observed among product types (Figure 2c). The highest Fe concentrations were observed in fortified unpolished split (196.7 ppm) and polished football (191.5 ppm) dal. Polished football dal, which is typically polished with water and/or vegetable oil after milling, performed best in the context of uniformity of mixing with the fortificant solution and drying in the shaker-when placed in the shaker, the polished football dal moved more and agitated more quickly in the mixing trays. This helped to distribute the heat over the surface of the dal, hence it dried more uniformly and did not stick to the tray surface when wet. Selection of dehulled lentil rather than whole lentil was important, because removal of the seed coat has a significant effect on reducing the levels of polyphenolic compounds, thereby increasing Fe bioavailability [21].

For commercial-scale fortification, any of the four lentil product types potentially could be fortified. Consumer demand and the relative cost and availability of the various processing techniques would be important considerations. Successful fortification to produce fortified food depends on the interactions among the food vehicle, fortificant and the fortification technique. Dehulled lentil dal is available in three colors—red, yellow and green. Red cotyledon lentil was selected for fortification since it is the most widely consumed form of lentil dal, with wide acceptability in South Asia and the Middle

East [28]. Consumers from some countries in these regions consume lentil as an essential component of their typical daily diet. Yellow and green lentil dal samples also were fortified and no significant differences were observed for final Fe concentration when fortified with similar concentrations of Fe fortificants (data not shown). Hence, any of red, yellow or green lentil dal could be fortified with the Fe fortificants.

3.2. Selection and Evaluation of the Most Suitable Fe Fortificant for Lentil

The success of food fortification programs is based on the chemistry between food vehicles and the fortificant selected to fortify foods [29]. Different food vehicles may contain different moisture levels and oxidizing agents that can react with fortificants and develop rancidity, metallic taste, off-color or degradation of vitamins, all factors that can influence bioavailability [30,31].

NaFeEDTA was shown previously to be two to four times more effective for increasing absorption of dietary Fe in humans compared to $FeSO_4$ and ferrous fumarate [32]. It also was reported that Fe absorption was increased by using a mixture of $FeSO_4$ and NaFeEDTA, instead of NaFeEDTA alone [33]. In another study, NaFeEDTA was proven to be a promising cost effective, water-soluble and highly bioavailable Fe fortificant that improved the Fe status of Vietnamese woman when consumed for 6 months (10 mg Fe for 6 days/week) [33]. These authors also reported that the prevalence of Fe deficiency and Fe deficiency anemia were reduced from 62.5% to 32.8% and from 58.3% to 20.3%, respectively.

The effect of NaFeEDTA-fortified wheat flour on urinary zinc extraction was studied and no effect was found in children [34]. Another study revealed no significant negative effects of NaFeEDTA-fortified bread (bread made with 100 g of NaFeEDTA-fortified wheat flour that contained 5 mg of Fe and was consumed as a single meal per day) consumption on Zn and Ca metabolism, and that NaFeEDTA might increase Zn absorption and Fe bioavailability from the low bioavailability diets [35]. In another study, NaFeEDTA was shown to have no influence on absorption or urinary excretion of Mn [36]. NaFeEDTA-fortified fish sauces also increased significantly the amounts of Hb and serum ferritin when provided to iron-deficient, anemic school children in Cambodia [37].

The review of the safety and efficacy of different dietary strategies for improving Fe status revealed that there are no reported data that demonstrate specific adverse effects of iron-fortified food items [38]. Moreover, the daily dose of Fe is much lower from fortified food than on supplementation [39]. The joint FAO/WHO Expert Committee on Food Additives (JECFA) summarized data on the basis of acute and chronic toxicity, reproduction, carcinogenicity, genotoxicity and teratogenicity of EDTA and its salts, such as NaFeEDTA [40]. The Committee also evaluated biochemical and toxicological aspects of using NaFeEDTA as a fortificant and stated that: (i) Fe from NaFeEDTA is released from the chelate to the common non-heme iron pool before Fe absorption; (ii) a very small fraction (1–2%) of NaFeEDTA is absorbed intact and is rapidly and completely excreted via the kidneys in the urine; (iii) dietary Fe fortification with NaFeEDTA does not increase the risk of iron accumulation in iron-replete individuals, and has no negative influence on the absorption of other micronutrients, such as Zn; and (iv) NaFeEDTA has low oral toxicity and does not induce gene mutations when tested with bacterial and mammalian cells in vitro. In addition, considering the cost of fortificant, NaFeEDTA is more expensive compared to $FeSO_4 \cdot 7H_2O$ and $FeSO_4 \cdot H_2O$, but its extra cost can be offset by its higher bioavailability in phytate-rich foods such as lentil [14].

3.3. Selection of Appropriate Methods for Fortification

3.3.1. Techniques Used for Lentil Fortification

Significant variation in Fe concentration was found among the five methods used to fortify lentil dal. The highest concentrations of Fe were found with the DSD (lentil dal oven dried, soaked, followed by oven drying) and SSD (lentil dal sprayed with fortificant solution followed by shaking and drying) methods (Figure 3). Although the highest Fe absorption into the lentil seed was observed with DSD, the discoloration (increased darkness) of the final product may cause concern in the context of expected consumer preferences and longer fortification time (Figure 4). The homogeneity of Fe concentration was tested by randomly selecting six samples from the mixing tray. All samples contained similar amounts of Fe (215–220 ppm) after fortification.

3.3.2. HunterLab Colorimetric Measurements of Fe-Fortified Lentil Samples

The HunterLab results indicated significant variation for all three scales (L*, a* and b*), indicating off-color development due to fortification (Figure 4b-1–b-3). The highest values for all three scales were found for the unfortified control lentil dal sample. The lowest L* value was found for the DSD sample, whereas the lowest a* and b* values were found for the samples produced by the SD, RDSD and DSD methods. The L*, a* and b* values ranged from 46.3 to 52.8, 25.3 to 33.1 and 36.6 to 44.6, respectively. The shortest processing time was required with the SSD method (Figure 4b-4), which also generated off- color but significantly less compared to the SD, RDSD and DSD methods.

3.3.3. Assessment of Appropriate Temperature and Duration for Drying Fortified Lentil Dal

Temperature has been shown to have a significant effect on the drying time required to achieve a level of moisture suitable for safe storage [41]. The results from the assessment of appropriate temperature and duration for drying fortified lentil dal showed that with an increase in temperature caused by raising the light bulb wattage, there was an increase in the temperature (°C) of both the aluminum foil tray used for fortification and the fortified lentil seed. An inverse relationship was observed between total drying time and temperature (Figure S1). The temperature used to dry fortified lentil dal should be optimized to avoid off-color development, as a relationship between temperature and off-color development in fortified foods has been observed [30]. Using the 250-watt bulb, the temperature rose to 75 °C, which dried the fortified lentil dal in the shortest time (12–14 min). The moisture content of the fortified dal was approximately 14%, which is similar to the moisture content (%) of dehulled lentil dal (13–14)% that is commercially available in the local market [42]. During fortification, lentil dal was treated with fortificant solution and then heat was applied to dry the product. This process might reduce the level of phytate and phenolics level to some extent, and enhance the bioavailability of both Fe and Zn [43].

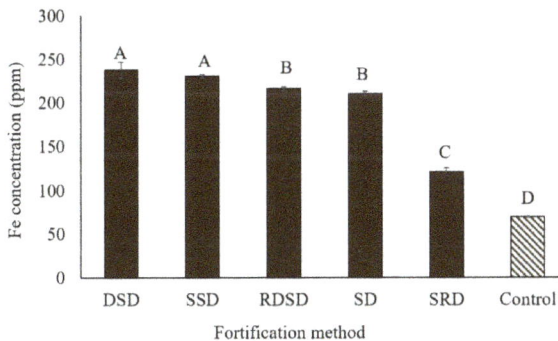

Figure 3. Iron concentration in polished football lentil dal fortified with $FeSO_4 \cdot 7H_2O$ solution (1600 ppm Fe) at 10 mL/100 g lentil dal using five different techniques. DSD = lentil dal oven dried for 10 minutes followed by soaking in fortificant solution and drying at 80 °C; SSD = lentil dal sprayed with fortificant solution followed by shaking and drying; RDSD = lentil dal rinsed, oven dried, followed by soaking in fortificant solution and then drying; SD = lentil dal directly soaked in fortificant solution followed by drying; SRD = lentil dal soaked in fortificant solution followed by rinsing with deionized water and drying. Different letters within the figure represent significant differences ($p < 0.05$).

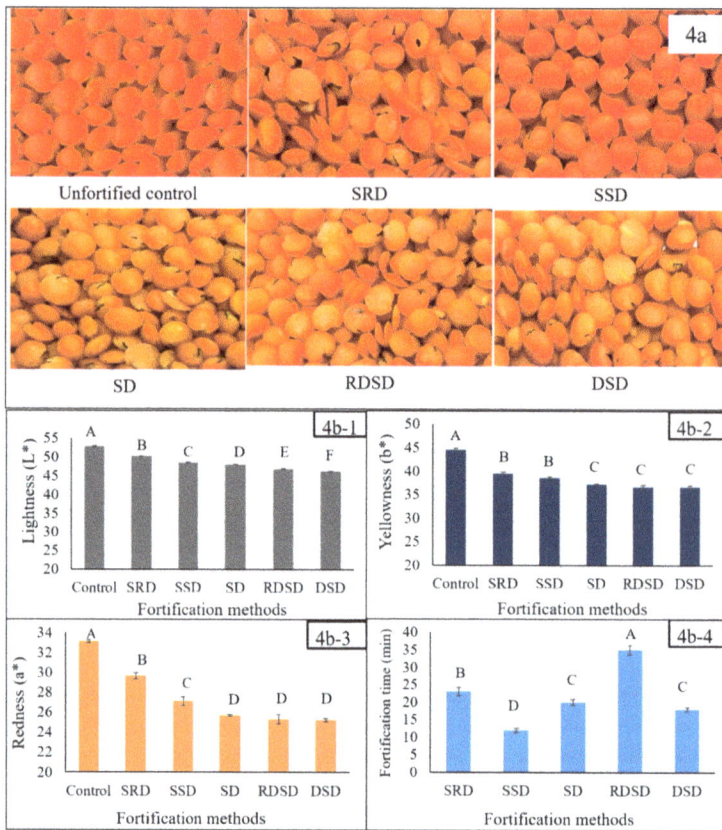

Figure 4. (**a**) Fe-fortified lentil developed by five different fortification methods: SRD = lentil dal soaked in fortificant solution followed by rinsing with deionized water and drying; SSD = lentil dal sprayed with fortificant solution followed by shaking and drying; SD = lentil dal directly soaked in fortificant solution followed by drying; RDSD = lentil dal rinsed, oven dried, followed by soaking in fortificant solution and then drying; DSD = lentil dal oven dried for 10 minutes followed by soaking in fortificant solution and drying at 80 °C; (**b1**–**b4**) Effect of different fortification methods on changes in lightness (L*), yellowness (b*) and redness (a*) score of Fe-fortified lentil dal and on the fortification process. Different letters within each figure represent significant differences ($p < 0.05$).

3.4. Assessment of the pH of Solutions Prepared with Three Fe Fortificants over a Range of Concentrations

Measurement of pH over a range of concentrations of the Fe fortificants showed an inverse relationship between pH and an increase in the concentration of Fe in the solution. The pHs of the three fortificant solutions were lower (<5) than that of deionized water (6.7). The rate of decrease of pH with an increase in Fe concentration was highest for $FeSO_4 \cdot H_2O$, followed by $FeSO_4 \cdot 7H_2O$ and NaFeEDTA (Figure 5). The pH of the fortificant solution would have an effect on the solubility of Fe [44]. Both pH and redox potential influence the oxidation state of Fe, and both the Fe^{+2} and the Fe^{+3} form are used for fortification. Both have unfilled orbits that can react with electron-rich components, thus influencing organoleptic attributes and bioavailability [45]. The oxidation-reduction reactions (redox potential) in fortified foods, due to the addition of Fe that can react with phenolic compounds, cause off-color development [43]. Ferrous ion oxidizes to the ferric form as redox potential increases, but remains constant at a lower redox potential [30,44]. The solubility of $FeSO_4$ in 0.1 M HCl was reported to decrease by 74% with changes in pH over the range of 2–6, but remained constant for NaFeEDTA [45]. In this study, an increase in $FeSO_4$ concentration resulted in a faster rate of pH reduction in comparison to NaFeEDTA. Moreover, to obtain a similar amount of soluble Fe at a specific pH, more $FeSO_4$ is required than NaFeEDTA. This may cause a major change in the organoleptic characteristics of lentil dal. This study showed that NaFeEDTA would be a better choice than $FeSO_4$ for fortification of lentil dal.

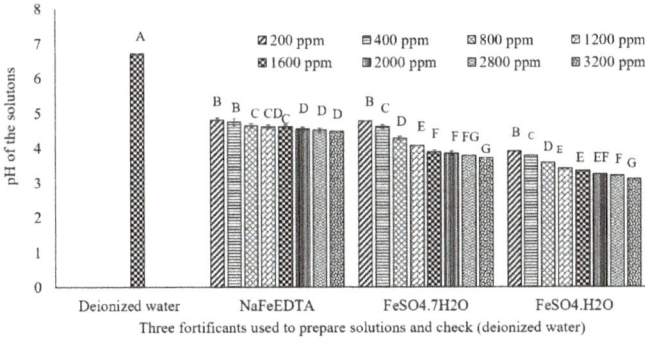

Figure 5. pH of Fe solutions prepared with three fortificants (NaFeEDTA, $FeSO_4 \cdot 7H_2O$, and $FeSO_4 \cdot H_2O$) ranging in concentration from 200 to 3200 ppm. Different letters within each figure represent significant differences ($p < 0.05$).

3.5. Estimation of Fe Concentration in Fortified Lentil Dal Samples Using F-AAS

The concentration of Fe in fortified lentil dal increased with an increase in Fe concentration in the fortificant solution (Table 1). Off-color development also increased gradually with an increase in the Fe concentration of the fortificant (Table 2).

Table 1. Fe concentration (ppm) in polished football lentil dal samples prepared using three fortificants ($FeSO_4 \cdot 7H_2O$, NaFeEDTA and $FeSO_4 \cdot H_2O$) at concentrations ranging from 100 to 3200 ppm.

Fe Concentration in Fortificant Solution (ppm)	Fe Concentration in Fortified Lentil Dal		
	$FeSO_4 \cdot 7H_2O$	NaFeEDTA	$FeSO_4 \cdot H_2O$
Control	69.0 ± 0.9 [a]	69.0 ± 0.9 [a]	65.6 ± 0.8 [a]
100	76.0 ± 1.9 [a]	83.7 ± 2.5 [a]	71.8 ± 0.7 [b]
400	132.5 ± 3.2 [b]	113.2 ± 4.2 [b]	108.6 ± 1.1 [c]
800	147.9 ± 4.7 [c]	182.9 ± 5.8 [c]	151.4 ± 2.8 [d]
1200	157.8 ± 4.3 [c]	185.3 ± 5.6 [c]	185.0 ± 6.6 [e]
1600	203.6 ± 3.9 [d]	205.3 ± 2.8 [d]	207.5 ± 3.9 [f]
2000	217.5 ± 8.2 [d]	274.7 ± 5.6 [e]	261.8 ± 3.9 [g]
2400	246.6 ± 9.3 [e]	309.7 ± 10.0 [f]	322.3 ± 3.7 [h]
2800	286.7 ± 6.0 [f]	346.7 ± 5.2 [g]	363.5 ± 6.2 [i]
3200	349.0 ± 1.8 [g]	326 ± 3.1 [h]	381.7 ± 3.6 [j]

[a] Mean ± SD. Mean scores for Fe concentration followed by different letters within columns are significantly different ($p < 0.001$).

Table 2. Lightness (L*), redness (a*) and yellowness (b*) scores of fortified lentil samples prepared using FeSO$_4$·7H$_2$O, NaFeEDTA and FeSO$_4$·H$_2$O at concentrations ranging from 100 to 3200 ppm after six months and after one year of storage.

Fe Concentration (ppm)	Lightness (L*)			Redness (a*)			Yellowness (b*)		
	Initial	After 6 Months	After One Year	Initial	After 6 Months	After One Year	Initial	After 6 Months	After One Year
FeSO$_4$·7H$_2$O fortified samples									
Control	50.6 ± 0.4 [a]	50.8 ± 0.2 [a]	51.0 ± 0.2 [a]	31.5 ± 0.2 [a]	31.3 ± 0.2 [a]	30.6 ± 0.6 [a]	41.6 ± 1.0 [a]	41.2 ± 1.0 [a]	40.3 ± 1.0 [a]
200	49.9 ± 0.6 [ab]	50.6 ± 0.6 [a]	52.0 ± 0.5 [b]	29.7 ± 0.8 [b]	29.4 ± 0.8 [b]	28.8 ± 0.8 [b]	40.5 ± 0.1 [b]	38.9 ± 0.1 [b]	37.9 ± 0.1 [b]
800	49.6 ± 0.2 [b]	50.3 ± 0.1 [a]	51.5 ± 0.0 [b]	27.4 ± 0.3 [c]	26.8 ± 0.2 [c]	25.8 ± 0.3 [ac]	37.8 ± 0.3 [c]	36.4 ± 0.3 [c]	34.6 ± 0.3 [c]
1600	46.2 ± 0.5 [c]	46.9 ± 0.5 [b]	48.5 ± 0.4 [c]	24.6 ± 0.7 [d]	24.9 ± 0.6 [d]	25.5 ± 1.2 [c]	36.4 ± 0.1 [d]	33.9 ± 0.1 [d]	34.0 ± 0.1 [c]
2400	43.9 ± 0.2 [d]	44.5 ± 0.1 [c]	45.8 ± 0.2 [c]	22.6 ± 0.2 [e]	22.2 ± 0.1 [e]	21.3 ± 0.2 [d]	32.0 ± 0.3 [e]	31.2 ± 0.1 [e]	30.0 ± 0.4 [d]
3200	42.1 ± 0.6 [e]	42.7 ± 0.6 [d]	43.9 ± 0.6 [d]	21.3 ± 0.8 [f]	34.4 ± 0.9 [f]	20.3 ± 1.2 [d]	30.0 ± 0.2 [f]	29.7 ± 0.7 [f]	28.6 ± 0.3 [e]
NaFeEDTA fortified samples									
Control	50.5 ± 0.4 [a]	50.8 ± 0.2 [a]	50.8 ± 0.2 [a]	31.5 ± 0.3 [a]	31.3 ± 0.3 [a]	30.6 ± 0.6 [a]	41.6 ± 0.3 [a]	41.2 ± 0.1 [a]	40.3 ± 0.7 [a]
200	50.4 ± 0.1 [a]	51.0 ± 0.2 [a]	51.0 ± 0.2 [a]	31.6 ± 0.7 [a]	31.1 ± 0.8 [a]	30.3 ± 0.8 [a]	41.9 ± 0.1 [a]	41.5 ± 0.1 [a]	40.6 ± 0.3 [a]
800	50.1 ± 0.2 [a]	50.6 ± 0.6 [a]	50.6 ± 0.6 [b]	31.1 ± 0.3 [a]	30.5 ± 0.2 [a]	29.0 ± 0.5 [b]	40.6 ± 0.9 [b]	39.3 ± 0.4 [a]	36.9 ± 0.8 [b]
1600	48.8 ± 0.1 [b]	52.0 ± 0.5 [b]	52.0 ± 0.5 [b]	29.4 ± 0.3 [b]	29.1 ± 0.2 [b]	28.6 ± 0.4 [b]	38.9 ± 0.2 [c]	38.2 ± 0.2 [b]	36.6 ± 0.5 [b]
2400	47.5 ± 0.2 [c]	50.3 ± 0.1 [c]	50.3 ± 0.1 [c]	27.5 ± 1.3 [c]	27.0 ± 1.2 [c]	26.1 ± 1.1 [c]	36.3 ± 0.7 [d]	35.8 ± 0.6 [c]	34.6 ± 0.6 [c]
3200	46.4 ± 0.5 [d]	51.5 ± 0.0 [d]	51.5 ± 0.0 [c]	27.8 ± 0.4 [c]	27.4 ± 0.4 [c]	26.5 ± 0.4 [c]	36.9 ± 0.7 [d]	36.4 ± 0.8 [c]	35.2 ± 0.9 [c]
FeSO$_4$·H$_2$O fortified samples									
Control	50.5 ± 0.4 [a]	50.5 ± 0.4 [a]	50.8 ± 0.2 [a]	51.2 ± 0.3 [a]	31.5 ± 0.2 [a]	31.3 ± 0.2 [a]	30.6 ± 0.6 [a]	41.6 ± 0.3 [a]	41.2 ± 0.1 [a]
200	51.1 ± 0.5 [a]	51.1 ± 0.5 [a]	51.3 ± 0.3 [b]	51.7 ± 0.3 [b]	30.0 ± 0.7 [b]	29.9 ± 0.7 [a]	29.8 ± 0.7 [b]	39.9 ± 0.1 [b]	39.6 ± 0.1 [b]
800	49.3 ± 0.7 [b]	49.7 ± 0.7 [b]	50.4 ± 0.5 [b]	27.9 ± 0.3 [c]	27.6 ± 0.4 [c]	27.1 ± 0.4 [a]	37.3 ± 0.9 [c]	36.9 ± 0.4 [c]	36.5 ± 0.8 [c]
1600	46.9 ± 0.7 [c]	47.3 ± 0.4 [c]	48.1 ± 0.2 [c]	25.4 ± 0.3 [d]	25.4 ± 0.3 [d]	25.4 ± 0.4 [c]	34.6 ± 0.2 [d]	34.6 ± 0.2 [d]	34.6 ± 0.5 [d]
2400	44.4 ± 0.6 [d]	44.7 ± 0.4 [d]	45.4 ± 0.4 [d]	23.3 ± 0.7 [e]	22.8 ± 0.7 [e]	21.9 ± 0.9 [d]	32.2 ± 0.7 [e]	31.9 ± 0.6 [e]	30.2 ± 0.6 [e]
3200	42.6 ± 0.3 [e]	42.6 ± 0.3 [e]	42.7 ± 0.5 [e]	22.7 ± 0.7 [e]	22.1 ± 0.7 [e]	21.1 ± 0.8 [d]	31.5 ± 0.7 [f]	30.9 ± 0.8 [f]	29.8 ± 0.9 [f]

[a] Mean ± SD. Mean scores for lightness (L*), redness (a*) and yellowness (b*) score followed by different letters within columns are significantly different ($p < 0.001$).

3.6. Assessment of the Appropriate Dose of Fe

Consideration of the appropriate dose of Fe is important for optimizing the amount of fortificant required to provide a major part of the estimated average requirement (EAR) for available Fe. The WHO has suggested suitable iron compounds to fortify specific food vehicles [13]. For instance, NaFeEDTA was suggested to fortify high extraction wheat flour, sugar, soy sauce, and fish at different rates. The bioavailability of Fe depends on the levels of various compounds present in the food vehicle, e.g., phytate, dietary fiber, tannins and other polyphenols [25,46]. These components can reduce the absorption of micronutrients, e.g., Fe, Zn. Moreover, Fe of plant origin is exclusively non-heme Fe, which is less bioavailable than the heme Fe from animal sources [46,47]. In this study, lentil dal fortified with three different fortificants showed an increase in Fe concentration with an increase in the Fe concentration in the fortificant solution. Lentil seed may exhibit a wide range in Fe concentration [7]. According to the FAO and WHO, EARs for iron having 10% bioavailability are 29.4 and 10.8 mg Fe day^{-1} for females and males, 19–50 years of age, respectively [13]. Therefore, 50 g of unfortified dehulled lentil could provide approximately 3.5 mg of Fe, based on the Fe concentration in the control lentil dal sample. The bioavailability may decrease if the dal is prepared with spices or condiments and is eaten with other foods such as rice, bread or vegetables, which may contain phytate, polyphenols or other components that reduce the absorption of Fe. To obtain a major portion of daily Fe from food fortificants, an optimum dose should be recommended. In this study, it was shown that lentil dal fortified with 1600 ppm of Fe could provide approximately 130–140 ppm of Fe per 100 g of lentil. Therefore, 50 g of fortified lentil could provide approximately 10 mg of Fe (6.5–7 mg of Fe from the fortificant + 3.5 mg from the lentil). This could provide a major portion of the EAR. Currently, 30–45 mg kg^{-1} ferrous sulphate and 250 mg kg^{-1} NaFeEDTA are used to fortify wheat flour and soy/fish sauce, respectively [13].

3.7. HunterLab Colorimeter Measurements of Stored Fe-Fortified Dal Samples

Color attributes influence the acceptability of a food product to consumers. The L*, a* and b* scores were significantly decreased with an increase in Fe concentration provided by any of the fortificants. Significant variation in color was observed among lentil dal samples fortified with the three fortificants at any concentration. Samples fortified with NaFeEDTA had higher L*, a* and b* scores, similar to those of the control, indicating less off-color development when compared to dal samples fortified with $FeSO_4 \cdot 7H_2O$ or $FeSO_4 \cdot H_2O$ (Figure 6).

The usual expectation for any Fe-fortified food product is that it does not exhibit any off-color. The dark color of the micropylar area of fortified lentil dal possibly could be used as an indicator to help consumers distinguish between fortified and unfortified lentil dal, where the micropylar region is white. The L*, a* and b* color values for the fortified lentil dal samples showed some inverse relationships with the progress of storage time (Table 2). Lightness (L*) increased slightly, but a* and b* decreased in all of the fortified lentil dal samples over time. Initially, just after fortification, the L* value ranged from 50.6 (unfortified control) to 42.2 (fortified with 3200 ppm of $FeSO_4 \cdot 7H_2O$), which was similar to the samples fortified with $FeSO_4 \cdot H_2O$ (42.6). The range was narrower for the L* value of samples fortified with NaFeEDTA (50.6 to 46.4) (Table 2). For all three fortificants, after 6 months and one year of storage of fortified lentil dal, there was an increasing trend in L*, but a decreasing trend for the a* and b* values (Table 2). The non-significant differences in the L*, a* and b* scores for the unfortified and fortified lentil samples provides assurance that the minor changes observed will not influence consumer acceptability. The L*, a* and b* values for fortified lentil dal, prepared with the three fortificants at 1600 ppm of Fe, showed numerical decreases, but these were not significant for the three storage periods, except for the L* and b* scores for the $FeSO_4 \cdot 7H_2O$-fortified and the NaFeEDTA-fortified samples, respectively (Figure 7). These small changes may be caused by the presence of very small amounts of lipid (1.52–2.95%) [48] that could increase the likelihood of lipid oxidation and result in off-color development over time.

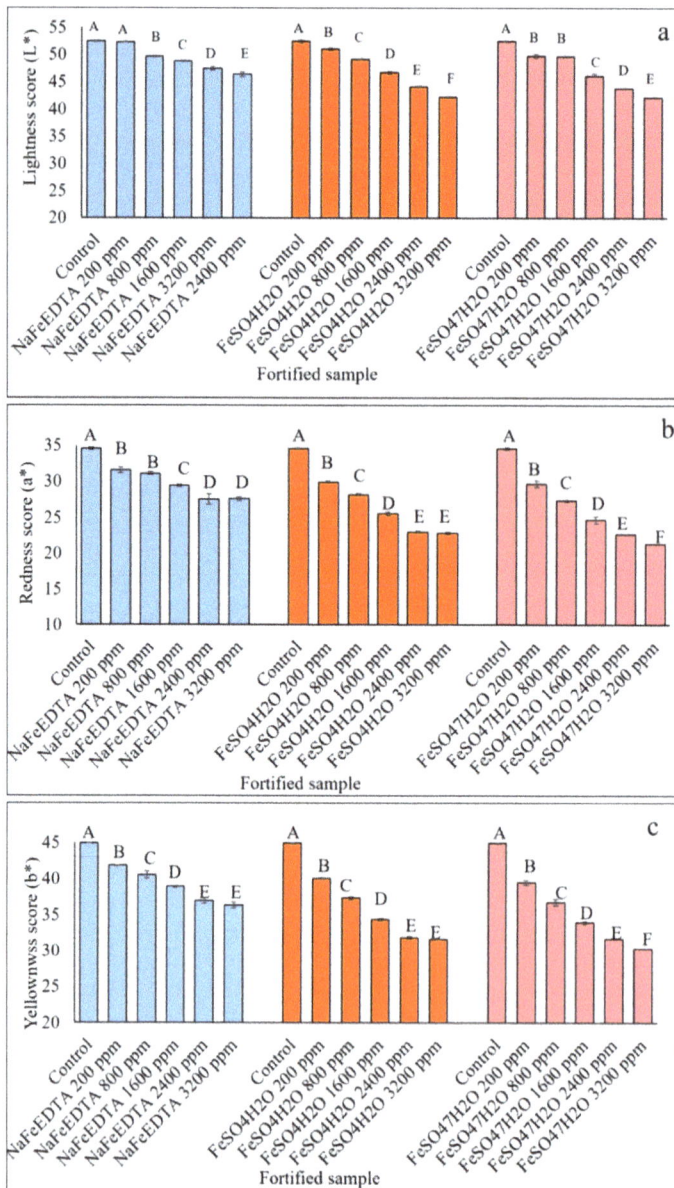

Figure 6. Effect of increasing Fe concentration on lightness (L*), redness (a*) and yellowness scores (b*) of lentil dal samples fortified with $FeSO_4 \cdot 7H_2O$, NaFeEDTA and $FeSO_4 \cdot H_2O$ at five different concentrations ranging from 200 to 3200 ppm. Different letters within each figure represent significant differences ($p < 0.05$).

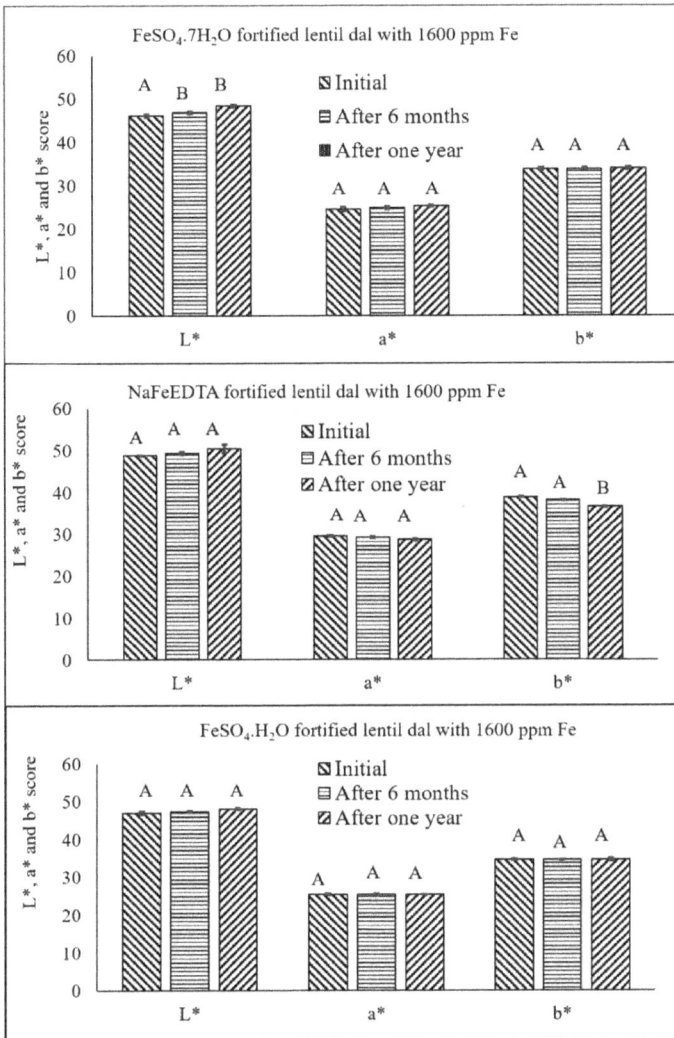

Figure 7. Effect of storage time on changes in L*, a* and b* score of football lentil samples fortified with 1600 ppm of Fe using $FeSO_4 \cdot 7H_2O$, NaFeEDTA and $FeSO_4 \cdot H_2O$. Different letters within each figure represent significant differences ($p < 0.05$).

3.8. Boiling Time Estimation of Fortified Samples Compared to the Unfortified Control

The boiling time of lentil dal is important and may influence consumer acceptability due to energy and time consumption during cooking. Compared to unfortified lentil dal, the fortified lentil dal should take equal or less time to cook, and have similar texture, taste and appearance after cooking. Among the four samples that were cooked to determine the variability in boiling time, all had similar cooking times (Figure S2). Fortification had no significant influence on the boiling time of $FeSO_4 \cdot 7H_2O$-, $FeSO_4 \cdot H_2O$- or NaFeEDTA-fortified samples compared to the control.

3.9. Iron Concentration, Relative Fe Bioavailability and Phytic Acid Concentration of Fortified Lentils

Significant differences were observed among fortified and unfortified lentil samples in Fe concentration, relative Fe bioavailability and phytic acid concentration (Table 3). Similar iron and phytic acid concentrations were observed in $FeSO_4·7H_2O$- and NaFeEDTA- fortified samples. The unfortified lentil samples were statistically different than the three fortified samples for all four measurements. The relative bioavailability was similar for all three fortified lentil dal samples. Iron concentration and relative Fe bioavailability ranged from 68.7 to 238.5 ppm and 68.3 to 104.9, respectively. The relative Fe bioavailability of the three cooked fortified lentil dal samples was 1.4 to 1.5 times higher than that of unfortified cooked lentil sample (control). Phytic acid concentration ranged from 7.2 to 8.0 mg g^{-1}.

Table 3. Mean iron (Fe) concentration (ppm), relative bioavailability (ng ferritin (mg protein)$^{-1}$) and phytic acid concentration (mg g^{-1}) of four cooked freeze-dried lentil samples.

Cooked Lentil Sample	Fe Concentration (ppm) [a]	Ferritin Formation (ng Ferritin (mg Protein)$^{-1}$) [a]	Relative Fe Bioavailability (% Control Lentil) [a]	Phytic Acid (mg g^{-1}) [a]
Unfortified dehulled lentil	68.7 ± 0.3 [a]	12.7 ± 1.0 [a]	68.3 ± 14.8 [a]	8.0 ± 0.1 [a]
NaFeEDTA fortified (1600 ppm Fe)	230.8 ± 8.5 [b]	17.4 ± 2.7 [b]	100.5 ± 7.5 [b]	8.0 ± 0.2 [a]
$FeSO_4·H_2O$ fortified (1600 ppm Fe)	220.5 ± 2.1 [c]	17.6 ± 2.2 [b]	104.9 ± 16.7 [b]	7.2 ± 0.1 [c]
$FeSO_4·7H_2O$ fortified (1600 ppm Fe)	238.5 ± 4.7 [b]	21.2 ± 1.9 [b]	103.4 ± 10.4 [b]	7.4 ± 0.1 [b]

[a] Mean ± SD. Mean scores for Fe concentration, bioavailability (ng ferritin (mg protein)$^{-1}$), relative Fe bioavailability (% control lentil) and phytic acid (mg g^{-1}) followed by different letters within columns are significantly different ($p < 0.001$).

Fortification of lentil dal is more complex than fortifying flour, beverages and most other food products due to the requirement to apply fortificant solution to the surface of the dal. Considering all of the results from the various experiments, it was concluded that lentil dal could be used as a vehicle for Fe fortification and that NaFeEDTA was the most suitable Fe fortificant for lentil dal. These results represent baseline data for the commercial production of Fe-fortified lentil dal. This research is unique in the context of lentil dal fortification, and will be followed by sensory evaluation to select the most appropriate fortificant after evaluation of overall acceptability. Results from sensory evaluation with both uncooked and cooked fortified lentil dal compared favorably with the control and will be described in a subsequent manuscript. Community-based efficacy and effectiveness studies with fortified lentil in the target populations will be required. The bioavailability of fortified lentil in a large-scale human trial also could be evaluated to obtain an empirical estimate of the amount of Fe required to provide a major portion of the EARs for Fe in regions where Fe deficiency exists.

Supplementary Materials: The following are available online at www.mdpi.com/2072-6643/9/8/863/s1, Figure S1: Effect of increasing light bulb wattage on temperature (°C) and drying time (min) of fortified lentil samples, Figure S2: Effect of the three fortificants solution used to prepare three fortified lentil samples ($FeSO_4·7H_2O$, NaFeEDTA and $FeSO_4·H_2O$) on boiling time compared with one unfortified control sample. Different letters within each figure are significantly different ($p < 0.05$).

Acknowledgments: The authors would like to acknowledge financial assistance received from The Saskatchewan Ministry of Agriculture (Agriculture Development Fund) and Grand Challenges Canada. The authors are grateful for technical assistance provided by B. Goetz, Crop Development Centre, University of Saskatchewan and Chowdhury Jalal, Micronutrient Initiative, Ottawa for invaluable guidance during manuscript preparation.

Author Contributions: R. Podder and A. Vandenberg conceived and designed the study. R. Podder, B. Tar'an and D. DellaValle analysed the data. R. Podder prepared the draft manuscript. B. Tar'an, R. T. Tyler, C. J. Henry, D. M. DellaValle and A. Vandenberg reviewed all documents critically and approved the final manuscript for submission in the Journal.

Conflicts of Interest: The authors declare no conflict of interest.

References

1. Podder, R.; Banniza, S.; Vandenberg, A. Screening of wild and cultivated lentil germplasm for resistance to stemphylium blight. *Plant Genet. Resour.* **2013**, *11*, 26–35. [CrossRef]
2. Thavarajah, D.; Thavarajah, P.; Wejesuriya, A.; Rutzke, M.; Glahn, R.P.; Combs, G.F.; Vandenberg, A. The potential of lentil (*Lens culinaris* L.) as a whole food for increased selenium, iron, and zinc intake: Preliminary results from a 3 year study. *Euphytica* **2011**, *180*, 123–128. [CrossRef]
3. Thavarajah, D.; Thavarajah, P.; Sarker, A.; Vandenberg, A. Lentils (*Lens culinaris* Medikus Subspecies culinaris): A Whole Food for Increased Iron and Zinc Intake. *J. Agric. Food Chem.* **2009**, *57*, 5413–5419. [CrossRef] [PubMed]
4. Wang, N.; Daun, J.K. Effects of variety and crude protein content on nutrients and anti-nutrients in lentils (*Lens culinaris*). *Food Chem.* **2006**, *95*, 493–502. [CrossRef]
5. Hoover, R.; Hughes, T.; Chung, H.J.; Liu, Q. Composition, molecular structure, properties, and modification of pulse starches: A review. *Food Res. Int.* **2010**, *43*, 399–413. [CrossRef]
6. Huang, J.; Schols, H.A.; van Soest, J.J.G.; Jin, Z.; Sulmann, E.; Voragen, A.G.J. Physicochemical properties and amylopectin chain profiles of cowpea, chickpea and yellow pea starches. *Food Chem.* **2007**, *101*, 1338–1345. [CrossRef]
7. DellaValle, D.M.; Glahn, R.P.; Shaff, J.E.; O'Brien, K.O. Iron Absorption from an Intrinsically Labeled Lentil Meal Is Low but Upregulated in Women with Poor Iron Status. *J. Nutr.* **2015**, *145*, 2253–2257. [CrossRef] [PubMed]
8. Lynch, S.R.; Beard, J.L.; Dassenko, S.A.; Cook, J.D. Iron absorption from legumes in humans. *Am. J. Clin. Nutr.* **1984**, *40*, 42–47. [PubMed]
9. Li, S.; Zhou, X.; Huang, Y.; Zhu, L.; Zhang, S.; Zhao, Y.; Guo, J.; Chen, J.; Chen, R. Identification and characterization of the zinc-regulated transporters, iron-regulated transporter-like protein (ZIP) gene family in maize. *BMC Plant Biol.* **2013**, *13*, 114. [CrossRef] [PubMed]
10. Bermejo, F.; Garcia-Lopez, S. A guide to diagnosis of iron deficiency and iron deficiency anemia in digestive diseases. *World J. Gastroenterol.* **2009**, *15*, 4638–4643. [CrossRef] [PubMed]
11. Detzel, P.; Wieser, S. Food fortification for addressing iron deficiency in filipino children: Benefits and cost-effectiveness. *Ann. Nutr. Metab.* **2015**, *66*, 35–42. [CrossRef] [PubMed]
12. Boccio, J.R.; Iyengar, V. Iron deficiency: Causes, consequences, and strategies to overcome this nutritional problem. *Biol. Trace Elem. Res.* **2003**, *94*, 1–32. [CrossRef]
13. Allen, L.; de Benoist, B.; Dary, O.; Hurrell, R. Guidelines on Food Fortification with Micronutrients. Available online: http://www.unscn.org/layout/modules/resources/files/fortification_eng.pdf (accessed on 21 April 2017).
14. Northrop-Clewes, C.A. Food fortification. In *Nutrition in Infancy*; Humana Press: Totowa, NJ, USA, 2013; pp. 359–381.
15. Dary, O. The importance and limitations of food fortification for the management of nutritional anemias. In *The Guidebook Nutritional Anemia*; Badham, J., Micheal, B., Zimmermann, K.K., Eds.; Sight and Life Press: Basel, Switzerland, 2007; pp. 315–336. ISBN 3-906412-35-0.
16. Nilson, A.; Piza, J. Food fortification: A tool for fighting hidden hunger. *Food Nutr. Bull.* **1998**, *19*, 49–60. [CrossRef]
17. Darnton-Hill, I.; Nalubola, R. Fortification strategies to meet micronutrient needs: Successes and failures. *Proc. Nutr. Soc.* **2002**, *61*, 231–241. [CrossRef] [PubMed]
18. Dwyer, J.T.; Wiemer, K.L.; Dary, O.; Keen, C.L.; King, J.C.; Miller, K.B.; Philbert, M.A.; Tarasuk, V.; Taylor, C.L.; Gaine, P.C.; et al. Fortification and Health: Challenges and Opportunities. *Adv. Nutr. Int. Rev. J.* **2015**, *6*, 124–131. [CrossRef] [PubMed]
19. Pachón, H.; Spohrer, R.; Mei, Z.; Serdula, M.K. Evidence of the effectiveness of flour fortification programs on iron status and anemia: A systematic review. *Nutr. Rev.* **2015**, *73*, 780–795. [CrossRef] [PubMed]
20. Martînez-Navarrete, N.; Camacho, M.; Martînez-Lahuerta, J.; Martînez-Monzó, J.; Fito, P. Iron deficiency and iron fortified foods—A review. *Food Res. Int.* **2002**, *35*, 225–231. [CrossRef]
21. DellaValle, D.M.; Thavarajah, D.; Thavarajah, P.; Vandenberg, A.; Glahn, R.P. Lentil (*Lens culinaris* L.) as a candidate crop for iron biofortification: Is there genetic potential for iron bioavailability? *Field Crop. Res.* **2013**, *144*, 119–125. [CrossRef]

22. Wrolstad, R.E.; Smith, D.E. Color analysis. In *Food Analysis*; Nielson, S.S., Ed.; Springer International Publishing: Cham, Switzerland, 2010; pp. 545–555, ISBN 978-1-4419-1477-4.
23. Diapari, M.; Sindhu, A.; Bett, K.; Deokar, A.; Warkentin, T.D.; Tar'an, B.; Francki, M. Genetic diversity and association mapping of iron and zinc concentrations in chickpea (*Cicer arietinum* L.). *Genome* **2014**, *57*, 459–468. [CrossRef] [PubMed]
24. Kohinoor, H.; Siddiqua, A.; Akhtar, S.; Hossain, M.G.; Podder, R.; Hossain, M.A. *Nutrition and Easy Cooking of Pulses*; Bangladesh Agricultural Research Institute Press: Gazipur, Bangladesh; Print Valley Printing Press: Gazipur, Bangladesh, 2010.
25. DellaValle, D.M.; Glahn, R.P. Differences in relative iron bioavailability in traditional Bangladeshi meal plans. *Food Nutr. Bull.* **2014**, *35*, 431–439. [CrossRef] [PubMed]
26. Glahn, R. Use of Caco-2 cells in defining nutrient bioavailability: Application to iron bioavailability of foods. In *Designing Functional Foods: Measuring and Controlling Food Structure Breakdown and Nutrient Absorption*; McClements, D.J., Eric, A.D., Eds.; Woodhead Publishing Limited Press: Cambridge, UK; CRC Press: Boca Raton, FL, USA, 2009; pp. 340–361, ISBN 9781845696603.
27. Mckie, V.A.; Mccleary, B.V. A novel and rapid colorimetric method for measuring total phosphorus and phytic acid in foods and animal feeds. *J. AOAC Int.* **2016**, *99*, 738–743. [CrossRef] [PubMed]
28. Erskine, W. Origin, phylogeny, domestication and spread. In *The Lentil: Botany, Production and Uses*; Erskine, W., Muehlbauer, J.F., Sarker, A., Sharma, B., Eds.; CAB International: Oxfordshire, UK, 2009; pp. 13–33, ISBN 9781845934873.
29. Mellican, R.I.; Li, J.; Mehansho, H.; Nielsen, S.S. The role of iron and the factors affecting off-color development of polyphenols. *J. Agric. Food Chem.* **2003**, *51*, 2304–2316. [CrossRef] [PubMed]
30. Hurrell, R.F. Preventing iron deficiency through food fortification. *Nutr. Rev.* **1997**, *55*, 210–222. [CrossRef] [PubMed]
31. Hurrell, R.F.; Cook, J.D. Strategies for iron fortification of foods. *Trends Food Sci. Technol.* **1990**, *1*, 56–61. [CrossRef]
32. Hurrell, R.F.; Reddy, M.B.; Burri, J.; Cook, J.D. An evaluation of EDTA compounds for iron fortification of cereal-based foods. *Br. J. Nutr.* **2000**, *84*, 903–910. [PubMed]
33. Van Thuy, P.; Berger, J.; Davidsson, L.; Khan, N.C.; Lam, N.T.; Cook, J.D.; Hurrell, R.F.; Khoi, H.H. Regular consumption of NaFeEDTA-fortified fish sauce improves iron status and reduces the prevalence of anemia in anemic Vietnamese women. *Am. J. Clin. Nutr.* **2003**, *78*, 284–290.
34. Amalrajan, V.; Thankachan, P.; Selvam, S.; Kurpad, A. Effect of wheat flour fortified with sodium iron EDTA on urinary zinc excretion in school-aged children. *Food Nutr. Bull.* **2012**, *33*, 177–179. [CrossRef] [PubMed]
35. Davidsson, L.; Kastenmayer, P.; Hurrell, R.F. Sodium iron EDTA [NaFe(III)EDTA] as a food fortificant: The effect on the absorption and retention of zinc and calcium in women. *Am. J. Clin. Nutr.* **1994**, *60*, 231–237. [PubMed]
36. Davidsson, L.; Almgren, A.; Hurrell, R.F. Sodium iron EDTA [NaFe(III)EDTA] as a food fortificant does not influence absorption and urinary excretion of manganese in healthy adults. *J. Nutr.* **1998**, *128*, 1139–1143. [PubMed]
37. Longfils, P.; Monchy, D.; Weinheimer, H.; Chavasit, V.; Nakanishi, Y.; Schümann, K.A. Comparative intervention trial on fish sauce fortified with NaFe-EDTA and FeSO4+ citrate in iron deficiency anemic school children in Kampot, Cambodia. *Asia Pac. J. Clin. Nutr.* **2008**, *17*, 250–257. [PubMed]
38. Prentice, A.M.; Mendoza, Y.A.; Pereira, D.; Cerami, C.; Wegmuller, R.; Constable, A.; Spieldenner, J. Dietary strategies for improving iron status: Balancing safety and efficacy. *Nutr. Rev.* **2017**, *75*, 49–60. [CrossRef] [PubMed]
39. Eichler, K.; Wieser, S.; Rüthemann, I.; Brügger, U. Effects of micronutrient fortified milk and cereal food for infants and children: A systematic review. *BMC Public Health* **2012**, *12*, 506. [CrossRef] [PubMed]
40. FAO; WHO. Evaluation of Certain Food Additives and Contaminants. Available online: http://apps.who. int/iris/bitstream/10665/43870/1/9789241209472_eng.pdf (accessed on 12 June 2017).
41. Hayma, J. *The Storage of Tropical Agricultural Products*; Van Otterloo-Butler, S., Ed.; Agromisa: Wageningen, The Netherlands, 2003; ISBN 9077073604.
42. McVicar, R.; McCall, P.; Brenzil, C.; Hartley, S.; Panchuk, K.; Mooleki, P. Lentils in Saskatchewan. Available online: http://publications.gov.sk.ca/documents/20/86381-LentilsinSaskatchewan.pdf (accessed on 12 June 2017).

43. Oghbaei, M.; Prakash, J. Effect of primary processing of cereals and legumes on its nutritional quality: A comprehensive review. *Cogent Food Agric.* **2016**, *2*. [CrossRef]

44. Mehansho, H. Iron fortification technology development: New approaches. *J. Nutr.* **2006**, *136*, 1059–1063. [PubMed]

45. García-Casal, M.N.; Layrisse, M. The effect of change in pH on the solubility of iron bis-glycinate chelate and other iron compounds. *Arch. Latinoam. Nutr.* **2001**, *51*, 35–36. [PubMed]

46. Hurrell, R.; Egli, I. Iron bioavailability and dietary reference values. *Am. J. Clin. Nutr.* **2010**, *91*, 1461S–1467S. [CrossRef] [PubMed]

47. Marie Minihane, A.; Rimbach, G. Iron absorption and the iron binding and anti-oxidant properties of phytic acid. *Int. J. Food Sci. Technol.* **2002**, *37*, 741–748. [CrossRef]

48. Zhang, B.; Deng, Z.; Tang, Y.; Chen, P.; Liu, R.; Ramdath, D.D.; Liu, Q.; Hernandez, M.; Tsao, R. Fatty acid, carotenoid and tocopherol compositions of 20 Canadian lentil cultivars and synergistic contribution to antioxidant activities. *Food Chem.* **2014**, *161*, 296–304. [CrossRef] [PubMed]

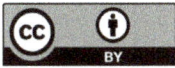

nutrients

MDPI

Article

Dietary Factors Modulate Iron Uptake in Caco-2 Cells from an Iron Ingot Used as a Home Fortificant to Prevent Iron Deficiency

Ildefonso Rodriguez-Ramiro *,†, Antonio Perfecto † and Susan J. Fairweather-Tait

Norwich Medical School, University of East Anglia, Norwich NR4 7UQ, UK; a.perfecto@uea.ac.uk (A.P.);
s.fairweather-tait@uea.ac.uk (S.J.F.-T.)
* Correspondence: i.rodriguez-ramiro@uea.ac.uk
† These authors contributed equally to this work.

Received: 7 August 2017; Accepted: 7 September 2017; Published: 12 September 2017

Abstract: Iron deficiency is a major public health concern and nutritional approaches are required to reduce its prevalence. The aim of this study was to examine the iron bioavailability of a novel home fortificant, the "Lucky Iron Fish™" (LIF) (www.luckyironfish.com/shop, Guelph, Canada) and the impact of dietary factors and a food matrix on iron uptake from LIF in Caco-2 cells. LIF released a substantial quantity of iron (about 1.2 mM) at pH 2 but this iron was only slightly soluble at pH 7 and not taken up by cells. The addition of ascorbic acid (AA) maintained the solubility of iron released from LIF (LIF-iron) at pH 7 and facilitated iron uptake by the cells in a concentration-dependent manner. In vitro digestion of LIF-iron in the presence of peas increased iron uptake 10-fold. However, the addition of tannic acid to the digestion reduced the cellular iron uptake 7.5-fold. Additionally, LIF-iron induced an overproduction of reactive oxygen species (ROS), similar to ferrous sulfate, but this effect was counteracted by the addition of AA. Overall, our data illustrate the major influence of dietary factors on iron solubility and bioavailability from LIF, and demonstrate that the addition of AA enhances iron uptake and reduces ROS in the intestinal lumen.

Keywords: iron bioavailability; iron fortification; simulated gastrointestinal digestion

1. Introduction

The World Health Organization (WHO) estimated in 2010 that iron deficiency anemia (IDA) affects one third of the world's population [1]. IDA is particularly prevalent in developing countries [2] and therefore represents a heavy economic burden. Amongst the strategies used to reduce the prevalence of iron deficiency, food-based or home fortification strategies can be very cost-effective [3].

Cooking in iron pots has been proposed as a strategy for improving the iron status of iron deficient populations [4]. However, its effectiveness is somewhat reduced by a lack of acceptability [5]. A recent study carried out in three refugee camps in Tanzania reported low acceptability for using iron and iron-alloy cooking pots due to a number of factors including rusting, heavy weight, difficulty in use and cleaning [6]. A new home fortification approach uses an iron ingot, the "Lucky Iron Fish™" (LIF), and has recently been tested in a Cambodian population [7–9]. It is based on the principle of releasing iron during cooking, as occurs with iron pots, but the LIF is much smaller, only weighing approximately 200 g, and has been shaped as a fish, a symbol of luck in Cambodian culture, in an attempt to improve its acceptability in this population [10]. Three randomised clinical trials (RCT) have been performed evaluating the effectiveness of LIF in reducing iron deficiency [7,8,11], with conflicting results. Apart from compliance issues related to its acceptability, other parameters, such as the composition of the diet or genotype, may have influenced the outcome of those trials. Therefore, there is a need to study the cellular iron bioavailability of this novel home fortificant and potential interactions with dietary factors.

The in vitro digestion/Caco-2 cell model has been extensively used to predict iron bioavailability from food and iron supplements and to investigate the intestinal cellular mechanisms of iron uptake [12–15]. Therefore, the aims of the present study were to use this model to evaluate the potential bioavailability of iron from LIF, taking into consideration the impact of dietary factors, and to examine oxidative stress initiated by the iron released from LIF, in order to provide new insights into this novel home iron fortificant.

2. Materials and Methods

2.1. Samples and Reagents

The iron-ingot, Lucky Iron Fish™ (Figure 1), was purchased through an e-commerce online shop (www.luckyironfish.com/shop, Guelph, Canada). The same iron ingot was used for all experiments, cleaned in Milli-Q H_2O, and dried at the end of each experiment. Chemicals, enzymes and hormones were purchased from Sigma-Aldrich, (Gillingham, UK) unless otherwise stated. Frozen *petit pois* peas (*Pisum sativum*) were obtained from a local supermarket, microwaved, lyophilized, finely ground and stored in a desiccator at 4 °C over silica gel.

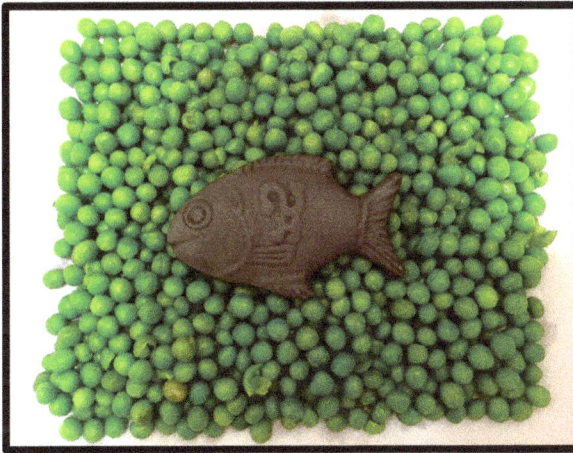

Figure 1. Iron ingot (Lucky Iron Fish™ (LIF)) used to treat iron deficiency. The selected picture background shows the relative size of LIF compared to *petit pois* peas.

2.2. Cell Culture and LIF Treatments

Caco-2 cells (HTB-37) were obtained from the American Type Culture Collection (Manassas, VA, USA) at passage 20 and stored in liquid nitrogen. Cells were grown in Dulbecco's modified Eagle's medium (DMEM), supplemented with 25 mM HEPES solution, 10% fetal bovine serum, 1% penicillin (5000 μ/mL), 1% L-glutamine (200 mM) (ThermoFisher Scientific, Loughborough, UK) and 1% MEM non-essential amino acids solution (Sigma-Aldrich, Gillingham, UK). Cells were maintained at 37 °C in a humidified incubator containing 5% CO_2 and 95% air. Cells between passages 30–36 were seeded onto collagen-coated 6-, 12-, 24- or 96-well plates (Bio-Greiner, Stonehouse, UK) at a density of 5×10^4 cells/cm^2 depending on the experiment and the media was replaced every 2 days. For all experiments, cells were post-confluent and used at 13–15 days post-seeding. In order to ensure low basal iron levels, 24 h prior to the initiation of the experiments, the DMEM medium was replaced with Eagle's minimum essential medium (MEM), without fetal bovine serum, and supplemented with 10 mmol/L PIPES (piperazine-*N*,*N*′-bis-(2-ethanesulfonic acid)), 26.1 mM NaHCO$_3$, 19.4 mmol/L glucose, 1% antibiotic-antimycotic solution, 11 μmol/L hydrocortisone, 0.87 μmol/L insulin, 0.02 μmol/L sodium selenite (Na$_2$SeO$_3$), 0.05 µmol/L triiodothyronine and 20 µg/L epidermal growth factor as previously reported [16].

LIF was boiled for 10 min in 1 L of Milli-Q (18.2 MΩ) H$_2$O at acidic pH (pH 2) for maximal iron release. An acid-washed beaker was used to avoid external iron contamination. Samples of 25 mL were placed in polypropylene tubes, cooled to room temperature, and ascorbic acid (AA) added to obtain a final concentration of 0, 1 and 10 mM, respectively. The pH of the solutions was gradually increased to 7 with 0.1 M NaHCO$_3$. The iron released from LIF (LIF-Iron) with or without added AA was determined at this stage prior to further dilution in MEM (LIF-Iron:MEM, 1:1, 1:3, or 1:10, depending on the nature of each experiment). Subsequently, cells were exposed to the different treatments for the indicated times. For iron uptake experiments, Caco-2 cells were subjected to the LIF-iron treatments and to a set of controls including blanks with/without AA and a positive control (0.05 mM FeSO$_4$ plus 0.5 mM AA, (FeSO$_4$)). When simulated digestion was performed, different methods were used (see next section).

2.3. In Vitro Simulated Gastrointestinal Digestion

The simulated gastrointestinal digestion was performed as described by Glahn et al. [16] with minor modifications to adjust for the addition of iron from LIF. A pH 2 saline solution (140 mmol/L NaCl, 5 mmol/L KCl) was used to initiate the simulated digestions. For all the experiments, the saline solution without any added iron was used as a blank digestion control to ensure no iron contamination in the in vitro digestion/cellular system. Additionally, 1 g of freeze-dried peas (containing 51 µg Fe/g dry weight, analysed by ICP-OES as previously described [13]) was added to the saline solution as a reference digestion of the pea matrix sample. To ensure that all of the iron released from the peas during digestion remained in solution when the pH was increased to duodenal levels, ascorbic acid (AA) was added at the gastric step of digestion at a final concentration of 0.5 mM (molar ratio of 1:10, Fe:AA). LIF was boiled for 10 min in 1 L of the pH 2 saline solution and samples of 10 mL were used for digestions (see below). To evaluate the effect of the pea matrix on LIF-iron bioavailability, 10 mL of LIF-iron samples was added to 1 g of pea sample. The impact of dietary iron inhibitors (as found in a meal) on LIF-iron bioavailability was examined by adding tannic acid (TA) or phytic acid (PA) at 0.05 and 0.5 mM, as indicated.

To simulate gastric conditions, pepsin (0.04 g/mL) was added and the samples were incubated for 60 min on a rolling table at 37 °C. After 60 min, the pH of the samples was gradually adjusted to pH 5.5 with 0.1 M NaHCO$_3$, and bile (0.007 g/mL) and pancreatin (0.001 g/mL) enzymes were added. The samples were further readjusted to pH 7, and incubated for 30 min on a rolling table at 37 °C to mimic intestinal conditions. At the end of the simulated gastrointestinal digestion, 1.5 mL of the digestate was placed on top of an upper chamber consisting of a Transwell insert fitted with a 15 KDa molecular weight cut-off dialysis membrane (Spectra/Por 7 dialysis tubing, Spectrum laboratories, Europe) suspended over Caco-2 cell monolayers grown in collagen-coated 6-well plates. The digestates were incubated with the cells for 2 h at 37 °C in a humidified incubator containing 5% CO$_2$ and 95% air. Inserts were removed, an additional 1 mL of supplemented MEM was added, and cells were incubated for a further 22 h prior to harvesting for ferritin analysis.

2.4. Analysis of Soluble and Total Iron Released from LIF

The total iron content of freshly prepared LIF-iron solution was measured using Ferene-S (3-(2-Pyridyl)-5,6-bis(5-sulfo-2-furyl)-1,2,4-triazine disodium salt hydrate), which binds ferrous iron, forming a deep blue complex. Freshly prepared solutions of LIF-iron were used to determine total iron. The soluble iron content was determined by centrifuging 1 mL aliquots of LIF-iron solution at 10,000 g for 5 min, and supernatants were collected for iron analysis. Samples (100 µL) were digested in 100 µL 1% HCl for 10 min in a shaker water bath at 80 °C. After 10 min, samples were briefly cooled on ice and the following reagents were added sequentially and vortexed after each addition: 500 µL 7.5% ammonium acetate, 100 µL AA, 100 µL 2.5% sodium dodecylsulphate (SDS), and 100 µL 1.5%

ferene. Samples were centrifuged at 13,400× g for 5 min and the absorbance of the supernatant was measured at 593 nm against an iron standard curve (0–20 nmol Fe as ammonium iron (II) sulfate).

2.5. Determination of Ferritin Formation

Ferritin formation was measured 24 h after treatment. Cells were rinsed with Milli-Q (18.2 MΩ) H_2O and subsequently lysed by scraping in 100 μL (12-well plates) or 200 μL (6-well plates) of CelLytic M (Sigma-Aldrich, Gillingham, UK). Cell lysates were kept on ice for 15 min and stored at −80 °C. For analysis, samples were thawed and centrifuged at 14,000× g for 15 min. Cellular debris was discarded and the supernatant containing the proteins was analysed for ferritin using the Spectro Ferritin ELISA assay (Ramco Laboratories Inc., Stafford, TX, USA). The ferritin concentration in the samples was determined using a microplate reader at an excitation wavelength of 500 nm according to the manufacturer's protocol. Ferritin concentrations were normalized to total cell protein using the Pierce Protein BCA protein assay (ThermoFisher Scientific, Loughborough, UK).

2.6. Determination of Cellular Viability

Cell viability was determined using the CellTiter 96® Aqueous One Solution colorimetric assay (Promega, Southampton, UK) according to the manufacturer's protocol. This method is based on the measurement of the colored product of MTS tetrazolium, which is bio-reduced by cells into formazan. NADPH or NADH produced by dehydrogenase enzymes facilitates the bio-reduction in metabolically active cells. Briefly, Caco-2 cells seeded in 96-well plates and grown for 14 days, were treated with the LIF treatments for 24 h. A cell lysis solution, Triton-X (10%), was used as a positive control to produce physical disruption of cell membranes and subsequent cell death. After 24 h, treatments were removed, replenished with fresh MEM containing 20% MTS solution, and cells were incubated for 15 min, prior to reading the absorbance of each well using a microplate reader at 490 nm.

2.7. Determination of the Reactive Oxygen Species (ROS) Generation

Cellular ROS generation was determined using the dichlorofluorescin-diacetate (DCFH) assay as previously described [17] with minor modifications. Caco-2 cells were seeded in collagen-coated 24-well plates and grown for 12 days. On the day prior to LIF treatments, the media was replaced with MEM. On the day of the experiment, 10 μM of DCFH was added to each well for 30 min at 37 °C. Cells were washed with PBS and treated with LIF-iron (with or without AA) diluted in MEM (LIF-iron:MEM, 1:10) or $FeSO_4$ in equimolar concentrations (100 μM Fe). After being oxidized by intracellular oxidants, DCFH converts to dichlorofluorescein and becomes fluorescent. ROS generation was measured over time (up to 2 h) using a fluorescent microplate reader with an excitation of 485 nm and an emission of 530 nm.

2.8. Analysis of Iron Content in the Cellular Lysates Samples

The content of iron in the cellular lysates were determined using an Inductively Coupled Plasma Optical Emission Spectroscopy (Varian Vista Pro CCD Axial simultaneous ICP-OES) equipped with a glass expansion Seaspray concentric nebulizer (2 mL/min sample flow rate), a 50 mL glass cyclonic spray chamber and an Axial torch with a 2.3 mm i.d. quartz injector. Sample solutions were introduced using a SDS5 Autosampler. White/white and Blue/Blue PVC acct pump tubing was used. Running conditions are described in Supplementary Table S1. The cellular lysates were 4-fold diluted HNO_3 (10%) to a final acid concentration of 7.5%. Then, samples were centrifuged 14,500× g for 10 min and the supernatants were used for the analysis. Blank controls and internal quality controls were prepared alongside the cell lysates and analysed with the samples. A series of external calibration standards containing iron were prepared from commercial standard stock solutions (Centi Prep), with final concentrations ranging from 0 to 1000 ppb in a diluent with a final concentration of 7.5% HNO_3. The iron concentrations were calculated against the linear regression obtained from the calibration standards at wavelength of 259.9 nm.

2.9. Statistical Analysis

Data are presented as mean values with the standard errors of the means (SEM). Homogeneity of variances was evaluated by the test of Levene. For multiple comparisons, one-way ANOVA followed by a Bonferroni test was used when variances were homogeneous or by Tamhane test when variances were non-homogeneous. Statistical significance was set at $p \leq 0.05$. The statistical analysis was performed using the SPSS package (version 23; SPSS Inc., Chicago, IL, USA).

3. Results

3.1. Effect of pH and AA on the Quantity of Iron Released from LIF

To evaluate the reproducibility of iron released from LIF, four independent iron extractions were performed in 1 L of water at pH 2. As shown in Figure 2a, similar iron concentrations with a mean of 1.2 mM were obtained at pH 2. However, when the LIF solution was increased to pH 7, a 25% reduction was observed in the total iron concentration. The addition of AA at 1 and 10 mM produced a concentration-dependent increase in the soluble iron in water treated with LIF, from 2.5 to 5.4 fold respectively (Figure 2b). In addition, when the pH of the water was increased from 2 to 7, the addition of 10 mM of AA prevented the precipitation of iron from LIF.

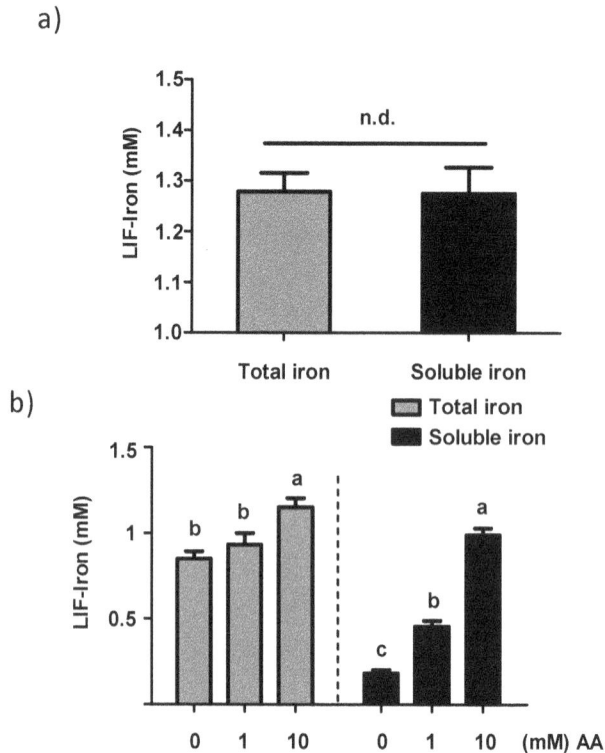

Figure 2. Concentration of total and soluble iron from the iron ingot (Lucky Iron Fish™ (LIF)) at (**a**) pH 2 and (**b**) pH 7 with or without AA. Data represent means ± SEM (*n* = 4). Means without a common letter differ (*p* < 0.05). n.d. means not statistically different.

3.2. Effect of Iron Released from LIF on Cell Viability

Next, we investigated whether the soluble iron released from LIF in water resulted in changes to the viability of the Caco-2 cell monolayer. As shown in Figure 3, the addition of iron from LIF with AA at different molar ratios Fe:AA, (1:0, 1:1 and 1:10) did not induce changes in cell viability when the LIF treatments were 10-fold diluted in MEM (LIF:MEM, 1:10). However, a modest increase in cell proliferation (30% and 16%) was observed when cells were treated at higher concentrations of LIF-iron with AA (molar ratio, Fe:AA (1:10)) using less diluted treatments (dilution LIF:MEM, 1:3 and 1:1). This increase in cell proliferation was even more pronounced in cells treated only with AA at the highest concentration (5 mM), highlighting the proliferative effects of AA on differentiated Caco-2 cells. Therefore, subsequent experiments using AA were performed at concentrations $\leq$1 mM to avoid any effects on cellular proliferation.

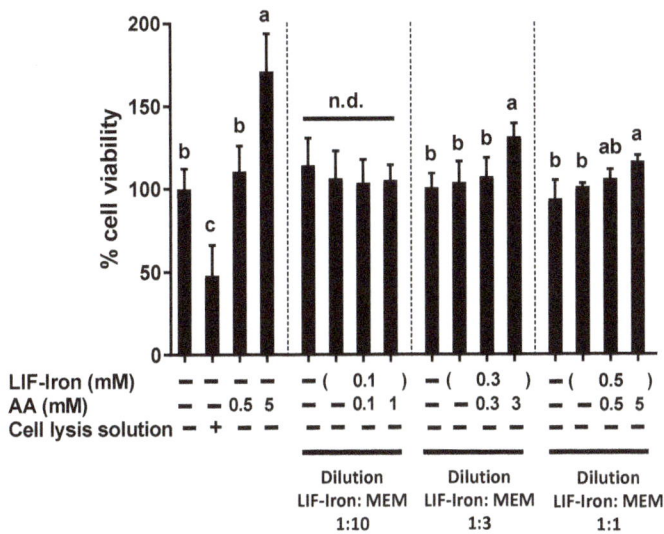

Figure 3. Effect of iron ingot (Lucky Iron Fish™ (LIF)) on cellular viability. Caco-2 cells were treated with the iron released from LIF (LIF-iron) plus the final indicated concentration of ascorbic acid (AA) diluted in MEM (LIF-iron:MEM, 1:10, 1:3 and 1:1) for 24 h. Data represent means $\pm$ SEM (n = 8). Different letters indicate statistically significant differences ($p < 0.05$). n.d. means not statistically different.

3.3. Effect of AA on Cellular Iron Uptake from LIF

In order to investigate whether the increase in soluble iron associated with AA was bioavailable to intestinal cells, the cellular ferritin response, a surrogate marker of iron uptake, was measured in Caco-2 cells (Figure 4). No significant difference was found between blank controls with/without AA at 0, 0.1 and 1 mM, with 8.1, 9.1 and 17.1 ng/mg of protein respectively, whereas a high ferritin response (122 ng/mg of protein) was observed for $FeSO_4$. LIF treatment without AA did not result in a significant increase in the ferritin response (18.9 ng/mg of protein). However, the addition of AA in 0.1 and 1 mM amounts to LIF significantly increased the ferritin response by 100 and 480 ng/mg of protein respectively. In addition, the analysis of the iron content of the Caco-2 cell lysates by ICP-OES confirmed the effect of AA on the cellular iron uptake from LIF (Supplementary Figure S1).

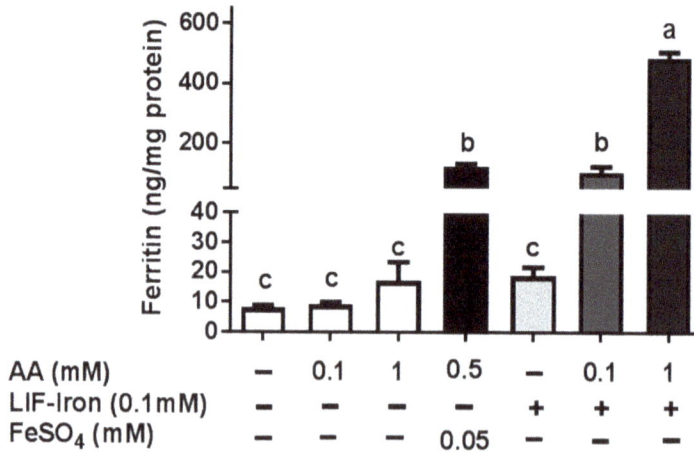

Figure 4. Cellular ferritin response, as a surrogate of the iron uptake, from the iron ingot (Lucky Iron Fish™ (LIF)) with or without ascorbic acid (AA). Caco-2 cells were exposed for 24 h to the LIF-iron (0.1 mM Fe) with the indicated concentration of AA. Data represent means ± SEM (n = 6–8). Different letters indicate statistically significant differences ($p < 0.05$).

3.4. Effect of Including Food Matrix Dietary Factors in a Simulated Gastrointestinal Digestion on Cellular Iron Uptake from LIF

LIF is designed for home fortification of cooked foods. We thus assessed the impact of a pea food matrix (a common staple food) on the iron uptake from LIF in Caco-2 cells after an in vitro digestion. Cells were exposed to digestates of LIF, peas or the combination of LIF plus peas as presented in Figure 5a. We found a significantly increased ferritin response with LIF and peas compared to the blank control (35 and 28 vs. 11 ng/mg of protein, respectively). Surprisingly, the combination of LIF plus peas produced an increase in ferritin response by about 10-fold compared to the treatment in isolation (Figure 5a and Supplementary Figure S2).

a)

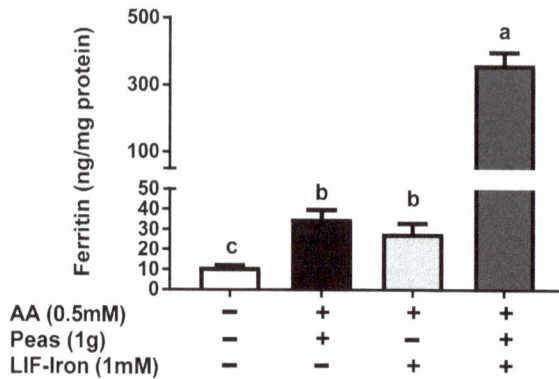

Figure 5. *Cont.*

b)

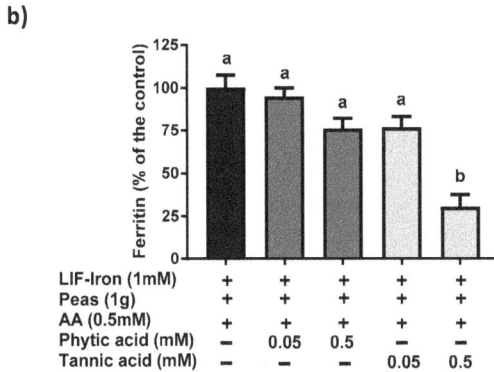

Figure 5. Iron uptake in Caco-2 cells exposed to simulated gastrointestinal digestates of peas and different dietary factors combined with the (Lucky Iron Fish™ (LIF))-iron. Cellular ferritin response exposed for 24 hour incubation with the in vitro gastrointestinal digestion containing LIF-iron plus ascorbic acid (0.5 mM) (**a**) with or without 1g of pea; and (**b**) with pea plus added tannic acid or phytic acid at the indicated concentrations. Data represent means $\pm$ SEM (n = 6–8). Means without a common letter differs ($p < 0.05$).

In order to simulate the effect of a mixed-diet containing iron chelators, we added phytic and tannic acid, two well-known dietary inhibitors of iron absorption, to the in vitro digestion containing the combination of LIF plus peas (Figure 5b). We found that tannic acid at 0.5 mM reduced the ferritin response from LIF plus peas by 75%, but no significant changes were observed at a lower concentration of tannic acid or at any concentration of phytic acid.

3.5. Effect of Iron Released from LIF on ROS Generation

Finally, we explored the possibility that the iron released from LIF could generate oxidative stress similar to $FeSO_4$, a widely used iron supplement. We observed that the addition of iron from LIF induced a 2-fold increase in ROS generation after 30 min, which was similar to $FeSO_4$ (added in a similar iron concentration (0.1 mM)). These levels were sustained for at least 2 h. However, the addition of AA, with its potent antioxidant behaviour, at a Fe:AA molar ratio of 1:1, significantly reduced oxidative stress caused by the iron released from LIF (Figure 6).

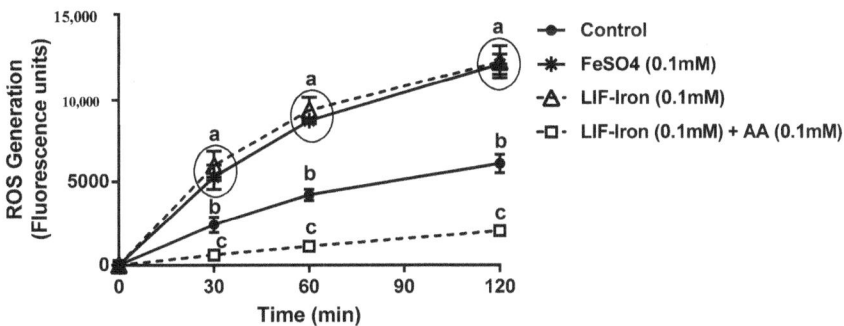

Figure 6. Effect of the iron ingot (Lucky Iron Fish™ (LIF)) on reactive oxygen species (ROS) generation. Cells were exposed to $FeSO_4$ (0.1 mM) or a similar LIF-iron concentration with or without AA. The intracellular ROS production was evaluated at 0, 30, 60 and 120 min. Data represent means $\pm$ SEM (n = 8). Different letters indicate statistically significant differences at each time point ($p < 0.05$).

4. Discussion

In this study, we provide the first direct evidence of the potential bioavailability of iron from the LIF home fortificant, using a widely used in vitro digestion/Caco-2 cell model for assessing iron uptake at the intestinal level. Furthermore, we explored the effect of dietary factors and an example of a food matrix on iron uptake from LIF. In particular, we found (1) a dose-response with AA in relation to iron solubility and iron uptake in Caco-2 cells from LIF; (2) a high ferritin response from LIF in the presence of peas when they were subjected to simulated digestion; and (3) a reduction in iron availability from LIF when tannic acid was added to the digestion. Finally, we demonstrated that LIF induced an overproduction of ROS, similar to FeSO$_4$, which was counteracted by AA without causing cellular cytotoxicity at the concentrations used in our cellular model.

Previous studies investigating the total iron released by LIF in water at different pH values reported that the amount of iron was higher at lower pH [9,10]. Armstrong et al. [10] reported that LIF released similar amounts of iron (about 80 µg/mL Fe) in acidic conditions (pH 3.5) towards more neutral pH conditions. However, at pH 7, the total iron released significantly decreased to 30 µg/mL Fe. The amount of iron released in our experiments was in agreement with this study, with 1.2 mM (67 µg/mL) and 0.85 mM (47 µg/mL) of iron at pH 2 and pH 7, respectively. There is also evidence that water weakly acidified (pH 3.2–4.5) with lemon juice or other foods, can have a differential effect on the quantity of iron released from LIF [9]. However, specific dietary factors or the extent to which these factors impact LIF iron solubility have not been investigated. We studied the influence of AA, an enhancer of iron absorption, on the soluble and total iron released from LIF in water. We observed that AA facilitated iron solubility in water with increasing pH (pH 2 to pH 7) in a concentration-dependent manner, providing further evidence for the potential efficacy of AA on maintaining LIF-iron in a form that can be absorbed in the small intestine.

Three RCTs [7,8,11] have been carried out in Cambodia investigating the effect of using the LIF ingot in food and drinking water. Results from these trials were conflicting. In the first trial, LIF significantly improved the hemoglobin levels of women after 3 months, but these levels reverted back to baseline after 6 months [8]. In the follow-up trial, both hemoglobin and serum ferritin were measured at 3, 6, 9 and 12 months. LIF increased hemoglobin levels after 9 months (118 vs. 123 g/L) and both hemoglobin (120 vs. 130 g/L) and serum ferritin (66 vs. 102 ng/mL) levels after 12 months [7]. The authors suggested that the lack of efficacy of LIF at 6 months in the first RCT might be due to seasonal variations in the water parameters that could reduce iron bioavailability. A third RCT reported no changes in hemoglobin after 6 or 12 months of using LIF [11]. However, in this trial the prevalence of structural hemoglobin variants was about 70%, and only 9% of participants had serum ferritin concentrations indicative of iron deficiency, which suggests that this population was not ideal for evaluating the efficacy of LIF.

As far as we are aware, no studies have examined whether the iron released from LIF itself is bioavailable in the small intestine after exposure to gastrointestinal digestion. This requires the use of in vitro models to assess the impact of different dietary factors on iron uptake from LIF. Here, we have demonstrated that while LIF released a high amount of iron in acidic conditions, it is poorly bioavailable in Caco-2 cells in the absence of iron enhancers at neutral pH conditions found in the intestine. Nevertheless, the addition of AA increased the amount of soluble iron and iron uptake in Caco-2 cells. Yun et al. [15] examined the effect of AA on iron bioavailability, comparing the Caco-2 cell response with previously published human absorption data. In their study, AA ranging from 25 to 500 mg added to semisynthetic meals, increased iron absorption in Caco-2 cells and was predictive of its effect in human trials. Hence, we suggest that the addition of AA to LIF during food preparation can have a major role in improving iron absorption in vivo, especially in iron-deficient populations.

In order to determine the impact of the food matrix on iron bioavailability from LIF, we undertook a simulated gastrointestinal digestion with peas (a staple food) plus LIF-iron. We observed that this combination produced a much greater (10-fold) ferritin response in cells compared to pea and LIF-iron individually. According to its nutritional composition [18], peas contain about 0.22 mg/g of AA, so it is highly unlikely that the quantity of endogenous AA provided from the peas could account for more than 0.5 mM in our simulated digestion. Therefore, we suggest that other dietary factors from the pea matrix contributed to the increase in iron uptake of the digestate with LIF-iron and peas. For example, peas contain a high amount of sucrose (66 mg/g fresh weight) [18]. There is evidence for an enhancing effect from sugars, and in particular fructose, on iron uptake in Caco-2 cells [19]. Thus, it is possible that some sucrose could be hydrolysed into glucose and fructose by the sucrase activity of differentiated Caco-2 monolayers [20] thereby enhancing iron absorption. However, we cannot rule out other dietary factors from the pea matrix, which can result in promoting iron absorption. Considering the high levels of total iron from LIF in the digestates (approximately 1 mM), even a small amount of enhancer would result in a considerable quantity of iron being taken into the cells. Further research is warranted to elucidate the reasons for the unexpected positive interaction between peas and LIF. The addition of exogenous (0.5 mM) tannic acid but not phytic acid to the simulated digestion mixture reduced iron uptake by 75%, which is in agreement with studies which showed that tannic acid is a much more potent inhibitor of non-heme iron uptake than phytic acid in Caco-2 cells [21]. All of these data suggest that the iron bioavailability from LIF can be modulated differently depending on the dietary factors present in the food matrix during cooking and digestion.

The manufactured LIF ingot contains a mixture of predominately ferrous iron, trace amounts of ferric iron, and iron complexed to other minerals [10]. Forms of ferrous iron are widely used as oral supplements due to their relative high bioavailability. However, they are also associated with gastrointestinal side effects, which result in non-adherence to the treatment [22,23]. Oxidative stress generated by ferrous iron salts has been proposed as one of the main reasons for GI intolerance [22,23]. Cellular death was not evident with LIF when cells were exposed to our iron uptake treatments with or without AA. However, we observed that the addition of LIF-iron generated an overproduction of ROS to the same extent as $FeSO_4$, which indicates that they have similar iron chemistry. In contrast, the addition of AA (in a molar ratio Fe:AA 1:1) ameliorated the increase in ROS generation. There is evidence suggesting that intracellular ROS generation induced by iron could be modulating divalent metal transporter-1 (DMT-1) internalization as a redox sensor to control iron uptake [24]. Esparza et al. [24] demonstrated that DMT-1 internalization induced by Fe^{2+} was prevented by pre-incubation with the antioxidant N-acetyl-L-cysteine (NAC), suggesting that iron-induced ROS was counteracted by NAC. This is in agreement with our results. Thus, the most plausible explanation is that free iron transported inside the cells produced an increase in ROS, which in turn internalised DMT-1 and reduced iron uptake. However, by complexing/binding ferrous iron [25] or neutralising free radicals [23], AA is likely to have prevented the intracellular environment from further oxidation, resulting in the increase in iron uptake. Therefore, all the above suggests that AA could enhance iron uptake not only through an increase in soluble iron but also through intracellular redox mechanisms that are DMT-1 dependent.

Despite the fact that LIF could ameliorate iron deficiency in the short term, especially if our findings are taken into account when providing instructions for the use of LIF, further studies on the long-term effect of this iron fortificant must be performed to assess possible adverse consequences. For example, the daily use of micronutrient powders for four months as an in-home fortification strategy has been associated with changes in the gut microbiome profile of weaning infants and an increased abundance of enteropathogens bacteria, which in turn was associated with inflammation [26]. Likewise, the use of home-fortification strategies should be very tightly controlled in anemic populations where genetic hemoglobin disorders (i.e., mild thalassemia) or inflammation, rather than dietary iron deficiency, are the main causes of anemia, as in such cases it could lead to iron overload [27–29].

In conclusion, this study demonstrates that dietary factors can modulate the solubility and bioavailability of LIF-iron forms. The addition of AA resulted in greater iron solubility, was associated with lower ROS production, and enhanced iron uptake in Caco-2 cells. The wider use of AA and the selection of foods with recognised iron enhancing properties in the guidelines for LIF might help to make this strategy more effective for reducing iron deficiency.

Supplementary Materials: The following are available online at www.mdpi.com/2072-6643/9/9/1005/s1, Figure S1: Iron content in cellular lysates of Caco-2 cells after treatment with the iron ingot (Lucky Iron Fish™ (LIF)) with or without ascorbic acid (AA), Figure S2: Iron content in cellular lysates of Caco-2 cells exposed to simulated gastrointestinal digestates of peas combined with the (Lucky Iron Fish™ (LIF))-iron, Table S1: Running conditions used for ICP-OES.

Acknowledgments: This study was supported by a Biotechnology and Biological Sciences Research Council (BBSRC)-Diet and Health Research Industry Club (DRINC) 2 grant (BB/L025396/1 and BB/L025515/1). I.R.R. is currently funded by a BBSRC DRINC2 Post-Doctoral fellowship grant. We thank Graham Chilvers, UEA SCI Faculty Analytical Facility, for assistance with ICP-OES.

Author Contributions: The experimental work described was part of AP's PhD project, supervised by S.J.F.-T. I.R.R., A.P. and S.J.F.-T. conceived and designed the experiments; I.R.R. and A.P. performed the experiments and analysed the data; I.R.R. wrote the paper and all authors read and approved the final version of the manuscript.

Conflicts of Interest: The authors declare no conflict of interest.

References

1. Lopez, A.; Cacoub, P.; Macdougall, I.C.; Peyrin-Biroulet, L. Iron deficiency anaemia. *Lancet* **2016**, *387*, 907–916. [CrossRef]

2. McLean, E.; Cogswell, M.; Egli, I.; Wojdyla, D.; de Benoist, B. Worldwide prevalence of anaemia, who vitamin and mineral nutrition information system, 1993–2005. *Public Health Nutr.* **2009**, *12*, 444–454. [CrossRef] [PubMed]

3. Pasricha, S.R.; Drakesmith, H.; Black, J.; Hipgrave, D.; Biggs, B.A. Control of iron deficiency anemia in low-and middle-income countries. *Blood* **2013**, *121*, 2607–2617. [CrossRef] [PubMed]

4. Geerligs, P.D.; Brabin, B.J.; Omari, A.A. Food prepared in iron cooking pots as an intervention for reducing iron deficiency anaemia in developing countries: A systematic review. *J. Hum. Nutr. Diet.* **2003**, *16*, 275–281. [CrossRef] [PubMed]

5. Geerligs, P.P.; Brabin, B.; Mkumbwa, A.; Broadhead, R.; Cuevas, L.E. The effect on haemoglobin of the use of iron cooking pots in rural malawian households in an area with high malaria prevalence: A randomized trial. *Trop. Med. Int. Health* **2003**, *8*, 310–315. [CrossRef] [PubMed]

6. Tripp, K.; Mackeith, N.; Woodruff, B.A.; Talley, L.; Mselle, L.; Mirghani, Z.; Abdalla, F.; Bhatia, R.; Seal, A.J. Acceptability and use of iron and iron-alloy cooking pots: Implications for anaemia control programmes. *Public Health Nutr.* **2010**, *13*, 123–130. [CrossRef] [PubMed]

7. Charles, C.V.; Dewey, C.E.; Hall, A.; Hak, C.; Channary, S.; Summerlee, A.J. A randomized control trial using a fish-shaped iron ingot for the amelioration of iron deficiency anemia in rural Cambodian women. *Trop. Med. Surg.* **2015**, *3*. [CrossRef]

8. Charles, C.V.; Dewey, C.E.; Daniell, W.E.; Summerlee, A.J. Iron-deficiency anaemia in rural cambodia: Community trial of a novel iron supplementation technique. *Eur. J. Public Health* **2011**, *21*, 43–48. [CrossRef] [PubMed]

9. Charles, C.V.; Summerlee, A.J.; Dewey, C.E. Iron content of cambodian foods when prepared in cooking pots containing an iron ingot. *Trop. Med. Int. Health* **2011**, *16*, 1518–1524. [CrossRef] [PubMed]

10. Armstrong, G.R.; Dewey, C.E.; Summerlee, A.J.S. Iron release from the lucky iron fish (r): Safety considerations. *Asia Pac. J. Clin. Nutr.* **2017**, *26*, 148–155. [PubMed]

11. Rappaport, A.I.; Whitfield, K.C.; Chapman, G.E.; Yada, R.Y.; Kheang, K.M.; Louise, J.; Summerlee, A.J.; Armstrong, G.R.; Green, T.J. Randomized controlled trial assessing the efficacy of a reusable fish-shaped iron ingot to increase hemoglobin concentration in anemic, rural Cambodian women. *Am. J. Clin. Nutr.* **2017**, *106*, 667–674. [CrossRef] [PubMed]

12. Fairweather-Tait, S.; Lynch, S.; Hotz, C.; Hurrell, R.; Abrahamse, L.; Beebe, S.; Bering, S.; Bukhave, K.; Glahn, R.; Hambidge, M.; et al. The usefulness of in vitro models to predict the bioavailability of iron and zinc: A consensus statement from the harvestplus expert consultation. *Int. J. Vitam. Nutr. Res.* **2005**, *75*, 371–374. [CrossRef] [PubMed]

13. Rodriguez-Ramiro, I.; Brearley, C.A.; Bruggraber, S.F.; Perfecto, A.; Shewry, P.; Fairweather-Tait, S. Assessment of iron bioavailability from different bread making processes using an in vitro intestinal cell model. *Food Chem.* **2017**, *228*, 91–98. [CrossRef] [PubMed]

14. Perfecto, A.; Elgy, C.; Valsami-Jones, E.; Sharp, P.; Hilty, F.; Fairweather-Tait, S. Mechanisms of iron uptake from ferric phosphate nanoparticles in human intestinal caco-2 cells. *Nutrients* **2017**, *9*, 359. [CrossRef] [PubMed]

15. Yun, S.; Habicht, J.P.; Miller, D.D.; Glahn, R.P. An in Vitro digestion/caco-2 cell culture system accurately predicts the effects of ascorbic acid and polyphenolic compounds on iron bioavailability in humans. *J. Nutr.* **2004**, *134*, 2717–2721. [PubMed]

16. Glahn, R.P.; Lee, O.A.; Yeung, A.; Goldman, M.I.; Miller, D.D. Caco-2 cell ferritin formation predicts nonradiolabeled food iron availability in an in vitro digestion/caco-2 cell culture model. *J. Nutr.* **1998**, *128*, 1555–1561. [PubMed]

17. Rodriguez-Ramiro, I.; Ramos, S.; Bravo, L.; Goya, L.; Martin, M.A. Procyanidin B2 and a cocoa polyphenolic extract inhibit acrylamide-induced apoptosis in human Caco-2 cells by preventing oxidative stress and activation of JNK pathway. *J. Nutr. Biochem.* **2011**, *22*, 1186–1194. [CrossRef] [PubMed]

18. Finglas, P.M.; Roe, M.A.; Pinchen, H.M.; Berry, R.; Church, S.M.; Dodhia, S.K.; Farron-Wilson, M.; Swang, G. *Mccance and Widdowson's the Composition of Foods*, 7th Summary ed.; Royal Society of Chemistry: Cambridge, UK, 2015.

19. Christides, T.; Sharp, P. Sugars increase non-heme iron bioavailability in human epithelial intestinal and liver cells. *PLoS ONE* **2013**, *8*, e83031. [CrossRef] [PubMed]

20. Ferruzza, S.; Rossi, C.; Scarino, M.L.; Sambuy, Y. A protocol for in situ enzyme assays to assess the differentiation of human intestinal Caco-2 cells. *Toxicol. In Vitro* **2012**, *26*, 1247–1251. [CrossRef] [PubMed]

21. Engle-Stone, R.; Yeung, A.; Welch, R.; Glahn, R. Meat and ascorbic acid can promote fe availability from fe-phytate but not from Fe-tannic acid complexes. *J. Agric. Food Chem.* **2005**, *53*, 10276–10284. [CrossRef] [PubMed]

22. Tolkien, Z.; Stecher, L.; Mander, A.P.; Pereira, D.I.; Powell, J.J. Ferrous sulfate supplementation causes significant gastrointestinal side-effects in adults: A systematic review and meta-analysis. *PLoS ONE* **2015**, *10*, e0117383. [CrossRef] [PubMed]

23. Koskenkorva-Frank, T.S.; Weiss, G.; Koppenol, W.H.; Burckhardt, S. The complex interplay of iron metabolism, reactive oxygen species, and reactive nitrogen species: Insights into the potential of various iron therapies to induce oxidative and nitrosative stress. *Free Radic. Biol. Med.* **2013**, *65*, 1174–1194. [CrossRef] [PubMed]

24. Esparza, A.; Gerdtzen, Z.P.; Olivera-Nappa, A.; Salgado, J.C.; Nunez, M.T. Iron-induced reactive oxygen species mediate transporter dmt1 endocytosis and iron uptake in intestinal epithelial cells. *Am. J. Physiol. Cell Physiol.* **2015**, *309*, C558–C567. [CrossRef] [PubMed]

25. Scheers, N.; Andlid, T.; Alminger, M.; Sandberg, A.S. Determination of Fe^{2+} and Fe^{3+} in aqueous solutions containing food chelators by differential pulse anodic stripping voltammetry. *Electroanal* **2010**, *22*, 1090–1096. [CrossRef]

26. Jaeggi, T.; Kortman, G.A.; Moretti, D.; Chassard, C.; Holding, P.; Dostal, A.; Boekhorst, J.; Timmerman, H.M.; Swinkels, D.W.; Tjalsma, H.; et al. Iron fortification adversely affects the gut microbiome, increases pathogen abundance and induces intestinal inflammation in Kenyan infants. *Gut* **2015**, *64*, 731–742. [CrossRef] [PubMed]

27. Karakochuk, C.D.; Barker, M.K.; Whitfield, K.C.; Barr, S.I.; Vercauteren, S.M.; Devlin, A.M.; Hutcheon, J.A.; Houghton, L.A.; Prak, S.; Hou, K.; et al. The effect of oral iron with or without multiple micronutrients on hemoglobin concentration and hemoglobin response among nonpregnant cambodian women of reproductive age: A 2 × 2 factorial, double-blind, randomized controlled supplementation trial. *Am. J. Clin. Nutr.* **2017**, *106*, 233–244. [CrossRef] [PubMed]

28. Musallam, K.M.; Rivella, S.; Vichinsky, E.; Rachmilewitz, E.A. Non-transfusion-dependent thalassemias. *Haematologica* **2013**, *98*, 833–844. [CrossRef] [PubMed]
29. Karakochuk, C.D.; Whitfield, K.C.; Barr, S.I.; Lamers, Y.; Devlin, A.M.; Vercauteren, S.M.; Kroeun, H.; Talukder, A.; McLean, J.; Green, T.J. Genetic hemoglobin disorders rather than iron deficiency are a major predictor of hemoglobin concentration in women of reproductive age in rural Prey Veng, Cambodia. *J. Nutr.* **2015**, *145*, 134–142. [CrossRef] [PubMed]

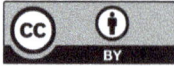

nutrients

MDPI

Review

Rational Management of Iron-Deficiency Anaemia in Inflammatory Bowel Disease

Ole Haagen Nielsen [1,*]**, Christoffer Soendergaard** [1]**, Malene Elbaek Vikner** [1] **and Günter Weiss** [2,3]

[1]   Department of Gastroenterology, Herlev Hospital, University of Copenhagen, Herlev, DK-2730, Denmark;
     christoffer.soendergaard@regionh.dk (C.S.); malene.elbaek@mail.dk (M.E.V.)
[2]   Department of Internal Medicine II, Medical University Hospital of Innsbruck, Innsbruck, A-6020, Austria;
     Guenter.Weiss@i-med.ac.at
[3]   Christian Doppler Laboratory for Iron Metabolism and Anemia Research, University of Innsbruck,
     Innsbruck, A-6020, Austria.
*   Correspondence: ohn@dadlnet.dk; Tel.: +45-386-83621

Received: 6 December 2017; Accepted: 11 January 2018; Published: 13 January 2018

Abstract: Anaemia is the most frequent, though often neglected, comorbidity of inflammatory bowel disease (IBD). Here we want to briefly present (1) the burden of anaemia in IBD, (2) its pathophysiology, which mostly arises from bleeding-associated iron deficiency, followed by (3) diagnostic evaluation of anaemia, (4) a balanced overview of the different modes of iron replacement therapy, (5) evidence for their therapeutic efficacy and subsequently, (6) an updated recommendation for the practical management of anaemia in IBD. Following the introduction of various intravenous iron preparations over the last decade, questions persist about when to use these preparations as opposed to traditional and other novel oral iron therapeutic agents. At present, oral iron therapy is generally preferred for patients with quiescent IBD and mild iron-deficiency anaemia. However, in patients with flaring IBD that hampers intestinal iron absorption and in those with inadequate responses to or side effects with oral preparations, intravenous iron supplementation is the therapy of choice, although information on the efficacy of intravenous iron in patients with active IBD and anaemia is scare. Importantly, anaemia in IBD is often multifactorial and a careful diagnostic workup is mandatory for optimized treatment. Nevertheless, limited information is available on optimal therapeutic start and end points for treatment of anaemia. Of note, neither oral nor intravenous therapies seem to exacerbate the clinical course of IBD. However, additional prospective studies are still warranted to determine the optimal therapy in complex conditions such as IBD.

Keywords: anaemia; Crohn's disease; IBD; iron deficiency; therapy; ulcerative colitis

---

1. Introduction

Anaemia and iron deficiency are global health issues and a recent analysis estimated that approximately one-third (i.e., >2.5 billion individuals) of the world's population is anaemic [1]. Furthermore, it is assumed that more than half the cases of anaemia are caused by an iron-deficient erythropoiesis [1]. Iron deficiency is therefore considered one of the most prevalent global nutritional deficiencies [2]. However, there is a huge geographic variation in prevalence due to a range of sociodemographic factors (i.e., industrialized versus developing countries) [1]. Nevertheless, in addition to anaemia, iron deficiencies cause decrements in energy metabolism, daily activities, quality of life, cognitive and sexual function, cardiac performance and work productivity. However, excess iron can cause cellular oxidative stress and damage by catalysing the formation of toxic radicals via Fenton chemistry [1–6].

1.1. Anaemia in Inflammatory Bowel Disease

In inflammatory bowel disease (IBD) [7,8], which shows increasing worldwide incidence and prevalence rates [9–11] and which affects up to 0.5% of the population in some countries [12], anaemia is a frequent comorbidity. A recent nationwide Portuguese cross-sectional study of 1287 patients with either Crohn's disease (CD) (*n* = 775) or ulcerative colitis (UC) (*n* = 512) revealed that flaring disease is the parameter most consistently related to the presence of anaemia, with no differences between CD and UC, although anaemia is more frequent among women [13], especially in CD [14]. Further, an analysis of 171 adult patients with CD showed that iron deficiency was present in 78% with active inflammation but in only 21% with quiescent disease (*p* < 0.001) [15]. It was noticed that markers of CD severity, such as stricturing disease and the need for tumour necrosis factor (TNF) inhibitors and surgery, appeared to be significantly associated with iron deficiency [15]. Moreover, a 2014 systematic review of tertiary referral centres showed a prevalence of anaemia in patients with CD of 27% (95% confidence interval (CI) 19–35%) and in patients with UC of 21% (95% CI 15–27%) [7]. The observed variation mirrored differences in the study populations (e.g., hospitalized patients versus outpatients) as well as the applied definition of anaemia in the studies included. Hence iron deficiency deserves attention in IBD, where the mean prevalence is shown to be 20% among outpatients [16] and 68% among hospitalized patients [17], exceeding by far the frequencies of other extraintestinal manifestations (e.g., rheumatic, dermatologic and ophthalmologic) commonly associated with IBD [18,19].

The pathogenesis of anaemia in IBD is multifactorial and results mainly from intestinal blood loss in inflamed mucosa and impaired dietary iron absorption [20]. The chronic inflammatory state impairs duodenal iron uptake via induction of hepcidin expression in the liver [21] but inflammatory cytokines also have a negative impact on the duodenal uptake of nutrients. Moreover, loss of appetite during flaring disease and a range of other factors such as medications used for IBD treatment (e.g., proton pump inhibitors, sulfasalazine, methotrexate and thiopurines) also have a negative effect on iron absorption and erythropoiesis [22,23]. Vitamin deficiencies, concomitant medical conditions (e.g., renal insufficiency, congestive heart failure, haemolysis, diabetes and innate hemoglobinopathies) [24,25], inflammatory cytokines and acute-phase reactants during flaring disease additionally impair iron availability for erythropoiesis and/or aggravate anaemia by other mechanisms. This blunts the biological response to erythropoietin as well and drives an inflammation-dependent impairment of erythroid progenitor cell proliferation [26–28]. Additionally, a predisposition to the development of anaemia may be caused by polymorphisms of iron metabolism genes as well as hormonal factors [29–31]. In essence, if the absorptive capacity of iron from the diet does not meet the body's requirement, iron deficiency develops.

1.2. Anaemia in Other Chronic Diseases

Apart from IBD, anaemia is observed in a number of chronic inflammatory disorders. These include autoimmune disorders (e.g., rheumatoid arthritis and celiac disease), cancer and infections. This so-called anaemia of chronic disease (ACD) or anaemia of inflammation is more prevalent in patients with advanced disease and in those responding poorly to therapy [28].

1.3. General Health Effects of Anaemia

Treatment of iron-deficiency anaemia in IBD is of importance because of the possible consequences on multiple organs and biological processes. These include cellular dysfunctions comprising impaired mitochondrial respiratory capacity and metabolic impairments that translate into specific organ dysfunctions, for example, in the central nervous system (e.g., impaired cognitive function, fatigue, restless legs syndrome and depression), immune system (e.g., immune cell proliferation and differentiation and regulation of innate and adaptive immune responses), cardiorespiratory system (e.g., reduced exercise capacity, exertional dyspnea, tachycardia, palpitations, cardiac hypertrophy, systolic ejection murmur and risk of cardiac failure), vascular system (e.g., hypothermia and skin pallor), genital tract (e.g., loss of libido and menstrual problems) and gastrointestinal tract (e.g., anorexia, nausea and motility disorders) [32,33]. Collectively, anaemia has a direct impact on the quality of life of affected patients [34–37].

The perception that anaemia in IBD needs specific treatment apart from regular control of IBD is still underdeveloped. Thus anaemia is neither diagnostically worked up nor do the majority of anaemic patients receive any specific treatment [17], although such an approach is strongly recommended by expert boards and clinical societies [25,38,39]. At present, a great many physicians are uncertain about applicable diagnostic procedures and treatment regimens for their patients with IBD and iron-deficiency anaemia [40]. The aims of this paper therefore are to explore the latest knowledge concerning the pathophysiology of anaemia, diagnostic evaluations, available iron replacement methods and evidence of clinical efficacy in order to provide updated recommendations for the management of iron-deficiency anaemia in IBD.

2. Pathophysiology of Anaemia in IBD

Iron constitutes a key part of haemoglobin in erythrocytes and of myoglobin in muscles, which in combination contain approximately two-thirds of the total body iron. In addition, iron is crucial to a wide range of biological processes [41,42]. The average adult harbours more than 3–4 g of iron, which is balanced between physiologic iron loss and dietary uptake. About 20–25 mg of iron is needed daily for the synthesis of heme. Thus approximately 1–2 mg originates from dietary intake and the remainder is acquired by recycling of iron from senescent erythrocytes by macrophages [41,43]. The total loss of iron averages 1–2 mg/day, mostly through desquamation of intestinal enterocytes or skin, whereas much higher amounts are lost during menstruation [44,45].

2.1. Structure of Iron

Dietary iron is available in two forms: heme and non-heme-bound iron. Within heme, iron is complexed as ferrous iron (Fe^{2+}) to the protoporphyrin ring, which is abundant in animal food products such as meat, poultry and seafood [46]. Most dietary iron is abundant as nonheme iron (Fe^{3+} or ferric iron) and is present in foods of vegetable origin (e.g., nuts, beans, vegetables and fortified grain products). Heme iron is assumed to constitute 10–15% of total iron intake in meat-eating populations but because of its higher bioavailability (estimated absorption rate of 15–35%) than nonheme iron (5–15%), it accounts for more than 30% of the total absorbed iron [47].

2.2. Iron Homeostasis

Body iron homeostasis is regulated systemically by several mechanisms, among which is the pivotal interaction of the liver-derived peptide hormone hepcidin with the major cellular iron exporter ferroportin [48]. Ferroportin is found primarily on intestinal epithelium (mostly in the duodenum), macrophages and hepatocytes, which constitute the major cellular iron stores. Ferroportin thus enables the transport of iron from cells into the circulation to maintain adequate systemic iron levels (Figure 1) [49]. Targeting of ferroportin by hepcidin results in ferroportin internalization, degradation and blockage of cellular iron egress into the serum, thus resulting in a reduced availability of iron for erythroid progenitor cells [49]. Synthesis and release of hepcidin and therefore cellular accumulation of iron and development of a low serum iron concentration, are induced by both a high concentration of iron in the liver and plasma and by inflammatory cytokines such as IL-1 (IL: interleukin) and IL-6 [50]. In contrast, during states of iron deficiency, hypoxia and anaemia, the synthesis of hepcidin is blocked in order to increase serum iron levels [29,49,51]. Of note, sexual hormones, alcohol, hepatic function and hypoxia-derived factor all affect hepcidin expression and thus the circulating iron levels [41–43]. The efficacy of orally administered iron therapy depends on circulating hepcidin levels. Thus, high hepcidin concentrations may predict nonresponsiveness to oral iron therapy [52]. Hepcidin levels may also control the response to intravenous iron administration, including high-molecular-weight preparations, which are taken up by macrophages and then delivered to the circulation via ferroportin-mediated iron export (Figure 1) [2,21,53]. This is in line with experimental data demonstrating reduced ferroportin expression in the duodenum and decreased iron absorption in individuals with increased hepcidin levels—primarily as a consequence of inflammation [21]. The development of inflammatory anaemia is thus characterized by low circulating iron levels and an iron-restricted erythropoiesis in the presence of high iron stores in the reticuloendothelial system, reflected by normal or elevated levels of ferritin.

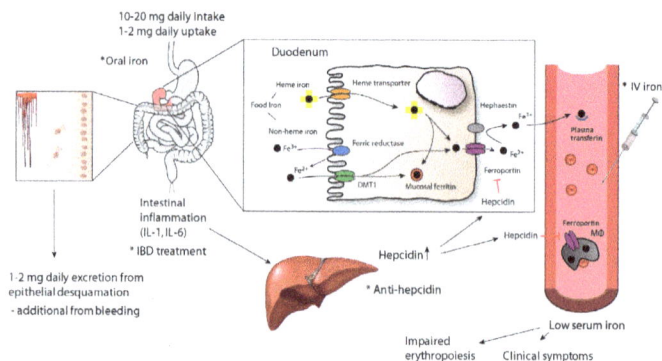

Figure 1. Pathogenesis of iron-deficiency anaemia and methods for supplementation and treatment in inflammatory bowel disease (IBD). IL: interleukin; DMT1: divalent metal-ion transporter 1; MΦ: macrophage; IV: intravenous.

Between 1 and 2 mg of iron is taken up daily from the diet, which is balanced by its secretion mainly through intestinal and skin epithelial desquamation. Intestinal bleeding in patients with IBD increases iron loss. With the majority of iron being taken up in the duodenum through heme and nonheme iron transporters (elementary iron is reduced to Fe^{2+} before uptake) with animal data showing some absorption from the large bowel as well [54], the iron enters the epithelial cells. Iron might be stored in the cells as mucosal ferritin or is exported to the circulation through the transporter, ferroportin and oxidized to Fe^{3+}. Circulating iron forms complexes with transferrin and is delivered as transferrin-bound iron to cells and tissues. Most of the iron needed for metabolic purposes and erythropoiesis (approximately 20–30 mg/day) originates from macrophages that engulf senescent erythrocytes and reuse iron that is returned to the circulation via ferroportin. During systemic inflammation and increased levels of inflammation-induced hepatic hepcidin secretion, the iron transporter ferroportin found in cells of the reticuloendothelial system and in enterocytes is degraded and cellular iron export is reduced. This results in iron retention in cells of the reticuloendothelial system and impaired dietary iron absorption, subsequently resulting in low serum iron levels with all the clinical consequences mentioned in the text. To overcome iron deficiency in patients with IBD, iron supplementation in the form of oral or intravenous iron can be applied. Novel approaches include inhibition of hepcidin itself or its expression. The most important preventive intervention for long-term well-being of the patients, however, is to efficiently treat the underlying condition, in this case the intestinal inflammatory process. The asterisk indicates points of therapeutic intervention.

2.3. Inflammatory Modulators in Anaemia

Cytokine-driven induction of hepcidin expression and the direct effects of cytokines on iron trafficking in macrophages and duodenal enterocytes play a decisive role in the development of ACD) or anaemia of inflammation by retaining iron in the reticuloendothelial system and blocking iron absorption, causing an iron-limited erythropoiesis [28,55]. Thus, ACD is more prevalent in patients with advanced disease and in those responding poorly to therapy [28]. In addition, cytokines and chemokines further contribute to anaemia by negatively influencing the biological activity of erythropoietin, by inhibiting the proliferation and differentiation of erythroid progenitor cells and by reducing the circulatory half-life of erythrocytes [28].

However, patients with flaring IBD experience chronic blood loss due to intestinal mucosal bleeding, which often causes true iron deficiency in conjunction with inflammatory anaemia (mirrored by low to normal ferritin levels) [22,56]. Of note, while hepcidin levels are increased in patients with ACD, concomitant true iron deficiency results in hepcidin suppression [21]. On the one hand, this is due to the fact that iron deficiency inhibits SMAD-mediated signalling pathways in hepatocytes, thereby blocking hepcidin expression even in the presence of inflammatory stimuli such as IL-6 [57]. On the other hand, anaemia and hypoxia result in activation of hormones that have a negative impact on hepcidin formation. These include erythroferrone produced by erythroblasts in response to erythropoeitic stress [58], as well as other mechanisms, including growth differentiation factor 15 (GDF-15), which is seen mainly in patients with hemoglobinopathies. Further, a hypoxia-driven blockade of hepcidin formation is induced via platelet-derived growth factor-BB (PDGF-BB) and/or hypoxia-inducible factors (HIFs) [58–62]. Together these mechanisms result in increased circulating iron levels via stimulation of iron absorption and redelivery from macrophages. Thus, in the presence of both inflammation and true iron deficiency due to intestinal bleeding in IBD, circulating hepcidin levels decrease because anaemia and iron-deficiency regulatory signals dominate over inflammation-driven hepcidin induction [62,63]. Therefore, truly iron-deficient patients, even in the presence of systemic inflammation, are able to absorb considerable amounts of iron from the intestine [21,49].

Finally, vitamin deficiencies (e.g., vitamin B_{12}, folic acid and vitamin D) due to either intestinal inflammation or extensive bowel resection can also contribute to the development of anaemia [22,64], as do specific medications for the treatment of IBD (as listed earlier).

3. Diagnostic Investigations

According to the World Health Organization (WHO), adult males and females with a blood haemoglobin concentration below 13 and 12 g/dL, respectively, are considered anaemic (<11 g/dL during pregnancy) [31]. Thresholds for defining the state of anaemia apart from sex and pregnancy, however, depend on such factors as age, altitude and ethnicity. The diagnosis of iron deficiency and anaemia is based on measurements of the blood haemoglobin concentration but some additional basic analyses are required for a diagnostic workup and for tailoring optimal therapy in patients with IBD [29,38,65]. During flaring IBD, measurements of iron status may be difficult to interpret because parameters relating to iron metabolism are influenced by the inflammation per se [66].

3.1. Transferrin and Transferrin Saturation

As a consequence of chronic inflammation, patients with active IBD may show reduced levels of transferrin, which is contrary to the definition of patients with iron deficiency [67]. Importantly, patients with inflammatory anaemia with or without true iron deficiency are characterized by reduced serum iron and a low transferrin saturation (TfS) (i.e., the quotient of iron concentration (μmol/L) divided by transferrin concentration (mg/dL) in fasting blood samples multiplied by 70.9 and stated as a percentage) [68]. Accordingly, a number of studies have used TfS as an indicator for low iron status and for determining appropriate initiation of iron supplementation therapy [37,38,69–71]. A TfS of 16% is generally used as a threshold when screening for iron deficiency, although a 20% threshold is often applied in the context of coexisting inflammatory disorders [65].

3.2. Ferritin

Serum ferritin concentration, which generally correlates with body iron stores, is the most widely used surrogate marker of stored iron and works nicely in patients without any concomitant inflammatory condition. Circulating ferritin levels, however, are influenced by inflammation; in fact, several proinflammatory cytokines stimulate ferritin expression, leading to measurements in the normal or even elevated range during chronic inflammation, even in the presence of true iron deficiency [66,72,73]. Thus, in situations of concomitant inflammation, chronic liver disease, or malignancy, ferritin levels may increase independently of iron status. Thus, independent of inflammation, a ferritin concentration below 30 μg/L is indicative of true iron deficiency [74,75], whereas this threshold may be higher in patients with inflammation, although prospective and interventional studies examining this issue in detail are lacking. In clinical practice, a ferritin level of up to 100 μg/L in the setting of an inflammatory disease and anaemia may be associated with true iron deficiency, whereas functional iron deficiency may be present with ferritin levels exceeding 100 μg/L in such conditions [68]. Currently, no standard clinical tests exist for the assessment of true iron deficiency in patients with concomitant inflammation and thus a combination of various paraclinical tests is often required to provide clinical evidence of iron deficiency and to guide therapy [68,76].

3.3. Soluble Transferrin Receptor

Serum-soluble transferrin receptor (sTfR), a proteolytic derivative of the membrane-bound transferrin receptor, is another marker of iron status. With true iron deficiency, increased synthesis of transferrin receptors is observed along with a corresponding increase in sTfR levels. Nevertheless, the sTfR concentration might also rise during disorders associated with increased erythropoiesis, including chronic lymphatic leukaemia, whereas it can be reduced by the actions of cytokines during inflammation. Therefore, no consensus currently exists as to a standardized cut-off value for sTfR [77]. To distinguish between patients with inflammation-driven ACD and patients with ACD and concomitant true iron deficiency, determination of the ratio between sTfR and the logarithm of serum ferritin concentration (i.e., the sTfR-F index) has been recommended [78]. A sTfR-F index above two is indicative of true iron deficiency among ACD patients, whereas a ratio below one is suggestive of ACD alone without concomitant iron deficiency [68,77].

3.4. Red Cell Indices

Based on erythrocyte analyses of full blood samples from anaemic patients, information about mean cellular haemoglobin concentration (MCHC, hypochromia) and mean cell volume (MCV, microcytosis) can be obtained. The values of these indices are decreased by iron deficiency. In the case of microcytosis in patients with an appropriate ethnic background, haemoglobin electrophoresis may be considered to rule out hemoglobinopathies such as sickle-cell disease and thalassemia [77]. Microcytosis or MCHC reductions thus may indicate true iron deficiency in patients with inflammation-associated ACD because classical ACD is characterized as normochromic and normocytic [66,67,70,76]. Among patients with chronic kidney disease, measuring the percentage of circulating hypochromic red cells as a proportion of total red blood cells can indicate the presence of iron deficiency using a cut-off value of 6% [79]. Unfortunately, freshly drawn blood samples and specific equipment are required for this analysis [80]. Accordingly, prospective evaluations of this parameter, as well as of the reticulocyte haemoglobin content in clinical situations, including patients with anaemia and inflammatory disorders, are scarce [68,81].

3.5. Bone Marrow Analyses

Bone marrow aspiration for diagnosing iron deficiency appears to be the gold standard. This method is thought to be unaffected by inflammation but it is invasive in nature, uncomfortable for the patient, expensive and might be affected by concomitant treatment with recombinant erythropoietin. Thus, bone marrow aspiration should be reserved for specific situations where other techniques are either unavailable or conflicting [77].

3.6. Hepcidin

Hepcidin has a key regulatory role in iron homeostasis as an inhibitor of cellular iron export [77]. Measurements of hepcidin may be an attractive tool to diagnose true iron deficiency in patients with inflammation-driven anaemia because its expression in vivo appears to be more affected by iron deficiency than by the inflammatory response [62,82]. Recently, commercially available tests have been introduced into clinical practice [83] but the usefulness of hepcidin determination to correctly indicate iron deficiency in patients with inflammation needs to be tested prospectively in future studies. Of note, concomitant pathologies that may contribute to the development and severity of anaemia, including folic acid, cobalamin, or vitamin D deficiency and haemolysis and erythropoietin deficiency per se, as well as any renal insufficiency, must be identified and treated properly, if possible.

It is of great importance to establish the presence of true iron-deficiency anaemia in patients to avoid any unnecessary treatment. The assessment should be guided by predictive serum parameters such as hepcidin, soluble transferrin receptor and others including red cell indices but no gold standard is available at present [76,84]. The success of treatment with either oral or intravenous iron is mirrored by an increase of haemoglobin levels or by increased levels of circulating ferritin.

4. Treatment of Anaemia

The primary treatment of ACD is to cure the underlying pathology or other easily treatable conditions contributing to anaemia, such as vitamin deficiency, which often leads to improvement in haemoglobin levels unless other pathophysiologic factors or deficiencies are present [14,25,28,29,33,85]. In cases of severe anaemia (i.e., haemoglobin < 7–8 g/dL) [2,86], especially when it is rapidly developing, as in association with acute gastrointestinal bleeding, or if the patient suffers from comorbidities such as coronary heart disease or chronic pulmonary disease, a rapid correction of haemoglobin levels may be indicated, which can best be achieved with red blood cell transfusions [25,28,33,87]. However, the use of blood transfusions must be considered carefully because negative effects are well documented [87,88] and a liberal application of transfusions is associated with higher mortality in patients with acute gastrointestinal bleeding [89]. Moreover, transfusions have been associated with an increased risk for nosocomial infections and mortality rates among intensive care patients [90], as well as a higher frequency of surgical-site infections [91]. Additionally, a risk of transfusion-related anaphylactic reaction, together with a small but residual risk for transmitting infectious disease, does exist [92–94].

5. Iron Replacement Formulations

Imbalances of iron homeostasis are the major reason for anaemia in patients with IBD. The currently available options for iron supplementation to balance iron intake and iron loss consist of oral and intravenous administration and their pros and cons are listed in Table 1.

Table 1. Main principles of iron supplementation and their pros and cons.

Iron Administration	Pros	Cons
Oral	Low cost Convenient Available over the counter Efficient when intestinal absorption is not impaired	Mucosal injury Alteration of microbiota Various disorders may impair uptake, e.g., celiac disease, ACD *, autoimmune gastritis High intestinal iron concentrations due to low bioavailability cause gastrointestinal side effects (nausea, vomiting, abdominal pain and constipation) and limit compliance
Intravenous	Fast repletion of iron stores Safe if formulations with dextran are avoided Effective even when intestinal absorption is impaired	Higher expenses, including need for administration by a healthcare professional Potential risk for iron overload that in excess may contribute to oxidative stress Potential risk for anaphylactic reactions using dextran-containing formulations Hypophosphatemia with some preparations

* Anaemia of chronic disease (ACD).

5.1. Oral Regimen

The bioavailability of "traditional" oral iron preparations is relatively low but nevertheless is the first-line therapy in iron-deficiency anaemia. Oral iron has a well-established safety profile, is easy to administer and comes with a generally low cost—with the latter being important in a pharmaco-economical setting [26]. Oral iron supplements are available as divalent Fe^{2+} (ferrous) or trivalent Fe^{3+} (ferric) salts coupled with sugar complexes or protein succinylate [95,96]. The most widely used preparations are ferrous sulphate, ferrous gluconate and ferrous fumarate, which all contain the ferrous form of iron, which has a better bioavailability than ferric-containing formulations [96]. Prior to absorption by enterocytes in the duodenum, iron is reduced to its ferrous state (Fe^{2+})—A process catalysed by membrane-bound ferric reductase. Divalent metal transporter-1 (DMT1) facilitates iron uptake in the acidic environment [97]. Ascorbic acid (or vitamin C) dose dependently facilitates absorption of oral iron [98] by providing reducing equivalents for ferric reductase, thus enhancing the reduction of Fe^{3+} to Fe^{2+} prior to epithelial uptake [99]. Further, vitamin C suppresses the negative effects on iron absorption of inhibitors such as phytate and calcium [47] (Figure 2).

Recently, a study in children has shown that supplementation of vitamin D facilitates increased haemoglobin levels. Here plasma concentrations of 25-hydroxyvitamin D (25(OH)D) below 30 ng/mL (i.e., vitamin D deficiency) were associated with increased hepcidin concentrations and reduced haemoglobin concentrations compared with individuals with plasma 25(OH)D concentrations above 30 ng/mL [100]. Because vitamin D deficiency is frequent in IBD [101] and because vitamin D has been shown to inhibit hepcidin expression [102] and to possess important immunologic effects of benefit in the clinical course of patients with IBD [103–105], normalization of vitamin D is important for elevating the haemoglobin level in these patients. Specifically, vitamin D binds to vitamin D response elements (VDREs) in the promoter region of hepcidin (hepcidin antimicrobial peptide, HAMP) and thereby reduces hepcidin expression [102,106–108]. Supplementing healthy adults with vitamin D decreased hepcidin levels by 73% [109] and significantly increased haemoglobin levels in critically ill patients following administration of up to 100,000 IU of vitamin D daily for 5 days [107]. These recent results highlight the importance of vitamin D in the context of anaemia (Figure 2).

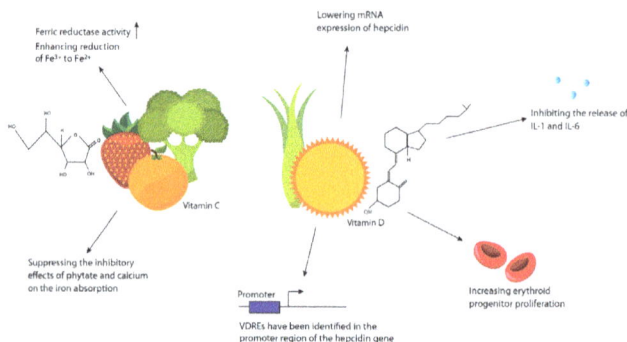

Figure 2. Importance of vitamins C and D in the treatment of iron-deficiency anaemia.

Dietary vitamin C enhances iron absorption by providing reducing equivalents for Fe^{3+} reduction by the enzyme ferric reductase to enhance its activity. Vitamin C also suppresses the inhibitory features of phytate and calcium on iron uptake. Vitamin D obtained from the diet or generated in the skin through ultraviolet-induced photolysis of vitamin D precursors augments iron absorption by lowering mRNA expression of hepcidin mediated by the presence of vitamin D response elements (VDREs) identified in the promoter region of the hepcidin gene. Additionally, vitamin D inhibits the release of IL-1 and IL-6 and increases erythroid progenitor proliferation.

Recently, new orally available products have been introduced into clinical practice. One of these, ferric maltol, has been successfully studied in a phase III trial in IBD patients with iron-deficiency anaemia who had previously been either intolerant or unresponsive to oral ferrous products [110].

Although the optimal dose of oral iron supplements in patients with IBD and iron deficiency has not been established, a dose of 50–200 mg/day of elemental iron is often recommended [111]. Only 10–25% of the dosed iron is expected to be absorbed in iron-deficient patients [71,97]. Because oral iron induces the expression of hepcidin, it appears reasonable to dose oral iron only once daily to circumvent the inhibitory effects of hepcidin on iron transfer from duodenal enterocytes to the circulation. A recent observational trial confirmed this notion. It was shown that oral administration of iron reduced the level of iron absorption on the following day and that application of iron twice daily resulted in a significant reduction in oral iron bioavailability. Of note, the relative percentage of absorbed iron could be increased even by administration every second day [112]. This observation, combined with a very recent study in women with depleted iron stores demonstrating that alternate-day administration of oral iron supplementation resulted in higher fractional as well as total iron absorption compared with daily administration [113], may alter the current practice of oral iron administration.

Given the low absorption of oral iron, a high proportion remains in the gut and is associated with the development of gastrointestinal side effects, including nausea, dyspepsia, diarrhoea, abdominal discomfort, vomiting and constipation in up to 20% of patients—often resulting in nonadherence to therapy [26,114]. Generally, nausea and abdominal discomfort occur within 1–2 h of drug intake and appear to be dose related, whereas other gastrointestinal side effects such as diarrhoea and constipation are idiosyncratic [71,111]. In patients reporting such intolerances, a delayed-release enteric-coated iron tablet may be prescribed. However, the bioavailability of iron from these formulations is reduced compared with standard preparations because almost all the iron is absorbed in the duodenum and not in distal part of the gastrointestinal tract [45,47]. Moreover, because oral iron is poorly absorbed in the setting of ongoing inflammation [21], IBD patients with increased C-reactive protein (CRP) levels often show a diminished response to oral iron therapy [115].

Most of the reservations regarding oral iron therapy in IBD come from studies in animal models, which have shown contradictory evidence regarding the impact of oral iron on ongoing intestinal inflammation [35,116]. In humans, the clinical evidence for the effects of oral iron in patients with flaring IBD is also controversial [38,117]. It is, however, established that iron therapy significantly affects the composition of the microbiome [118,119]. This is of interest because the composition of the microbiome is regarded as an important factor in the pathogenesis of IBD [120]. A recent open-label clinical trial showed a significant impact of iron supplementation (both oral and intravenous) on the phylogenetic composition and faecal metabolite landscape in patients with IBD and iron deficiency or anaemia [118]. A difference between the impact of orally and intravenously administered iron on bacterial phylotypes and faecal metabolites seems to exist and this may relate to differences in iron pharmacokinetics and iron availability for gut bacteria. Moreover, patients with CD appear to be more prone to changes in microbiome composition following iron replacement therapy and intravenous iron therapy might in fact benefit such anaemic patients with an unstable microbiota [118]. Based on these findings, iron ingestion may potentially influence the disease course in patients with IBD [118,121].

5.2. Intravenous Regimen

Parenteral iron administration more rapidly increases haemoglobin levels than oral delivery [122,123] and this option traditionally has been reserved for patients who are intolerant to or respond inadequately to oral iron supplementation, as well as for patients in whom a rapid iron replenishment is desired (e.g., patients scheduled for surgery) [25,85,114]. This approach is reflected by the indications approved by the U.S. Food and Drug Administration (FDA) and the European Medicines Agency (EMA) for a number of intravenous iron preparations [124,125]. In the past, when high-molecular-weight dextrans were used for intravenous iron therapy, infrequent severe or life-threatening anaphylactic reactions were reported following intravenous administration [126].

However, the risk of these severe adverse events is lower today with the currently used preparations including high-molecular-weight iron components [127]. Compared with oral administration, intravenous iron increases haemoglobin levels and iron storage and improves quality of life more rapidly but not always more effectively [119,128,129]. The disadvantages—apart from a higher cost of therapy—include a risk of infusion-related anaphylaxis, which means that equipment to manage such potentially life-threatening situations must be in place [127]. Moreover, intravenous iron has been recommended in favour of oral iron therapy in patients with more advanced inflammation to bypass the blockade of iron absorption by hepcidin, although clinical data are scarce in proof of concept of this suggestion. Patients with more advanced inflammation/severe disease activity have often been excluded from prospective clinical trials evaluating the efficacy of intravenous iron in IBD. Of note, a retrospective analysis of results from various clinical trials suggested that pre-treatment CRP levels are not significantly associated with therapeutic responses to intravenous iron [115].

Six intravenous iron preparations are available at present. These include iron dextran, iron gluconate and iron sucrose, as well as the more recently licensed high-molecular-weight compounds ferumoxytol, iron isomaltoside 1000 and ferric carboxymaltose [26,130,131]. The structural stability of these high-dose preparations is high and allows only the release of a low level of labile iron into the circulation, resulting in improved safety profiles and infusion of higher iron dosages. In most patients, the total iron dose required therefore can be provided in a single infusion.

5.2.1. Low-Molecular-Weight Iron

The iron dextran compounds exist in two forms that are stable: A low- (73 kDa) and a high-molecular-weight (165 kDa) complex. Because the latter has been linked to an increased risk of both anaphylactic and anaphylactoid reactions [132–135], only the low-molecular-weight iron dextran is currently marketed in Europe [136]. This form can be administered as a single dose of up to 200 mg over a minimum infusion period of 30 min [137]. Previously it was recommended first to administer a test dose to check for the risk of anaphylactic reactions (i.e., 0.5 mL over 2–5 min) before providing the full dose but this precaution is no longer recommended by the EMA [124].

The stability of both iron gluconate (37 kDa) and iron sucrose (43 kDa) is lower than that of iron dextran and these two iron compounds can be administered at a maximal single dose of 200 mg of iron gluconate (300 mg in some countries) over a minimum infusion time of 30 min [138] or 62.5 mg of iron sucrose (125 mg in some countries) over an infusion time of 5–10 min [139] without requiring a test dose. Increasing the dosages [140] or the infusion rates [53] enhances the risk of adverse events such as transient hypotension due to the release of labile iron. Accordingly, iron dextran, iron sucrose and iron gluconate preparations usually will require multiple rounds of administration with lower doses to replenish iron stores.

5.2.2. High-Molecular-Weight Iron Compounds

The introduction of more stable iron complex formulations for intravenous iron administration has permitted the infusion of higher single doses with minimal side effects and no need for test doses because of the marginal release of labile iron during administration. The highly stable 150 kDa complexes ferric carboxymaltose [141–145] and iron isomaltoside 1000 [146,147] allow for controlled and safe delivery of higher doses of molecular iron per infusion. Ferric carboxymaltose may be administered effectively at a dose up to 1000 mg over a period of at least 15 min once per week [146]. Iron isomaltoside 1000, because of its stable structure, can be administered in single doses of up to 20 mg/kg of body weight within a period of 15 min [146]. Currently, limited data exist on iron isomaltoside 1000 for the treatment of iron-deficiency anaemia in patients with IBD [129,147], although clinical trials are currently ongoing. Ferumoxytol has a molecular weight of 721 kDa, which allows for rapid dosing of relatively large doses [148]. A recent phase III randomized, double-blind, placebo-controlled trial conducted at 182 sites in the United States, India and Europe evaluated administration of 510 mg doses of ferumoxytol followed by a second dose 2–8 days later in 231 patients with various gastrointestinal conditions (including IBD, polyps and colon cancer). In this study, ferumoxytol was efficacious and generally well tolerated in patients with iron-deficiency anaemia along with underlying gastrointestinal disorders who had a history of unsatisfactory oral iron supplementation [149]. However, with respect to IBD, it has been suggested that the paramagnetic nature of ferumoxytol might lead to interference during magnetic resonance imaging (MRI) examinations [150] and such interference might hamper its use in a subset of IBD patients because MRI examinations are an important diagnostic tool in their management. Further, a comparison of different intravenous iron products in the United States showed that ferumoxytol, per sold unit, had the highest rate of adverse events [151], impeding its benefit-risk ratio. In addition, since March 2015, a boxed warning by the FDA has been attached to this product regarding potentially life-threatening allergic reactions.

Although different side-effect profiles are associated with various preparations of large-molecule iron complexes [133], the most frequently reported complaints after infusion are itching, dyspnea, wheezing and myalgia [152]. Moreover, it should be noted that acute myalgia following a first intravenous iron administration (without any other symptoms) ceases spontaneously within minutes (i.e., the so-called Fishbane reaction) and does not recur at re-challenge [152,153]. In addition, more specific side effects include hypotension, tachycardia, dyspepsia, diarrhoea, stridor, nausea, skin flushing and periorbital oedema. Serious side effects are rare following intravenous iron infusion [154] but can include cardiac arrest [155]. The risk is increased among elderly patients and has been observed most often following infusion of high-molecular-weight dextran-containing preparations that are no longer in clinical use [156]. Accordingly, an initial low infusion rate is advisable, as well as a close monitoring of patients for signs of hypersensitivity both during administration of an intravenous iron formulation and for at least 30 min thereafter [124].

Based on our expanding knowledge of the pathways underlying inflammatory anaemia and specifically the role of hepcidin, new therapeutic strategies are emerging that attempt to block hepcidin activity either by directly interfering with hepcidin synthesis by affecting different inflammation- or iron-driven signalling pathways that regulate hepcidin expression (such as SMAD, STAT3, BMP, BMPR, or TMPRSS6) or by neutralizing hepcidin in the circulation [57,157–160] (Figure 1). Such interventions are currently under clinical investigation but they can only be effective in patients with inflammation- or renal insufficiency- driven hepcidin elevation and subsequent iron retention in macrophages, where hepcidin antagonization will result in redistribution of iron to the circulation and delivery of the metal to erythroid progenitors. In patients with true iron deficiency in the setting of inflammation, which is often the case in IBD, such therapies will not work and iron supplementation will remain the treatment of choice. Another set of new drugs has arisen from the development of prolyl-hydroxylase inhibitors. These therapeutic agents cause stabilization of HIFs, resulting in increased endogenous erythropoietin formation and stimulation of iron uptake based on the regulatory effects of HIFs on the expression of transmembrane iron transporters. These agents are currently being investigated in clinical trials mainly to combat renal anaemia [161–163].

6. Evidence of Management

Members of our group previously performed a systematic search that yielded a total of 632 studies concerning iron therapy in IBD published from January 2004 to March 2015 (i.e., in a time frame with novel high-dose intravenous iron preparations), of which 13 prospective trials met the inclusion criteria as randomized, controlled trials and included 2906 patients in total [164]. This systematic review indicated that administration of intravenous iron in IBD patients with mild anaemia (haemoglobin $\geq$ 10 g/dL) frequently resulted in higher ferritin levels but not in higher haemoglobin concentrations compared with oral iron supplementation at short-term follow-up [129,144,145,165]. In more aggravated iron-deficiency anaemia, intravenous iron supplementation was superior to oral treatment when the evaluation was based on the increase in haemoglobin [128,134,145,165].

Comparative studies of intravenous versus oral iron supplementation in the systematic review did not demonstrate any significant difference in haemoglobin normalization favouring the use of intravenous iron therapy unless considered for patients with intolerance or an inadequate response to oral supplementation [164]. In patients undergoing biological therapy with TNF inhibitors, concomitant iron supplementation may be prescribed without affecting the disease course/activity. Moreover, another recent systematic review of randomized, controlled trials with the aim of assessing drug safety demonstrated that intravenous iron therapy may increase the risk of infection [166]. This issue has also been evaluated in predialysis and dialysis patients indicating differences in the risk of infection based on baseline ferritin levels, mode of administration (intermittent or bolus) and the specific drugs used [167–171].

It is known that apart from the WHO definitions of anaemia [31], a low TfS in fasting blood samples (<20%) and a serum ferritin concentration of less than 30 µg/L (with a serum CRP level within the normal range or a ferritin concentration of less than 100 µg/L with an elevated serum CRP level) are suitable laboratory tests for the diagnosis and assessment of iron deficiency in IBD used in the randomized, controlled studies [164].

Only nine randomized, controlled trials investigating oral iron supplementation in IBD patients were published between 2004 and 2017 [35,110,128,129,134,138,144,145,165]. Oral supplementation appears to be well tolerated and has a positive effect on both haemoglobin levels and body iron parameters. From these studies, it seems that milder side effects (i.e., abdominal discomfort, diarrhoea, nausea and vomiting) occur less often after intravenous therapy than after oral therapy [128,134,138,144,165], although one study did not report any differences [129]. No comparison of side effects based on the various forms of oral supplementation was, however, performed. From an examination of the available data, it was apparent that there are no indications that oral iron supplementation exacerbates symptoms of the underlying IBD. Only one study in this systematic review [164] reported worsening of disease activity in 2 of 33 patients with UC (but not in patients with CD). However, in this study, the IBD quality-of-life scores improved significantly ($p = 0.016$) at the same time [35] and when the eight studies using oral iron supplementation were evaluated, it was apparent that an adequate level of evidence is provided to verify the safety of oral iron supplementation in IBD. Of note, a study with oral ferric maltol has suggested that this drug may be an alternative for patients who are unresponsive to or intolerant of formulations containing ferrous salts [110], an observation that needs to be confirmed in future studies, though.

A very recent systematic review and Bayesian network meta-analysis performed on the five eligible randomized, controlled trials with a total population of 1143 patients has shown ferric carboxymaltose to be the most effective preparation for the treatment of iron-deficiency anaemia in IBD, followed by iron sucrose, iron isomaltoside and oral iron in fourth place [172]. This analysis incorporated all currently available evidence on intravenous iron replacements in IBD patients with iron-deficiency anaemia and is the first attempt to systematically and quantitatively review the literature in the field.

It is generally accepted that individuals with iron deficiency and coexisting anaemia need treatment. It is, however, a subject of debate whether treatment of iron deficiency should be initiated before the development of anaemia—a condition that recently was reported to occur in 37% of IBD patients in a Spanish outpatient cohort [173]—because data from clinical trials on this issue are scarce. Thus, a placebo-controlled, double-blinded, randomized study in women with iron deficiency but without anaemia indicated that intravenous iron administration resulted in an improvement of fatigue in 82% of patients in the intervention group compared with 47% in the placebo group and that the effect of iron supplementation on fatigue was most pronounced in women with an initial ferritin concentration of less than 15 ng/mL [174]. Similar beneficial effects of intravenous iron administration regarding quality of life in non-anaemic patients with IBD have recently been published [175,176]. Thus, none of these observational, single centre studies included a placebo control given the high incidence of placebo mediated benefits on quality of life in such patient cohorts [174,177]. Nevertheless, it has to be kept in mind that uncritical iron supplementation or iron overloading may have several adverse effects described herein, including allergic reactions, risk of infections or intravascular oxidative stress as well as impairment of mitochondrial function with subsequent fatigue [178]. This leads to the yet unsolved question of therapeutic start and end points in terms of target haemoglobin and/or sTfS/ferritin levels and whether or not full correction of anaemia is optimal for patients with inflammation-associated anaemia. Nevertheless, patients with concomitant diseases such as congestive heart failure and fatigue due to true iron deficiency may benefit from such iron supplementation [70].

7. Recommendations for Clinicians

The cause of anaemia and specifically of concomitant iron deficiency should be identified in every patient with IBD. Thus, the recurrence of iron deficiency following successful treatment is often due to persistence or relapse of the initial inciting cause (e.g., recurrent gastrointestinal or urogenital bleeding), which should be managed appropriately. Further, in patients who have failed to respond to either oral or parenteral iron therapy, the cause for this failure should be carefully determined.

Previously it was accepted that clinical symptoms of anaemia occurred only when the haemoglobin level dropped abruptly [37] and, conversely, that patients would adapt to low haemoglobin levels if the anaemia developed slowly. This led to the concept of asymptomatic anaemia. In truth, the term asymptomatic seems to reflect the fact that impairments in physical condition, quality of life, cardiovascular performance and cognitive function may have been neglected by both patients and their physicians. Therefore, the process of adaptation in chronic anaemia seems to be an acceptance/toleration of impaired quality of life [37] and chronic fatigue and reduced physical activity/cardiovascular performance caused by anaemia may actually debilitate and even worry patients with IBD as much as abdominal pain or diarrhoea [37]. Accordingly, the beneficial effect on quality of life and metabolic processes derived from the correction of anaemia in patients with IBD may be just as important as the control of their intestinal disease [37].

7.1. Oral versus Intravenous Iron Supplementation

Clinical guidelines often emphasize that because of the ease of treatment, patients with uncomplicated iron-deficiency anaemia should be treated with oral rather than intravenous iron formulations [179]. In this context, an appropriate dosage for treatment of iron deficiency in adults is usually recommended in the range of 100–200 mg/day of elemental iron but guidelines do not consider that a number of side effects are dose related and might be prevented by reducing the dosage to as low as 50 mg of elemental iron per day in selected patients, which, in fact, may be sufficient to correct mild iron-deficiency anaemia [180].

Indications for intravenous iron administration include severe anaemia (haemoglobin < 10 g/dL), intolerance of or inappropriate response to oral iron administration, severe intestinal disease activity and concomitant therapy with an erythropoiesis agent or patient preference. Oral iron supplements can be used if these indications for intravenous therapy are not met.

If intravenous iron supplementation is considered, the use of low-dose regimens is not recommended from the point of view of clinical efficacy because a number of infusions might be needed over several days or weeks. Instead, high-dose regimens that result in fewer infusions and increase both convenience and cost-effectiveness of intravenous iron repletion should be considered.

The optimal dosing strategy for intravenous iron compounds depends on the type of preparation, the body weight of the patient and the haemoglobin concentration. The amount of iron needed to correct the haemoglobin can be calculated using the Ganzoni equation [181], often regarded as the gold standard, although this formula might underestimate the iron needed when a target haemoglobin of 13 g/dL and stored iron of 500 mg are used to determine individual iron deficits [129]. Because this formula is inconvenient in clinical practice [129,144], simpler schemes for the estimation of total iron need have been published [38,182], including a simple regimen to predict individual iron requirements for ferric carboxymaltose [142] that may also be used in clinical practice for dosing of other intravenous iron preparations [38]. It should be mentioned that patients with iron-deficiency anaemia who are unresponsive even to intravenous iron supplementation (i.e., haemoglobin increase ≤ 2 g/dL within

4 weeks) may in addition need recombinant erythropoiesis-stimulating agents after ruling out other causes of anaemia such as vitamin deficiencies [183–185].

7.2. Surveillance of Patients Following Iron Supplementation

Last but not least, it should be kept in mind that iron deficiency in IBD often relapses after iron replenishment [143]. Consequently, periodic monitoring, for example, every 3 months during treatment and again after a year once the haemoglobin value is normalized and iron stores are replenished (i.e., preventive treatment), is essential to assess whether retreatment is required [73]. Such a proactive concept of anaemia management not only could improve the quality of life for patients with IBD but also could be of economic benefit. However, we lack solid data on when to stop iron supplementation therapy in order to avoid iron overloading, which may cause side effects due to iron-catalysed formation of toxic radicals [31]. Recent guidelines on the management of anaemia among dialysis patients suggest that ferritin levels of up to 500 ng/mL appear to be safe and this also might be a useful upper threshold in the management of patients with IBD and anaemia [186].

This leads to the questions of (1) therapeutic start and end points (i.e., when should iron supplementation therapy be initiated and when it should be discontinued?) and (2) whether or not iron-deficiency anaemia should be treated differently depending on the underlying disease? To start with the latter point, in general, subjects with pure iron-deficiency anaemia on the basis of an inadequate dietary iron intake and/or increased blood losses and iron-deficient IBD patients with no or minimal signs of inflammation should initially be recommended to oral iron therapy. However, such a recommendation might have some caveats. Oral iron replacement therapy may be of limited efficiency in the setting of concomitant inflammation, which is usually associated with increased hepcidin concentrations resulting in an impaired response to iron therapy [84,187]. Yet true iron deficiency in the setting of inflammation causes hepcidin reduction and enables duodenal iron absorption, although to a lesser extent than in healthy control individuals [21,62,63]. Second, iron supplementation may be a problem in areas with an endemic burden of infectious disease or in patients with active infections because iron is an essential growth factor for many microbes and also has an impact on antimicrobial immune responses [188]. Thus, dietary iron fortification strategies were associated with an increased risk of infections such as malaria, bacterial meningitis, bacterial pneumonia and viral diarrhoea along with a rise in infection-related mortality [189,190].

7.3. General Precautions for Iron Supplementation

While normalization of haemoglobin appears to be a reasonable readout in subjects with iron-deficiency anaemia in the absence of inflammation [31], retrospective data, mainly from patients with chronic kidney disease, who are also characterized by a low-grade inflammation, indicate that haemoglobin normalization seems to be associated with an increased mortality compared with subjects with mild anaemia [28,191,192]. This has resulted in recommendations from different societies that in the presence of an inflammatory disease, including cancer or autoimmune disorders, the target haemoglobin concentration should be slightly below normal [28,31]. However, this is an extrapolation of data from observational studies and it is still unknown whether this is also true for patients with IBD.

Importantly, life-threatening reactions possibly caused by release of free iron are rare after administration of intravenous iron supplementation therapies [127,193]. Thus, practical recommendations for minimizing the risk of hypersensitivity reactions, for example, by assessing any previous adverse reactions, multiple drug allergies, or severe atopy, should be applied. Also, decreasing the infusion rate as well as maintaining an appropriately staffed site equipped with resuscitation facilities may be considered [127]. An incompletely understood issue is the development of hypophosphatemia in some patients specifically in association with ferric-carboxymaltose administration. Infrequently, hypophosphatemia may become severe and life threatening and may be linked to alterations of the FWF23 and vitamin D pathways, although the details of that network, as well as measures to identify patients at risk, are not available thus far [194].

Patients with inflammatory diseases will respond poorly to oral iron therapy unless the iron deficiency is severe. Newer iron formulations, such as ferric maltose, have been shown to correct mild anaemia in patients with quiescent IBD [110] but whether this is also true in flaring IBD still remains to be established. Nevertheless, in patients with inflammation and anaemia based on iron-limited erythropoiesis and in patients with non-inflammatory-driven severe iron-deficiency anaemia, in whom a fast recovery of depleted iron stores is desired, intravenous iron appears to be the treatment of choice. Still, the evidence from studies in proof of this latter concept is rather scare [179] and we still lack data from prospective trials on the efficacy of intravenous iron preparations in patients with more advanced inflammation.

8. Conclusions

Here we have summarized the impact and pathophysiology of iron deficiency in the setting of IBD. Diagnostic criteria are provided as well as methods to differentiate between functional and true iron deficiency. We also discussed the currently available drugs and commented on issues that should be considered by physicians treating patients with IBD. Thus, treating physicians need to pay more attention to the management of anaemia and iron deficiency for improvement of the general well-being of their patients with IBD—a matter that actually does not gain the attention it deserves. Although we lack knowledge on the effects of iron repletion strategies on the course of IBD, the control of inflammation is pivotal in the management of anaemia in this intestinal disorder.

Given the novel intravenous high-dose iron replacement regimens introduced within the last decade, oral iron therapy should be preferred for IBD patients with mild and uncomplicated iron-deficiency anaemia (haemoglobin $\geq$ 10 g/dL) in quiescent disease stages unless previous complications have been observed, including an inadequate response (haemoglobin increase < 2 g/dL within 4 weeks) [195]. Intravenous iron supplementation may be of advantage in patients with aggravated iron-deficiency anaemia or flaring IBD (haemoglobin < 10 g/dL) because inflammation hampers intestinal iron absorption [27,196,197]. Further, based on the available data, iron therapy can be administered concomitantly with TNF inhibitors [198], a class of drugs widely used in the management of IBD [199]. When using intravenous iron preparations, physicians must be aware of infusion-related side effects and the risk of hypophosphatemia. Further, efficacy studies of intravenous iron preparations in patients with more advanced inflammation are urgently desired.

Finally, it should be emphasized that iron deficiency may relapse often after iron replenishment [143], specifically when IBD activity is not well controlled and consequently, periodic monitoring should be highlighted to assess whether retreatment is required [73]. However, we still lack solid data on when to stop iron supplementation therapy in order to avoid side effects due to iron overloading. Thus large, well-designed collaborative prospective trials involving scientists and physicians from different disciplines are warranted to assess the true impact on the management of IBD associated with iron-deficiency anaemia.

Author Contributions: O.H.N. wrote the first draft. C.S., M.E.V. and G.W. subsequently extracted, analysed and interpreted the data. All authors contributed to the various versions and approved the final version of the manuscript.

Conflicts of Interest: The authors declare no conflict of interest except that G.W. has received lecture honoraria from Vifor Pharma and AOP Orphan Pharmaceuticals.

References

1. Kassebaum, N.J.; Jasrasaria, R.; Naghavi, M.; Wulf, S.K.; Johns, N.; Lozano, R.; Regan, M.; Weatherall, D.; Chou, D.P.; Eisele, T.P.; et al. A systematic analysis of global anemia burden from 1990 to 2010. *Blood* **2014**, *123*, 615–624. [CrossRef] [PubMed]
2. Iron Deficinecy Anemia: Assessment, Prevention, and Control. A Guide for Programme Managers. Available online: http://www.who.int/nutrition/publications/en/ida_assessment_prevention_control.pdf (accessed on 11 November 2017).

3. Gulmez, H.; Akin, Y.; Savas, M.; Gulum, M.; Ciftci, H.; Yalcinkaya, S.; Yeni, E. Impact of iron supplementation on sexual dysfunction of women with iron deficiency anemia in short term: A preliminary study. *J. Sex. Med.* **2014**, *11*, 1042–1046. [CrossRef] [PubMed]

4. Haas, J.D.; Brownlie, T. Iron deficiency and reduced work capacity: A critical review of the research to determine a causal relationship. *J. Nutr.* **2001**, *131*, 676S–688S. [PubMed]

5. McClung, J.P.; Murray-Kolb, L.E. Iron nutrition and premenopausal women: Effects of poor iron status on physical and neuropsychological performance. *Annu. Rev. Nutr.* **2013**, *33*, 271–288. [CrossRef] [PubMed]

6. Bresgen, N.; Eckl, P.M. Oxidative stress and the homeodynamics of iron metabolism. *Biomolecules* **2015**, *5*, 808–847. [CrossRef] [PubMed]

7. Filmann, N.; Rey, J.; Schneeweiss, S.; Ardizzone, S.; Bager, P.; Bergamaschi, G.; Koutroubakis, I.; Lindgren, S.; Morena, F.L.; Moum, B.; et al. Prevalence of anemia in inflammatory bowel diseases in european countries: A systematic review and individual patient data meta-analysis. *Inflamm. Bowel Dis.* **2014**, *20*, 936–945. [CrossRef] [PubMed]

8. Fiorino, G.; Allocca, M.; Danese, S. Commentary: Anaemia in inflammatory bowel disease—The most common and ignored extra intestinal manifestation. *Aliment. Pharmacol. Ther.* **2014**, *39*, 227–228. [CrossRef] [PubMed]

9. Ng, S.C.; Shi, H.Y.; Hamidi, N.; Underwood, F.E.; Tang, W.; Benchimol, E.I.; Panaccione, R.; Ghosh, S.; Wu, J.C.Y.; Chan, F.K.L.; et al. Worldwide incidence and prevalence of inflammatory bowel disease in the 21st century: A systematic review of population-based studies. *Lancet* **2018**, *390*, 2769–2778. [CrossRef]

10. Eriksson, C.; Cao, Y.; Rundquist, S.; Zhulina, Y.; Henriksson, I.; Montgomery, S.; Halfvarson, J. Changes in medical management and colectomy rates: A population-based cohort study on the epidemiology and natural history of ulcerative colitis in Orebro, Sweden, 1963–2010. *Aliment. Pharmacol. Ther.* **2017**, *46*, 897–898. [CrossRef] [PubMed]

11. Molodecky, N.A.; Soon, I.S.; Rabi, D.M.; Ghali, W.A.; Ferris, M.; Chernoff, G.; Benchimol, E.I.; Panaccione, R.; Ghosh, S.; Barkema, H.W.; et al. Increasing incidence and prevalence of the inflammatory bowel diseases with time, based on systematic review. *Gastroenterology* **2012**, *142*, 46–54. [CrossRef] [PubMed]

12. Kaplan, G.G.; Jess, T. The Changing Landscape of Inflammatory Bowel Disease: East Meets West. *Gastroenterology* **2016**, *150*, 24–26. [CrossRef] [PubMed]

13. Portela, F.; Lago, P.; Cotter, J.; Goncalves, R.; Vasconcelos, H.; Ministro, P.; Lopes, S.; Eusebio, M.; Morna, H.; Cravo, M.; et al. Anaemia in patients with inflammatory bowel disease—A nationwide cross-sectional study. *Digestion* **2016**, *93*, 214–220. [CrossRef] [PubMed]

14. Hoivik, M.L.; Reinisch, W.; Cvancarova, M.; Moum, B. Anaemia in inflammatory bowel disease: A population-based 10-year follow-up. *Aliment. Pharmacol. Ther.* **2014**, *39*, 69–76. [CrossRef] [PubMed]

15. Azzopardi, N.; Ellul, P. Iron deficiency in Crohn's disease: Iron supplementation or disease control? *J. Crohn's Colitis* **2014**, *8*, 1333. [CrossRef] [PubMed]

16. Bager, P.; Befrits, R.; Wikman, O.; Lindgren, S.; Moum, B.; Hjortswang, H.; Dahlerup, J.F. High burden of iron deficiency and different types of anemia in inflammatory bowel disease outpatients in Scandinavia: A longitudinal 2-year follow-up study. *Scand. J. Gastroenterol.* **2013**, *48*, 1286–1293. [CrossRef] [PubMed]

17. Gisbert, J.P.; Gomollon, F. Common misconceptions in the diagnosis and management of anemia in inflammatory bowel disease. *Am. J. Gastroenterol.* **2008**, *103*, 1299–1307. [CrossRef] [PubMed]

18. Larsen, S.; Bendtzen, K.; Nielsen, O.H. Extraintestinal manifestations of inflammatory bowel disease: Epidemiology, diagnosis, and management. *Ann. Med.* **2010**, *42*, 97–114. [CrossRef] [PubMed]

19. Goodhand, J.R.; Kamperidis, N.; Rao, A.; Laskaratos, F.; McDermott, A.; Wahed, M.; Naik, S.; Croft, N.M.; Lindsay, J.O.; Sanderson, I.R.; et al. Prevalence and management of anemia in children, adolescents, and adults with inflammatory bowel disease. *Inflamm. Bowel Dis.* **2012**, *18*, 513–519. [CrossRef] [PubMed]

20. Vagianos, K.; Clara, I.; Carr, R.; Graff, L.A.; Walker, J.R.; Targownik, L.E.; Lix, L.M.; Rogala, L.; Miller, N.; Bernstein, C.N. What are adults with inflammatory bowel disease (IBD) eating? A closer look at the dietary habits of a population-based Canadian IBD cohort. *J. Parenter. Enter. Nutr.* **2015**, *2016*, 405–411. [CrossRef] [PubMed]

21. Theurl, I.; Aigner, E.; Theurl, M.; Nairz, M.; Seifert, M.; Schroll, A.; Sonnweber, T.; Eberwein, L.; Witcher, D.R.; Murphy, A.T.; et al. Regulation of iron homeostasis in anemia of chronic disease and iron deficiency anemia: Diagnostic and therapeutic implications. *Blood* **2009**, *113*, 5277–5286. [CrossRef] [PubMed]

22. Weiss, G.; Gasche, C. Pathogenesis and treatment of anemia in inflammatory bowel disease. *Haematologica* **2010**, *95*, 175–178. [CrossRef] [PubMed]

23. Hwang, C.; Ross, V.; Mahadevan, U. Micronutrient deficiencies in inflammatory bowel disease: From A to zinc. *Inflamm. Bowel Dis.* **2012**, *18*, 1961–1981. [CrossRef] [PubMed]

24. Murawska, N.; Fabisiak, A.; Fichna, J. Anemia of chronic disease and iron deficiency anemia in inflammatory bowel diseases: Pathophysiology, diagnosis, and treatment. *Inflamm. Bowel Dis.* **2016**, *22*, 1198–1208. [CrossRef] [PubMed]

25. Gasche, C.; Berstad, A.; Befrits, R.; Beglinger, C.; Dignass, A.; Erichsen, K.; Gomollon, F.; Hjortswang, H.; Koutroubakis, I.; Kulnigg, S.; et al. Guidelines on the diagnosis and management of iron deficiency and anemia in inflammatory bowel diseases. *Inflamm. Bowel Dis.* **2007**, *13*, 1545–1553. [CrossRef] [PubMed]

26. Goldberg, N.D. Iron deficiency anemia in patients with inflammatory bowel disease. *Clin. Exp. Gastroenterol.* **2013**, *6*, 61–70. [CrossRef] [PubMed]

27. Semrin, G.; Fishman, D.S.; Bousvaros, A.; Zholudev, A.; Saunders, A.C.; Correia, C.E.; Nemeth, E.; Grand, R.J.; Weinstein, D.A. Impaired intestinal iron absorption in Crohn's disease correlates with disease activity and markers of inflammation. *Inflamm. Bowel Dis.* **2006**, *12*, 1101–1106. [CrossRef] [PubMed]

28. Weiss, G.; Goodnough, L.T. Anemia of chronic disease. *N. Engl. J. Med.* **2005**, *352*, 1011–1023. [CrossRef] [PubMed]

29. Weiss, G.; Schett, G. Anaemia in inflammatory rheumatic diseases. *Nat. Rev. Rheumatol.* **2013**, *9*, 205–215. [CrossRef] [PubMed]

30. Nairz, M.; Schroll, A.; Demetz, E.; Tancevski, I.; Theurl, I.; Weiss, G. 'Ride on the ferrous wheel'—The cycle of iron in macrophages in health and disease. *Immunobiology* **2015**, *220*, 280–294. [CrossRef] [PubMed]

31. Camaschella, C. Iron-deficiency anemia. *N. Engl. J. Med.* **2015**, *372*, 1832–1843. [CrossRef] [PubMed]

32. Shander, A.; Goodnough, L.T.; Javidroozi, M.; Auerbach, M.; Carson, J.; Ershler, W.B.; Ghiglione, M.; Glaspy, J.; Lew, I. Iron deficiency anemia-bridging the knowledge and practice gap. *Transfus. Med. Rev.* **2014**, *28*, 156–166. [CrossRef] [PubMed]

33. Stein, J.; Hartmann, F.; Dignass, A.U. Diagnosis and management of iron deficiency anemia in patients with IBD. *Nat. Rev. Gastroenterol. Hepatol.* **2010**, *7*, 599–610. [CrossRef] [PubMed]

34. Pizzi, L.T.; Weston, C.M.; Goldfarb, N.I.; Moretti, D.; Cobb, N.; Howell, J.B.; Infantolino, A.; Dimarino, A.J.; Cohen, S. Impact of chronic conditions on quality of life in patients with inflammatory bowel disease. *Inflamm. Bowel Dis.* **2006**, *12*, 47–52. [CrossRef] [PubMed]

35. De Silva, A.D.; Tsironi, E.; Feakins, R.M.; Rampton, D.S. Efficacy and tolerability of oral iron therapy in inflammatory bowel disease: A prospective, comparative trial. *Aliment. Pharmacol. Ther.* **2005**, *22*, 1097–1105. [CrossRef] [PubMed]

36. Bager, P.; Befrits, R.; Wikman, O.; Lindgren, S.; Moum, B.; Hjortswang, H.; Hjollund, N.H.; Dahlerup, J.F. Fatigue in out-patients with inflammatory bowel disease is common and multifactorial. *Aliment. Pharmacol. Ther.* **2012**, *35*, 133–141. [CrossRef] [PubMed]

37. Gasche, C.; Lomer, M.C.; Cavill, I.; Weiss, G. Iron, anaemia, and inflammatory bowel diseases. *Gut* **2004**, *53*, 1190–1197. [CrossRef] [PubMed]

38. Dignass, A.U.; Gasche, C.; Bettenworth, D.; Birgegard, G.; Danese, S.; Gisbert, J.P.; Gomollon, F.; Iqbal, T.; Katsanos, K.; Koutroubakis, I.; et al. European consensus on the diagnosis and management of iron deficiency and anaemia in inflammatory bowel diseases. *J. Crohn's Colitis* **2015**, *9*, 211–222. [CrossRef] [PubMed]

39. Martin, J.; Radeke, H.H.; Dignass, A.; Stein, J. Current evaluation and management of anemia in patients with inflammatory bowel disease. *Expert Rev. Gastroenterol. Hepatol.* **2017**, *11*, 19–32. [CrossRef] [PubMed]

40. Stein, J.; Bager, P.; Befrits, R.; Gasche, C.; Gudehus, M.; Lerebours, E.; Magro, F.; Mearin, F.; Mitchell, D.; Oldenburg, B.; et al. Anaemia management in patients with inflammatory bowel disease: Routine practice across nine European countries. *Eur. J. Gastroenterol. Hepatol.* **2013**, *25*, 1456–1463. [CrossRef] [PubMed]

41. Hentze, M.W.; Muckenthaler, M.U.; Galy, B.; Camaschella, C. Two to tango: Regulation of Mammalian iron metabolism. *Cell* **2010**, *142*, 24–38. [CrossRef] [PubMed]

42. Zhang, C. Essential functions of iron-requiring proteins in DNA replication, repair and cell cycle control. *Protein Cell* **2014**, *5*, 750–760. [CrossRef] [PubMed]

43. Pantopoulos, K.; Porwal, S.K.; Tartakoff, A.; Devireddy, L. Mechanisms of mammalian iron homeostasis. *Biochemistry* **2012**, *51*, 5705–5724. [CrossRef] [PubMed]

44. Coad, J.; Conlon, C. Iron deficiency in women: Assessment, causes and consequences. *Curr. Opin. Clin. Nutr. Metab. Care* **2011**, *14*, 625–634. [CrossRef] [PubMed]
45. Andrews, N.C. Disorders of iron metabolism. *N. Engl. J. Med.* **1999**, *341*, 1986–1995. [CrossRef] [PubMed]
46. McDermid, J.M.; Lonnerdal, B. Iron. *Adv. Nutr.* **2012**, *3*, 532–533. [CrossRef] [PubMed]
47. Hurrell, R.; Egli, I. Iron bioavailability and dietary reference values. *Am. J. Clin. Nutr.* **2010**, *91*, 1461S–1467S. [CrossRef] [PubMed]
48. Ganz, T.; Nemeth, E. Hepcidin and iron homeostasis. *Biochim. Biophys. Acta* **2012**, *1823*, 1434–1443. [CrossRef] [PubMed]
49. Nemeth, E.; Tuttle, M.S.; Powelson, J.; Vaughn, M.B.; Donovan, A.; Ward, D.M.; Ganz, T.; Kaplan, J. Hepcidin regulates cellular iron efflux by binding to ferroportin and inducing its internalization. *Science* **2004**, *306*, 2090–2093. [CrossRef] [PubMed]
50. Ruchala, P.; Nemeth, E. The pathophysiology and pharmacology of hepcidin. *Trends Pharmacol. Sci.* **2014**, *35*, 155–161. [CrossRef] [PubMed]
51. Ganz, T.; Nemeth, E. Hepcidin and disorders of iron metabolism. *Annu. Rev. Med.* **2011**, *62*, 347–360. [CrossRef] [PubMed]
52. Bregman, D.B.; Morris, D.; Koch, T.A.; He, A.; Goodnough, L.T. Hepcidin levels predict nonresponsiveness to oral iron therapy in patients with iron deficiency anemia. *Am. J. Hematol.* **2013**, *88*, 97–101. [CrossRef] [PubMed]
53. Koskenkorva-Frank, T.S.; Weiss, G.; Koppenol, W.H.; Burckhardt, S. The complex interplay of iron metabolism, reactive oxygen species, and reactive nitrogen species: Insights into the potential of various iron therapies to induce oxidative and nitrosative stress. *Free Radic. Biol. Med.* **2013**, *65*, 1174–1194. [CrossRef] [PubMed]
54. Carvalho, L.; Brait, D.; Vaz, M.; Lollo, P.; Morato, P.; Oesterreich, S.; Raposo, J.; Freitas, K. Partially hydrolyzed guar gum increases ferroportin expression in the colon of anemic growing rats. *Nutrients* **2017**, *9*, 228. [CrossRef] [PubMed]
55. Ludwiczek, S.; Aigner, E.; Theurl, I.; Weiss, G. Cytokine-mediated regulation of iron transport in human monocytic cells. *Blood* **2003**, *101*, 4148–4154. [CrossRef] [PubMed]
56. Munoz, M.; Garcia-Erce, J.A.; Remacha, A.F. Disorders of iron metabolism. Part II: Iron deficiency and iron overload. *J. Clin. Pathol.* **2011**, *64*, 287–296. [CrossRef] [PubMed]
57. Theurl, I.; Schroll, A.; Sonnweber, T.; Nairz, M.; Theurl, M.; Willenbacher, W.; Eller, K.; Wolf, D.; Seifert, M.; Sun, C.C.; et al. Pharmacologic inhibition of hepcidin expression reverses anemia of chronic inflammation in rats. *Blood* **2011**, *118*, 4977–4984. [CrossRef] [PubMed]
58. Kautz, L.; Jung, G.; Valore, E.V.; Rivella, S.; Nemeth, E.; Ganz, T. Identification of erythroferrone as an erythroid regulator of iron metabolism. *Nat. Genet.* **2014**, *46*, 678–684. [CrossRef] [PubMed]
59. Peyssonnaux, C.; Zinkernagel, A.S.; Schuepbach, R.A.; Rankin, E.; Vaulont, S.; Haase, V.H.; Nizet, V.; Johnson, R.S. Regulation of iron homeostasis by the hypoxia-inducible transcription factors (HIFs). *J. Clin. Investig.* **2007**, *117*, 1926–1932. [CrossRef] [PubMed]
60. Sonnweber, T.; Nachbaur, D.; Schroll, A.; Nairz, M.; Seifert, M.; Demetz, E.; Haschka, D.; Mitterstiller, A.M.; Kleinsasser, A.; Burtscher, M.; et al. Hypoxia induced downregulation of hepcidin is mediated by platelet derived growth factor BB. *Gut* **2014**, *63*, 1951–1959. [CrossRef] [PubMed]
61. Tanno, T.; Bhanu, N.V.; Oneal, P.A.; Goh, S.H.; Staker, P.; Lee, Y.T.; Moroney, J.W.; Reed, C.H.; Luban, N.L.; Wang, R.H.; et al. High levels of GDF15 in thalassemia suppress expression of the iron regulatory protein hepcidin. *Nat. Med.* **2007**, *13*, 1096–1101. [CrossRef] [PubMed]
62. Theurl, I.; Schroll, A.; Nairz, M.; Seifert, M.; Theurl, M.; Sonnweber, T.; Kulaksiz, H.; Weiss, G. Pathways for the regulation of hepcidin expression in anemia of chronic disease and iron deficiency anemia in vivo. *Haematologica* **2011**, *96*, 1761–1769. [CrossRef] [PubMed]
63. Lasocki, S.; Baron, G.; Driss, F.; Westerman, M.; Puy, H.; Boutron, I.; Beaumont, C.; Montravers, P. Diagnostic accuracy of serum hepcidin for iron deficiency in critically ill patients with anemia. *Intensive Care Med.* **2010**, *36*, 1044–1048. [CrossRef] [PubMed]
64. Mullin, G.E. Micronutrients and inflammatory bowel disease. *Nutr. Clin. Pract.* **2012**, *27*, 136–137. [CrossRef] [PubMed]
65. Thomas, C.; Thomas, L. Anemia of chronic disease: Pathophysiology and laboratory diagnosis. *Lab. Hematol.* **2005**, *11*, 14–23. [CrossRef] [PubMed]

66. Oldenburg, B.; Koningsberger, J.C.; Van Berge Henegouwen, G.P.; Van Asbeck, B.S.; Marx, J.J. Iron and inflammatory bowel disease. *Aliment. Pharmacol. Ther.* **2001**, *15*, 429–438. [CrossRef] [PubMed]

67. Theurl, I.; Mattle, V.; Seifert, M.; Mariani, M.; Marth, C.; Weiss, G. Dysregulated monocyte iron homeostasis and erythropoietin formation in patients with anemia of chronic disease. *Blood* **2006**, *107*, 4142–4148. [CrossRef] [PubMed]

68. Weiss, G. Anemia of chronic disorders: New diagnostic tools and new treatment strategies. *Semin. Hematol.* **2015**, *52*, 313–320. [CrossRef] [PubMed]

69. Anker, S.D.; Comin, C.J.; Filippatos, G.; Willenheimer, R.; Dickstein, K.; Drexler, H.; Luscher, T.F.; Bart, B.; Banasiak, W.; Niegowska, J.; et al. Ferric carboxymaltose in patients with heart failure and iron deficiency. *N. Engl. J. Med.* **2009**, *361*, 2436–2448. [CrossRef] [PubMed]

70. Jankowska, E.A.; Malyszko, J.; Ardehali, H.; Koc-Zorawska, E.; Banasiak, W.; von Haehling, S.; Macdougall, I.C.; Weiss, G.; McMurray, J.J.; Anker, S.D.; et al. Iron status in patients with chronic heart failure. *Eur. Heart J.* **2013**, *34*, 827–834. [CrossRef] [PubMed]

71. Cook, J.D. Diagnosis and management of iron-deficiency anaemia. *Best Pract. Res. Clin. Haematol.* **2005**, *18*, 319–332. [CrossRef] [PubMed]

72. Arosio, P.; Levi, S. Ferritin, iron homeostasis, and oxidative damage. *Free Radic. Biol. Med.* **2002**, *33*, 457–463. [CrossRef]

73. Goddard, A.F.; McIntyre, A.S.; Scott, B.B. Guidelines for the management of iron deficiency anaemia. *Gut* **2000**, *46*, iv1–iv5. [CrossRef] [PubMed]

74. Lipschitz, D.A.; Cook, J.D.; Finch, C.A. A clinical evaluation of serum ferritin as an index of iron stores. *N. Engl. J. Med.* **1974**, *290*, 1213–1216. [CrossRef] [PubMed]

75. Mast, A.E.; Blinder, M.A.; Gronowski, A.M.; Chumley, C.; Scott, M.G. Clinical utility of the soluble transferrin receptor and comparison with serum ferritin in several populations. *Clin. Chem.* **1998**, *44*, 45–51. [PubMed]

76. Van Santen, S.; de Mast, Q.; Oosting, J.D.; van Ede, A.; Swinkels, D.W.; van der Ven, A.J.A.M. Hematologic parameters predicting a response to oral iron therapy in chronic inflammation. *Haematologica* **2014**, *99*, e171–e173. [CrossRef] [PubMed]

77. Archer, N.M.; Brugnara, C. Diagnosis of iron-deficient states. *Crit. Rev. Clin. Lab. Sci.* **2015**, *52*, 256–272. [CrossRef] [PubMed]

78. Punnonen, K.; Irjala, K.; Rajamaki, A. Serum transferrin receptor and its ratio to serum ferritin in the diagnosis of iron deficiency. *Blood* **1997**, *89*, 1052–1057. [PubMed]

79. Tessitore, N.; Solero, G.P.; Lippi, G.; Bassi, A.; Faccini, G.B.; Bedogna, V.; Gammaro, L.; Brocco, G.; Restivo, G.; Bernich, P.; et al. The role of iron status markers in predicting response to intravenous iron in haemodialysis patients on maintenance erythropoietin. *Nephrol. Dial. Transplant.* **2001**, *16*, 1416–1423. [CrossRef] [PubMed]

80. Brugnara, C.; Schiller, B.; Moran, J. Reticulocyte hemoglobin equivalent (Ret He) and assessment of iron-deficient states. *Clin. Lab. Haematol.* **2006**, *28*, 303–308. [CrossRef] [PubMed]

81. Goodnough, L.T.; Nemeth, E.; Ganz, T. Detection, evaluation, and management of iron-restricted erythropoiesis. *Blood* **2010**, *116*, 4754–4761. [CrossRef] [PubMed]

82. Van Santen, S.; van Dongen-Lases, E.C.; de Vegt, F.; Laarakkers, C.M.M.; van Riel, P.L.C.M.; van Ede, A.E.; Swinkels, D.W. Hepcidin and hemoglobin content parameters in the diagnosis of iron deficiency in rheumatoid arthritis patients with anemia. *Arthritis Rheum.* **2011**, *63*, 3672–3680. [CrossRef] [PubMed]

83. Girelli, D.; Nemeth, E.; Swinkels, D.W. Hepcidin in the diagnosis of iron disorders. *Blood* **2016**, *127*, 2809–2813. [CrossRef] [PubMed]

84. Prentice, A.M.; Doherty, C.P.; Abrams, S.A.; Cox, S.E.; Atkinson, S.H.; Verhoef, H.; Armitage, A.E.; Drakesmith, H. Hepcidin is the major predictor of erythrocyte iron incorporation in anemic African children. *Blood* **2012**, *119*, 1922–1928. [CrossRef] [PubMed]

85. Wilson, A.; Reyes, E.; Ofman, J. Prevalence and outcomes of anemia in inflammatory bowel disease: A systematic review of the literature. *Am. J. Med.* **2004**, *116*, 44–49. [CrossRef] [PubMed]

86. Gomollon, F.; Gisbert, J.P.; Garcia-Erce, J.A. Intravenous iron in digestive diseases: A clinical (re)view. *Ther. Adv. Chronic Dis.* **2010**, *1*, 67–75. [CrossRef] [PubMed]

87. Klein, H.G.; Spahn, D.R.; Carson, J.L. Red blood cell transfusion in clinical practice. *Lancet* **2007**, *370*, 415–426. [CrossRef]

88. Goodnough, L.T.; Bach, R.G. Anemia, transfusion, and mortality. *N. Engl. J. Med.* **2001**, *345*, 1272–1274. [CrossRef] [PubMed]

89. Villanueva, C.; Colomo, A.; Bosch, A.; Concepcion, M.; Hernandez-Gea, V.; Aracil, C.; Graupera, I.; Poca, M.; Alvarez-Urturi, C.; Gordillo, J.; et al. Transfusion strategies for acute upper gastrointestinal bleeding. *N. Engl. J. Med.* **2013**, *368*, 11–21. [CrossRef] [PubMed]

90. Taylor, R.W.; Manganaro, L.; O'Brien, J.; Trottier, S.J.; Parkar, N.; Veremakis, C. Impact of allogenic packed red blood cell transfusion on nosocomial infection rates in the critically ill patient. *Crit. Care Med.* **2002**, *30*, 2249–2254. [CrossRef] [PubMed]

91. Talbot, T.R.; D'Agata, E.M.; Brinsko, V.; Lee, B.; Speroff, T.; Schaffner, W. Perioperative blood transfusion is predictive of poststernotomy surgical site infection: Marker for morbidity or true immunosuppressant? *Clin. Infect. Dis.* **2004**, *38*, 1378–1382. [CrossRef] [PubMed]

92. Aubron, C.; Nichol, A.; Cooper, D.J.; Bellomo, R. Age of red blood cells and transfusion in critically ill patients. *Ann. Intensive Care* **2013**, *3*. [CrossRef] [PubMed]

93. Bihl, F.; Castelli, D.; Marincola, F.; Dodd, R.Y.; Brander, C. Transfusion-transmitted infections. *J. Transl. Med.* **2007**, *5*, 25. [CrossRef] [PubMed]

94. Guinet, F.; Carniel, E.; Leclercq, A. Transfusion-transmitted Yersinia enterocolitica sepsis. *Clin. Infect. Dis.* **2011**, *53*, 583–591. [CrossRef] [PubMed]

95. Cancelo-Hidalgo, M.J.; Castelo-Branco, C.; Palacios, S.; Haya-Palazuelos, J.; Ciria-Recasens, M.; Manasanch, J.; Perez-Edo, L. Tolerability of different oral iron supplements: A systematic review. *Curr. Med. Res. Opin.* **2013**, *29*, 291–303. [CrossRef] [PubMed]

96. Santiago, P. Ferrous versus ferric oral iron formulations for the treatment of iron deficiency: A clinical overview. *Sci. World J.* **2012**. [CrossRef] [PubMed]

97. Fuqua, B.K.; Vulpe, C.D.; Anderson, G.J. Intestinal iron absorption. *J. Trace Elem. Med. Biol.* **2012**, *26*, 115–119. [CrossRef] [PubMed]

98. Aspuru, K.; Villa, C.; Bermejo, F.; Herrero, P.; Lopez, S.G. Optimal management of iron deficiency anemia due to poor dietary intake. *Int. J. Gen. Med.* **2011**, *4*, 741–750. [PubMed]

99. Lane, D.J.; Richardson, D.R. The active role of vitamin C in mammalian iron metabolism: Much more than just enhanced iron absorption! *Free Radic. Biol. Med.* **2014**, *75*, 69–83. [CrossRef] [PubMed]

100. Syed, S.; Michalski, E.S.; Tangpricha, V.; Chesdachai, S.; Kumar, A.; Prince, J.; Ziegler, T.R.; Suchdev, P.S.; Kugathasan, S. Vitamin D Status is associated with hepcidin and hemoglobin concentrations in children with inflammatory bowel disease. *Inflamm. Bowel Dis.* **2017**, *23*, 1650–1658. [CrossRef] [PubMed]

101. Mouli, V.P.; Ananthakrishnan, A.N. Review article: Vitamin D and inflammatory bowel diseases. *Aliment. Pharmacol. Ther.* **2014**, *39*, 125–136. [CrossRef] [PubMed]

102. Bacchetta, J.; Zaritsky, J.J.; Sea, J.L.; Chun, R.F.; Lisse, T.S.; Zavala, K.; Nayak, A.; Wesseling-Perry, K.; Westerman, M.; Hollis, B.W.; et al. Suppression of iron-regulatory hepcidin by vitamin D. *J. Am. Soc. Nephrol.* **2014**, *25*, 564–572. [CrossRef] [PubMed]

103. Gubatan, J.; Mitsuhashi, S.; Zenlea, T.; Rosenberg, L.; Robson, S.; Moss, A.C. Low serum vitamin D during remission increases risk of clinical relapse in patients with ulcerative colitis. *Clin. Gastroenterol. Hepatol.* **2017**, *15*, 240–246. [CrossRef] [PubMed]

104. Kabbani, T.A.; Koutroubakis, I.E.; Schoen, R.E.; Ramos-Rivers, C.; Shah, N.; Swoger, J.; Regueiro, M.; Barrie, A.; Schwartz, M.; Hashash, J.G.; et al. Association of vitamin D level with clinical status in inflammatory bowel disease: A 5-year longitudinal study. *Am. J. Gastroenterol.* **2016**, *111*, 712–719. [CrossRef] [PubMed]

105. Winter, R.W.; Collins, E.; Cao, B.; Carrellas, M.; Crowell, A.M.; Korzenik, J.R. Higher 25-hydroxyvitamin D levels are associated with greater odds of remission with anti-tumour necrosis factor-alpha medications among patients with inflammatory bowel diseases. *Aliment. Pharmacol. Ther.* **2017**, *45*, 653–659. [CrossRef] [PubMed]

106. Smith, E.M.; Tangpricha, V. Vitamin D and anemia: Insights into an emerging association. *Curr. Opin. Endocrinol. Diabetes Obes.* **2015**, *22*, 432–438. [CrossRef] [PubMed]

107. Smith, E.M.; Jones, J.L.; Han, J.E.; Alvarez, J.A.; Sloan, J.H.; Konrad, R.J.; Zughaier, S.M.; Martin, G.S.; Ziegler, T.R.; Tangpricha, V. High-dose vitamin D_3 administration is associated with increases in hemoglobin concentrations in mechanically ventilated critically Ill adults: A pilot double-blind, randomized, placebo-controlled trial. *J. Parenter. Enter. Nutr.* **2018**. [CrossRef]

108. Zughaier, S.M.; Alvarez, J.A.; Sloan, J.H.; Konrad, R.J.; Tangpricha, V. The role of vitamin D in regulating the iron-hepcidin-ferroportin axis in monocytes. *J. Clin. Transl. Endocrinol.* **2014**, *1*, 19–25. [CrossRef] [PubMed]

109. Smith, E.M.; Alvarez, J.A.; Kearns, M.D.; Hao, L.; Sloan, J.H.; Konrad, R.J.; Ziegler, T.R.; Zughaier, S.M.; Tangpricha, V. High-dose vitamin D$_3$ reduces circulating hepcidin concentrations: A pilot, randomized, double-blind, placebo-controlled trial in healthy adults. *Clin. Nutr.* **2017**, *36*, 980–985. [CrossRef] [PubMed]
110. Gasche, C.; Ahmad, T.; Tulassay, Z.; Baumgart, D.C.; Bokemeyer, B.; Buning, C.; Howaldt, S.; Stallmach, A. Ferric maltol is effective in correcting iron deficiency anemia in patients with inflammatory bowel disease: Results from a phase-3 clinical trial program. *Inflamm. Bowel Dis.* **2015**, *21*, 579–588. [CrossRef] [PubMed]
111. Hallberg, L.; Ryttinger, L.; Solvell, L. Side-effects of oral iron therapy. A double-blind study of different iron compounds in tablet form. *J. Intern. Med.* **1966**, *180*, 3–10. [CrossRef]
112. Moretti, D.; Goede, J.S.; Zeder, C.; Jiskra, M.; Chatzinakou, V.; Tjalsma, H.; Melse-Boonstra, A.; Brittenham, G.; Swinkels, D.W.; Zimmermann, M.B. Oral iron supplements increase hepcidin and decrease iron absorption from daily or twice-daily doses in iron-depleted young women. *Blood* **2015**, *126*, 1981–1989. [CrossRef] [PubMed]
113. Stoffel, N.U.; Cercamondi, C.I.; Brittenham, G.; Zeder, C.; Geurts-Moespot, A.J.; Swinkels, D.W.; Moretti, D.; Zimmermann, M.B. Iron absorption from oral iron supplements given on consecutive versus alternate days and as single morning doses versus twice-daily split dosing in iron-depleted women: Two open-label, randomised controlled trials. *Lancet Haematol.* **2017**, *4*, e524–e533. [CrossRef]
114. Kulnigg, S.; Gasche, C. Systematic review: Managing anaemia in Crohn's disease. *Aliment. Pharmacol. Ther.* **2006**, *24*, 1507–1523. [CrossRef] [PubMed]
115. Iqbal, T.; Stein, J.; Sharma, N.; Kulnigg-Dabsch, S.; Vel, S.; Gasche, C. Clinical significance of C-reactive protein levels in predicting responsiveness to iron therapy in patients with inflammatory bowel disease and iron deficiency anemia. *Dig. Dis. Sci.* **2015**, *60*, 1375–1381. [CrossRef] [PubMed]
116. Erichsen, K.; Milde, A.M.; Arslan, G.; Helgeland, L.; Gudbrandsen, O.A.; Ulvik, R.J.; Berge, R.K.; Hausken, T.; Berstad, A. Low-dose oral ferrous fumarate aggravated intestinal inflammation in rats with DSS-induced colitis. *Inflamm. Bowel Dis.* **2005**, *11*, 744–748. [CrossRef] [PubMed]
117. Rizvi, S.; Schoen, R.E. Supplementation with oral vs. intravenous iron for anemia with IBD or gastrointestinal bleeding: Is oral iron getting a bad rap? *Am. J. Gastroenterol.* **2011**, *106*, 1872–1879. [CrossRef] [PubMed]
118. Lee, T.; Clavel, T.; Smirnov, K.; Schmidt, A.; Lagkouvardos, I.; Walker, A.; Lucio, M.; Michalke, B.; Schmitt-Kopplin, P.; Fedorak, R.; et al. Oral versus intravenous iron replacement therapy distinctly alters the gut microbiota and metabolome in patients with IBD. *Gut* **2017**, *66*, 863–871. [CrossRef] [PubMed]
119. Lee, T.W.; Kolber, M.R.; Fedorak, R.N.; van Zanten, S.V. Iron replacement therapy in inflammatory bowel disease patients with iron deficiency anemia: A systematic review and meta-analysis. *J. Crohn's Colitis* **2012**, *6*, 267–275. [CrossRef] [PubMed]
120. Kostic, A.D.; Xavier, R.J.; Gevers, D. The microbiome in inflammatory bowel disease: Current status and the future ahead. *Gastroenterology* **2014**, *146*, 1489–1499. [CrossRef] [PubMed]
121. Werner, T.; Wagner, S.J.; Martinez, I.; Walter, J.; Chang, J.S.; Clavel, T.; Kisling, S.; Schuemann, K.; Haller, D. Depletion of luminal iron alters the gut microbiota and prevents Crohn's disease-like ileitis. *Gut* **2011**, *60*, 325–333. [CrossRef] [PubMed]
122. Kulnigg, S.; Teischinger, L.; Dejaco, C.; Waldhor, T.; Gasche, C. Rapid recurrence of IBD-associated anemia and iron deficiency after intravenous iron sucrose and erythropoietin treatment. *Am. J. Gastroenterol.* **2009**, *104*, 1460–1467. [CrossRef] [PubMed]
123. Vadhan-Raj, S.; Strauss, W.; Ford, D.; Bernard, K.; Boccia, R.; Li, J.; Allen, L.F. Efficacy and safety of IV ferumoxytol for adults with iron deficiency anemia previously unresponsive to or unable to tolerate oral iron. *Am. J. Hematol.* **2014**, *89*, 7–12. [CrossRef] [PubMed]
124. New recommendations to manage risk of allergic reactions with intravenous iron-containing Medicines. Available online: http://www.ema.europa.eu/ema/index.jsp?curl=pages/news_and_events/news/2013/06/news_detail_001833.jsp&mid=WC0b01ac058004d5c1 (accessed on 27 November 2017).
125. Highlights of prescription information. Available online: http://www.accessdata.fda.gov/drugsatfda_docs/label/2013/203565s000lbl.pdf (accessed on 7 November 2017).
126. Auerbach, M.; Rodgers, G.M. Intravenous iron. *N. Engl. J. Med.* **2007**, *357*, 93–94. [CrossRef] [PubMed]
127. Rampton, D.; Folkersen, J.; Fishbane, S.; Hedenus, M.; Howaldt, S.; Locatelli, F.; Patni, S.; Szebeni, J.; Weiss, G. Hypersensitivity reactions to intravenous iron: Guidance for risk minimization and management. *Haematologia* **2014**, *99*, 1671–1676. [CrossRef] [PubMed]

128. Gisbert, J.P.; Bermejo, F.; Pajares, R.; Perez-Calle, J.L.; Rodriguez, M.; Algaba, A.; Mancenido, N.; de la Morena, F.; Carneros, J.A.; McNicholl, A.G.; et al. Oral and intravenous iron treatment in inflammatory bowel disease: Hematological response and quality of life improvement. *Inflamm. Bowel Dis.* **2009**, *15*, 1485–1491. [CrossRef] [PubMed]

129. Reinisch, W.; Staun, M.; Tandon, R.K.; Altorjay, I.; Thillainayagam, A.V.; Gratzer, C.; Nijhawan, S.; Thomsen, L.L. A randomized, open-label, non-inferiority study of intravenous iron isomaltoside 1000 (Monofer) compared with oral iron for treatment of anemia in IBD (PROCEED). *Am. J. Gastroenterol.* **2013**, *108*, 1877–1888. [CrossRef] [PubMed]

130. Auerbach, M.; Ballard, H. Clinical use of intravenous iron: Administration, efficacy, and safety. Hematology. *ASH Educ. Program Book* **2010**, *2010*, 338–347. [CrossRef] [PubMed]

131. Gomollon, F.; Gisbert, J.P. Intravenous iron in inflammatory bowel diseases. *Curr. Opin. Gastroenterol.* **2013**, *29*, 201–207. [CrossRef] [PubMed]

132. Gomollon, F.; Chowers, Y.; Danese, S.; Dignass, A.; Nielsen, O.H.; Lakatos, P.L.; Lees, C.W.; Lindgren, S.; Lukas, M.; Mantzaris, G.J.; et al. Letter: European Medicines Agency recommendations for allergic reactions to intravenous iron-containing medicines. *Aliment. Pharmacol. Ther.* **2014**, *39*, 743–744. [CrossRef] [PubMed]

133. Chertow, G.M.; Mason, P.D.; Vaage-Nilsen, O.; Ahlmen, J. Update on adverse drug events associated with parenteral iron. *Nephrol. Dial. Transplant.* **2006**, *21*, 378–382. [CrossRef] [PubMed]

134. Khalil, A.; Goodhand, J.R.; Wahed, M.; Yeung, J.; Ali, F.R.; Rampton, D.S. Efficacy and tolerability of intravenous iron dextran and oral iron in inflammatory bowel disease: A case-matched study in clinical practice. *Eur. J. Gastroenterol. Hepatol.* **2011**, *23*, 1029–1035. [CrossRef] [PubMed]

135. Koutroubakis, I.E.; Oustamanolakis, P.; Karakoidas, C.; Mantzaris, G.J.; Kouroumalis, E.A. Safety and efficacy of total-dose infusion of low molecular weight iron dextran for iron deficiency anemia in patients with inflammatory bowel disease. *Dig. Dis. Sci.* **2010**, *55*, 2327–2331. [CrossRef] [PubMed]

136. Rodgers, G.M.; Auerbach, M.; Cella, D.; Chertow, G.M.; Coyne, D.W.; Glaspy, J.A.; Henry, D.H. High-molecular weight iron dextran: A wolf in sheep's clothing? *J. Am. Soc. Nephrol.* **2008**, *19*, 833–834. [CrossRef] [PubMed]

137. Auerbach, M.; Pappadakis, J.A.; Bahrain, H.; Auerbach, S.A.; Ballard, H.; Dahl, N.V. Safety and efficacy of rapidly administered (one hour) one gram of low molecular weight iron dextran (INFeD) for the treatment of iron deficient anemia. *Am. J. Hematol.* **2011**, *86*, 860–862. [CrossRef] [PubMed]

138. Schroder, O.; Mickisch, O.; Seidler, U.; de Weerth, A.; Dignass, A.U.; Herfarth, H.; Reinshagen, M.; Schreiber, S.; Junge, U.; Schrott, M.; et al. Intravenous iron sucrose versus oral iron supplementation for the treatment of iron deficiency anemia in patients with inflammatory bowel disease—A randomized, controlled, open-label, multicenter study. *Am. J. Gastroenterol.* **2005**, *100*, 2503–2509. [CrossRef] [PubMed]

139. Reed, J. *Reed Book: Pharmacy's Fundamental Reference*, 114th ed.; Thompson Reuters: Montvale, NJ, USA, 2010; pp. 1–900.

140. Esposito, B.P.; Breuer, W.; Sirankapracha, P.; Pootrakul, P.; Hershko, C.; Cabantchik, Z.I. Labile plasma iron in iron overload: Redox activity and susceptibility to chelation. *Blood* **2003**, *102*, 2670–2677. [CrossRef] [PubMed]

141. Beigel, F.; Lohr, B.; Laubender, R.P.; Tillack, C.; Schnitzler, F.; Breiteneicher, S.; Weidinger, M.; Goke, B.; Seiderer, J.; Ochsenkuhn, T.; et al. Iron status and analysis of efficacy and safety of ferric carboxymaltose treatment in patients with inflammatory bowel disease. *Digestion* **2012**, *85*, 47–54. [CrossRef] [PubMed]

142. Evstatiev, R.; Marteau, P.; Iqbal, T.; Khalif, I.L.; Stein, J.; Bokemeyer, B.; Chopey, I.V.; Gutzwiller, F.S.; Riopel, L.; Gasche, C. FERGIcor, a randomized controlled trial on ferric carboxymaltose for iron deficiency anemia in inflammatory bowel disease. *Gastroenterology* **2011**, *141*, 846–853. [CrossRef] [PubMed]

143. Evstatiev, R.; Alexeeva, O.; Bokemeyer, B.; Chopey, I.; Felder, M.; Gudehus, M.; Iqbal, T.; Khalif, I.; Marteau, P.; Stein, J.; et al. Ferric carboxymaltose prevents recurrence of anemia in patients with inflammatory bowel disease. *Clin. Gastroenterol. Hepatol.* **2013**, *11*, 269–277. [CrossRef] [PubMed]

144. Kulnigg, S.; Stoinov, S.; Simanenkov, V.; Dudar, L.V.; Karnafel, W.; Garcia, L.C.; Sambuelli, A.M.; D'Haens, G.; Gasche, C. A novel intravenous iron formulation for treatment of anemia in inflammatory bowel disease: The ferric carboxymaltose (FERINJECT) randomized controlled trial. *Am. J. Gastroenterol.* **2008**, *103*, 1182–1192. [CrossRef] [PubMed]

145. Onken, J.E.; Bregman, D.B.; Harrington, R.A.; Morris, D.; Acs, P.; Akright, B.; Barish, C.; Bhaskar, B.S.; Smith-Nguyen, G.N.; Butcher, A.; et al. A multicenter, randomized, active-controlled study to investigate the efficacy and safety of intravenous ferric carboxymaltose in patients with iron deficiency anemia. *Transfusion* **2014**, *54*, 306–315. [CrossRef] [PubMed]

146. Gozzard, D. When is high-dose intravenous iron repletion needed? Assessing new treatment options. *Drug Des. Dev. Ther.* **2011**, *5*, 51–60. [CrossRef] [PubMed]

147. Nordfjeld, K.; Andreasen, H.; Thomsen, L.L. Pharmacokinetics of iron isomaltoside 1000 in patients with inflammatory bowel disease. *Drug Des. Dev. Ther.* **2012**, *6*, 43–51.

148. Auerbach, M.; Strauss, W.; Auerbach, S.; Rineer, S.; Bahrain, H. Safety and efficacy of total dose infusion of 1020 mg of ferumoxytol administered over 15 min. *Am. J. Hematol.* **2013**, *88*, 944–947. [CrossRef] [PubMed]

149. Ford, D.C.; Dahl, N.V.; Strauss, W.E.; Barish, C.F.; Hetzel, D.J.; Bernard, K.; Li, Z.; Allen, L.F. Ferumoxytol versus placebo in iron deficiency anemia: Efficacy, safety, and quality of life in patients with gastrointestinal disorders. *Clin. Exp. Gastroenterol.* **2016**, *9*, 151–162. [PubMed]

150. Schieda, N. Parenteral ferumoxytol interaction with magnetic resonance imaging: A case report, review of the literature and advisory warning. *Insights Imaging* **2013**, *4*, 509–512. [CrossRef] [PubMed]

151. Bailie, G.R. Comparison of rates of reported adverse events associated with i.v. iron products in the United States. *Am. J. Health Syst. Pharm.* **2012**, *69*, 310–320. [CrossRef] [PubMed]

152. Szebeni, J.; Fishbane, S.; Hedenus, M.; Howaldt, S.; Locatelli, F.; Patni, S.; Rampton, D.; Weiss, G.; Folkersen, J. Hypersensitivity to intravenous iron: Classification, terminology, mechanisms and management. *Br. J. Pharmacol.* **2015**, *172*, 5025–5028. [CrossRef] [PubMed]

153. Auerbach, M.; Ballard, H.; Glaspy, J. Clinical update: Intravenous iron for anaemia. *Lancet* **2007**, *369*, 1502–1504. [CrossRef]

154. Chertow, G.M.; Winkelmayer, W.C. On the relative safety of intravenous iron formulations: New answers, new questions. *Am. J. Hematol.* **2010**, *85*, 643–644. [CrossRef] [PubMed]

155. Fishbane, S.; Ungureanu, V.D.; Maesaka, J.K.; Kaupke, C.J.; Lim, V.; Wish, J. The safety of intravenous iron dextran in hemodialysis patients. *Am. J. Kidney Dis.* **1996**, *28*, 529–534. [CrossRef]

156. Auerbach, M.; Coyne, D.; Ballard, H. Intravenous iron: From anathema to standard of care. *Am. J. Hematol.* **2008**, *83*, 580–588. [CrossRef] [PubMed]

157. Boyce, M.; Warrington, S.; Cortezi, B.; Zollner, S.; Vauleon, S.; Swinkels, D.W.; Summo, L.; Schwoebel, F.; Riecke, K. Safety, pharmacokinetics and pharmacodynamics of the anti-hepcidin Spiegelmer Lexaptepid pegol in healthy subjects. *Br. J. Pharmacol.* **2016**, *173*, 1580–1588. [CrossRef] [PubMed]

158. Cooke, K.S.; Hinkle, B.; Salimi-Moosavi, H.; Foltz, I.; King, C.; Rathanaswami, P.; Winters, A.; Steavenson, S.; Begley, C.G.; Molineux, G.; et al. A fully human anti-hepcidin antibody modulates iron metabolism in both mice and nonhuman primates. *Blood* **2013**, *122*, 3054–3061. [CrossRef] [PubMed]

159. Sebastiani, G.; Wilkinson, N.; Pantopoulos, K. Pharmacological targeting of the hepcidin/ferroportin axis. *Front. Pharmacol.* **2016**, *7*, 160–170. [CrossRef] [PubMed]

160. Sun, C.C.; Vaja, V.; Chen, S.; Theurl, I.; Stepanek, A.; Brown, D.E.; Cappellini, M.D.; Weiss, G.; Hong, C.C.; Lin, H.Y.; et al. A hepcidin lowering agent mobilizes iron for incorporation into red blood cells in an adenine-induced kidney disease model of anemia in rats. *Nephrol. Dial. Transplant.* **2013**, *28*, 1733–1743. [CrossRef] [PubMed]

161. Gupta, N.; Wish, J.B. Hypoxia-inducible factor prolyl hydroxylase inhibitors: A potential new treatment for anemia in patients with CKD. *Am. J. Kidney Dis.* **2017**, *69*, 815–826. [CrossRef] [PubMed]

162. Haase, V.H. HIF-prolyl hydroxylases as therapeutic targets in erythropoiesis and iron metabolism. *Hemodial. Int.* **2017**, *21*, S110–S124. [CrossRef] [PubMed]

163. Simpson, R.J.; McKie, A.T. Iron and oxygen sensing: A tale of 2 interacting elements? *Metallomics* **2015**, *7*, 223–231. [CrossRef] [PubMed]

164. Nielsen, O.H.; Ainsworth, M.; Coskun, M.; Weiss, G. Management of iron-deficiency anemia in inflammatory bowel disease: A systematic review. *Medicine* **2015**, *94*, e963–e976. [CrossRef] [PubMed]

165. Lindgren, S.; Wikman, O.; Befrits, R.; Blom, H.; Eriksson, A.; Granno, C.; Ung, K.A.; Hjortswang, H.; Lindgren, A.; Unge, P. Intravenous iron sucrose is superior to oral iron sulphate for correcting anaemia and restoring iron stores in IBD patients: A randomized, controlled, evaluator-blind, multicentre study. *Scand. J. Gastroenterol.* **2009**, *44*, 838–845. [CrossRef] [PubMed]

166. Litton, E.; Xiao, J.; Ho, K.M. Safety and efficacy of intravenous iron therapy in reducing requirement for allogeneic blood transfusion: Systematic review and meta-analysis of randomised clinical trials. *BMJ* **2013**, *347*, f4822. [CrossRef] [PubMed]

167. Fishbane, S. Balance of benefit and risk in intravenous iron treatment in chronic kidney disease. *Semin. Nephrol.* **2016**, *36*, 119–123. [CrossRef] [PubMed]

168. Li, X.; Kshirsagar, A.V.; Brookhart, M.A. Safety of intravenous iron in hemodialysis patients. *Hemodial. Int.* **2017**, *21*, S93–S103. [CrossRef] [PubMed]

169. Macdougall, I.C.; Bircher, A.J.; Eckardt, K.U.; Obrador, G.T.; Pollock, C.A.; Stenvinkel, P.; Swinkels, D.W.; Wanner, C.; Weiss, G.; Chertow, G.M. Iron management in chronic kidney disease: Conclusions from a "Kidney Disease: Improving Global Outcomes" (KDIGO) Controversies Conference. *Kidney Int.* **2016**, *89*, 28–39. [CrossRef] [PubMed]

170. Miskulin, D.C.; Tangri, N.; Bandeen-Roche, K.; Zhou, J.; McDermott, A.; Meyer, K.B.; Ephraim, P.L.; Michels, W.M.; Jaar, B.G.; Crews, D.C.; et al. Intravenous iron exposure and mortality in patients on hemodialysis. *Clin. J. Am. Soc. Nephrol.* **2014**, *9*, 1930–1939. [CrossRef] [PubMed]

171. Zitt, E.; Sturm, G.; Kronenberg, F.; Neyer, U.; Knoll, F.; Lhotta, K.; Weiss, G. Iron supplementation and mortality in incident dialysis patients: An observational study. *PLoS ONE* **2014**, *9*. [CrossRef] [PubMed]

172. Aksan, A.; Isik, H.; Radeke, H.H.; Dignass, A.; Stein, J. Systematic review with network meta-analysis: Comparative efficacy and tolerability of different intravenous iron formulations for the treatment of iron deficiency anaemia in patients with inflammatory bowel disease. *Aliment. Pharmacol. Ther.* **2017**, *45*, 1303–1318. [CrossRef] [PubMed]

173. Gonzalez, A.C.; Pedrajas, C.C.; Marin, P.S.; Benitez, J.M.; Iglesias, F.E.; Salgueiro, R.; Medina, M.R.; Garcia-Sanchez, V. Prevalence of iron deficiency without anaemia in inflammatory bowel disease and impact on health-related quality of life. *Gastroenterol. Hepatol.* **2017**. [CrossRef]

174. Krayenbuehl, P.A.; Battegay, E.; Breymann, C.; Furrer, J.; Schulthess, G. Intravenous iron for the treatment of fatigue in nonanemic, premenopausal women with low serum ferritin concentration. *Blood* **2011**, *118*, 3222–3227. [CrossRef] [PubMed]

175. Cekic, C.; Iepk, S.; Aslan, F.; Akpinat, Z.; Arabul, M.; Topal, F.; Saritas-Yüksel, E.; Alper, E.; Ünsal, B. The effect of intravenous iron treatment on quality of life in inflammatory bowel disease patients with nonanemic iron deficiency. *Gastroenterol. Res. Pract.* **2015**, *2015*. [CrossRef] [PubMed]

176. Eliadou, E.; Kini, G.; Huang, J.; Champion, A.; Inns, S.J. Intrevenous iron replacement improves quality of life in hypoferritinemic inflammatory bowel disease patients with and without anemia. *Dig. Dis.* **2017**, *35*, 444–448. [CrossRef] [PubMed]

177. Favrat, B.; Balck, K.; Breymann, C.; Hedenus, M.; Keller, T.; Mezzacasa, A.; Gasche, C. Evaluation of a single dose of ferric carboxymaltose in fatigued, iron-deficient women—PREFER a randomized, placebo-controlled study. *PLoS ONE* **2014**, *9*, e94217. [CrossRef] [PubMed]

178. Volani, C.; Doerrier, C.; Demetz, E.; Haschka, D.; Paglia, G.; Lavdas, A.A.; Gnaiger, E.; Weiss, G. Dietary iron loading negatively affects liver mitochondrial function. *Metallomics* **2017**, *9*, 1634–1644. [CrossRef] [PubMed]

179. Nielsen, O.H.; Coskun, M.; Weiss, G. Iron replacement therapy: Do we need new guidelines? *Curr. Opin. Gastroenterol.* **2016**, *32*, 128–135. [CrossRef] [PubMed]

180. Rimon, E.; Kagansky, N.; Kagansky, M.; Mechnick, L.; Mashiah, T.; Namir, M.; Levy, S. Are we giving too much iron? Low-dose iron therapy is effective in octogenarians. *Am. J. Med.* **2005**, *118*, 1142–1147. [CrossRef] [PubMed]

181. Ganzoni, A.M. Intravenous iron-dextran: Therapeutic and experimental possibilities. *Schweiz. Med. Wochenschr.* **1970**, *100*, 301–303. [PubMed]

182. Reinisch, W.; Chowers, Y.; Danese, S.; Dignass, A.; Gomollon, F.; Nielsen, O.H.; Lakatos, P.L.; Lees, C.W.; Lindgren, S.; Lukas, M.; et al. The management of iron deficiency in inflammatory bowel disease—An online tool developed by the RAND/UCLA appropriateness method. *Aliment. Pharmacol. Ther.* **2013**, *38*, 1109–1118. [CrossRef] [PubMed]

183. Katsanos, K.H.; Tatsioni, A.; Natsi, D.; Sigounas, D.; Christodoulou, D.K.; Tsianos, E.V. Recombinant human erythropoietin in patients with inflammatory bowel disease and refractory anemia: A 15-year single center experience. *J. Crohn's Colitis* **2012**, *6*, 56–61. [CrossRef] [PubMed]

184. Liu, S.; Ren, J.; Hong, Z.; Yan, D.; Gu, G.; Han, G.; Wang, G.; Ren, H.; Chen, J.; Li, J. Efficacy of erythropoietin combined with enteral nutrition for the treatment of anemia in Crohn's disease: A prospective cohort study. *Nutr. Clin. Pract.* **2013**, *28*, 120–127. [CrossRef] [PubMed]

185. Solomon, S.D.; Uno, H.; Lewis, E.F.; Eckardt, K.U.; Lin, J.; Burdmann, E.A.; de Zeeuw, D.; Ivanovich, P.; Levey, A.S.; Parfrey, P.; et al. Erythropoietic response and outcomes in kidney disease and type 2 diabetes. *N. Engl. J. Med.* **2010**, *363*, 1146–1155. [CrossRef] [PubMed]

186. Drueke, T.B.; Parfrey, P.S. Summary of the KDIGO guideline on anemia and comment: Reading between the (guide)line(s). *Kidney Int.* **2012**, *82*, 952–960. [CrossRef] [PubMed]

187. Sonnweber, T.; Theurl, I.; Seifert, M.; Schroll, A.; Eder, S.; Mayer, G.; Weiss, G. Impact of iron treatment on immune effector function and cellular iron status of circulating monocytes in dialysis patients. *Nephrol. Dial. Transplant.* **2011**, *26*, 977–987. [CrossRef] [PubMed]

188. Weiss, G.; Carver, P.L. Role of divalent metals in infectious disease susceptibility and outcome. *Clin. Microbiol. Infect.* **2018**, *24*, 16–23. [CrossRef] [PubMed]

189. Sazawal, S.; Black, R.E.; Ramsan, M.; Chwaya, H.M.; Stoltzfus, R.J.; Dutta, A.; Dhingra, U.; Kabole, I.; Deb, S.; Othman, M.K.; et al. Effects of routine prophylactic supplementation with iron and folic acid on admission to hospital and mortality in preschool children in a high malaria transmission setting: Community-based, randomised, placebo-controlled trial. *Lancet* **2006**, *367*, 133–143. [CrossRef]

190. Soofi, S.; Cousens, S.; Iqbal, S.P.; Akhund, T.; Khan, J.; Ahmed, I.; Zaidi, A.K.; Bhutta, Z.A. Effect of provision of daily zinc and iron with several micronutrients on growth and morbidity among young children in Pakistan: A cluster-randomised trial. *Lancet* **2013**, *382*, 29–40. [CrossRef]

191. Besarab, A.; Bolton, W.K.; Browne, J.K.; Egrie, J.C.; Nissenson, A.R.; Okamoto, D.M.; Schwab, S.J.; Goodkin, D.A. The effects of normal as compared with low hematocrit values in patients with cardiac disease who are receiving hemodialysis and epoetin. *N. Engl. J. Med.* **1998**, *339*, 584–590. [CrossRef] [PubMed]

192. Locatelli, F.; Pisoni, R.L.; Combe, C.; Bommer, J.; Andreucci, V.E.; Piera, L.; Greenwood, R.; Feldman, H.I.; Port, F.K.; Held, P.J. Anaemia in haemodialysis patients of five European countries: Association with morbidity and mortality in the Dialysis Outcomes and Practice Patterns Study (DOPPS). *Nephrol. Dial. Transplant.* **2004**, *19*, 121–132. [CrossRef] [PubMed]

193. Bircher, A.J.; Auerbach, M. Hypersensitivity from intravenous iron products. *Immunol. Allergy Clin.* **2014**, *34*, 707–723. [CrossRef] [PubMed]

194. Schaefer, B.; Wurtinger, P.; Finkenstedt, A.; Braithwaite, V.; Viveiros, A.; Effenberger, M.; Sulzbacher, I.; Moschen, A.; Griesmacher, A.; Tilg, H.; et al. Choice of high-dose intravenous iron preparation determines hypophosphatemia risk. *PLoS ONE* **2016**, *11*, e0167146. [CrossRef] [PubMed]

195. Goldsmith, J.R.; Sartor, R.B. The role of diet on intestinal microbiota metabolism: Downstream impacts on host immune function and health, and therapeutic implications. *J. Gastroenterol.* **2014**, *49*, 785–798. [CrossRef] [PubMed]

196. Oustamanolakis, P.; Koutroubakis, I.E.; Messaritakis, I.; Malliaraki, N.; Sfiridaki, A.; Kouroumalis, E.A. Serum hepcidin and prohepcidin concentrations in inflammatory bowel disease. *Eur. J. Gastroenterol. Hepatol.* **2011**, *23*, 262–268. [CrossRef] [PubMed]

197. Ganz, T. Systemic iron homeostasis. *Physiol. Rev.* **2013**, *93*, 1721–1741. [CrossRef] [PubMed]

198. Katsanos, K.; Cavalier, E.; Ferrante, M.; Van Hauwaert, V.; Henckaerts, L.; Schnitzler, F.; Katsaraki, A.; Noman, M.; Vermeire, S.; Tsianos, E.V.; et al. Intravenous iron therapy restores functional iron deficiency induced by infliximab. *J. Crohn's Colitis* **2007**, *1*, 97–105. [CrossRef] [PubMed]

199. Nielsen, O.H.; Ainsworth, M.A. Tumor necrosis factor inhibitors for inflammatory bowel disease. *N. Engl. J. Med.* **2013**, *369*, 754–762. [CrossRef] [PubMed]

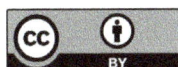

nutrients

MDPI

Review

Effects of an Acute Exercise Bout on Serum Hepcidin Levels

Raúl Domínguez [1,2,*], Antonio Jesús Sánchez-Oliver [3,4], Fernando Mata-Ordoñez [5], Adrián Feria-Madueño [6], Moisés Grimaldi-Puyana [4], Álvaro López-Samanes [7] and Alberto Pérez-López [2,8]

[1] College of Health Sciences, Alfonso X El Sabio University, 29691 Madrid, Spain
[2] College of Health Sciences, Isabel I University, 09004 Burgos, Spain; alberto_perez-lopez@hotmail.com
[3] Department of Sports, Faculty of Sports Sciences, University Pablo Olavide, 4103 Sevilla, Spain; asanchez@upo.es
[4] Department of Physical Education and Sports, Faculty of Educational Sciences, University of Seville, 41013 Sevilla, Spain; mgrimaldi@us.es
[5] NutriScience España, 14010 Córdoba, Spain; fmataor@gmail.com
[6] University Study Center Cardenal Spinola, CEU San Pablo University, 41930 Sevilla, Spain; aferia@ceuandalucia.es
[7] School of Physiotherapy, School of Health Sciences, Francisco de Vitoria, 28223 Pozuelo, Spain; alvaro.lopez@ufv.es
[8] Department of Medicine and Medical Specialties and Department of Biomedical Sciences, Faculty of Medicine and Health Sciences, University of Alcalá, 28871 Madrid, Spain
*   Correspondence: rdomiher@uax.es; Tel.: +34-695-182-853

Received: 26 December 2017; Accepted: 11 February 2018; Published: 14 February 2018

Abstract: Iron deficiency is a frequent and multifactorial disorder in the career of athletes, particularly in females. Exercise-induced disturbances in iron homeostasis produce deleterious effects on performance and adaptation to training; thus, the identification of strategies that restore or maintain iron homeostasis in athletes is required. Hepcidin is a liver-derived hormone that degrades the ferroportin transport channel, thus reducing the ability of macrophages to recycle damaged iron, and decreasing iron availability. Although it has been suggested that the circulating fraction of hepcidin increases during early post-exercise recovery (~3 h), it remains unknown how an acute exercise bout may modify the circulating expression of hepcidin. Therefore, the current review aims to determine the post-exercise expression of serum hepcidin in response to a single session of exercise. The review was carried out in the Dialnet, Elsevier, Medline, Pubmed, Scielo and SPORTDiscus databases, using hepcidin (and "exercise" or "sport" or "physical activity") as a strategy of search. A total of 19 articles were included in the review after the application of the inclusion/exclusion criteria. This search found that a single session of endurance exercise (intervallic or continuous) at moderate or vigorous intensity (60–90% VO_{2peak}) stimulates an increase in the circulating levels of hepcidin between 0 h and 6 h after the end of the exercise bout, peaking at ~3 h post-exercise. The magnitude of the response of hepcidin to exercise seems to be dependent on the pre-exercise status of iron (ferritin) and inflammation (IL-6). Moreover, oxygen disturbances and the activation of a hypoxia-induced factor during or after exercise may stimulate a reduction of hepcidin expression. Meanwhile, cranberry flavonoids supplementation promotes an anti-oxidant effect that may facilitate the post-exercise expression of hepcidin. Further studies are required to explore the effect of resistance exercise on hepcidin expression.

Keywords: iron metabolism; anemia; endurance; exercise; sport performance

1. Introduction

Iron deficiency is one of the most prevalent nutritional disturbances in the world [1]; in 2008, it affected 24.8% of the global population [2]. Exercise has been shown to play a regulative role in iron metabolism; in fact, the prevalence of iron deficiency is higher in physically active individuals and athletes, in comparison to the sedentary population [3,4]. Notably, higher deficiencies in iron storage have been reported in adolescents [5], and especially in female athletes [6], who exhibit a prevalence of iron disorders that is up to five to seven times higher than their male homologues [7].

Iron is an essential component of hemoglobin and myoglobin, which ensure oxygen supply to the skeletal muscle [8]. In the myocyte, iron is a component of several mitochondrial proteins that are integral parts of the electron transport chain, and facilitate the activation of oxidative phosphorylation [9]. Hence, the deficiency of this mineral may compromise the energy metabolism system by increasing the contribution of glycolysis [9], and reducing energy efficiency [10,11], performance [9–13], and adaptations to training [14–16].

The absorption–degradation rate determines iron status [17]. In humans, the dietary reference for iron intake is estimated to be 8 mg·day^{-1} and 18 mg·day^{-1} for adult males and females, respectively; while the degradation rate is ~0.896 mg·day^{-1} and ~1.42 mg·day^{-1} for men and women, respectively [18]. Nonetheless, both iron intake and degradation are affected by several factors, particularly in physically active individuals where hemolysis, hematuria, gastrointestinal bleeding and sweat are frequent and promote the loss and degradation of iron [19].

In response to hyperthermia, acidosis, hypoglycemia, and hemoconcentration, induced by exercise, an increase in osmotic resistance [20] and erythrocyte elasticity loss may occur [21]. Traditionally, exercise-induced hemolysis has been documented in those exercise modes or sports that involve a continuous mechanical impact, thus promoting the compression of red blood cells [22]. Nevertheless, some studies have found that hemolysis can be produced by other exercise activities, such as rowing [7] or cycling [23], which do not entail mechanical impacts. In hemolysis, iron is released from damaged erythrocytes, and although some can be recycled, a great amount is excreted [24]. This iron degradation increase the daily intake needed of this mineral to ensure the homeostasis of the absorption–degradation rate.

Furthermore, blood flow redistribution during exercise leads to hypoxia and necrosis of the digestive tract cells by stimulating iron degradation via gastrointestinal bleeding [25]. Exercise intensity and volume play a crucial role in iron loss through gastrointestinal bleeding [26] and hematuria [27]. Hence, exercise demands determine the iron degradation rate and subsequently modulate the necessity of increasing iron intake to ensure a homeostasis of iron concentration in the organism. The elevated iron demand during exercise apparently coincides with lower heme and non-heme iron absorption [28,29]; therefore, the identification of the mechanisms by which exercise regulates iron metabolism, particularly in physically active individuals, will enable the elaboration of strategies to restore or maintain the homeostasis of this mineral.

Dietary iron is absorbed in the duodenum by enterocytes of the duodenal lining, which is a process mediated by the heme carrier protein 1 (HCP1) [30]. Before being absorbed, a ferric reductase enzyme on the enterocyte brush border, the duodenal cytochrome B561 (DcytB), is required to reduce the ferric ions (Fe^{3+}) to a ferrous form (Fe^{2+}) [31]. Then, the protein divalent metal transporter 1 (DMT1) transports the Fe^{2+} across the enterocyte's cell membrane into the cell [32]. Inside the enterocyte, iron can be either be stored as ferritin [33] or transported across the cell membrane by ferroportin action [34,35] in cooperation with hephaestin (HP) [36] and possibly plasma homologue ceruloplasmin [37]. Once in circulation, iron is transported by transferrins that allow its uptake by different tissues. Among them, the red bone marrow uptakes iron via the transferrin receptor, and promotes red blood cells formation [38]. Moreover, iron derived from hemolysis caused by macrophages is recycled and returned into the circulation via HP, prior to the ferroportin reductase activity. All of these processes are mediated by hepcidin, which is an essential protein in human iron metabolism [39]. Hepcidin is an antimicrobial peptide hormone codified by the hepcidin antimicrobial peptide (HAMP) gene and mainly synthesized by hepatocytes, although macrophages, neutrophils, and cancerous cells can express hepcidin as well [40,41]. Hepcidin stimulates the degradation of ferroportin and the divalent metal transporter 1 (DMT1) by endocytosis [42], which reflects the ability of hepcidin to reduce iron absorption and recycling mechanisms [39,43], compromising the formation of new erythrocytes in the bone marrow. Consequently, a chronic elevation of hepcidin concentrations leads to iron-deficient states [44], while the decrease in this peptide hormone is associated with high levels of iron [45], as is found in hemochromatosis patients [44]. Therefore, hepcidin and iron storage work in a control feedback system by which the elevation of iron regulates the synthesis of hepcidin [46]; while a decrease in the concentrations of this mineral (e.g., anemia) promotes a reduction in hepcidin production, facilitating iron absorption from the diet and reutilization from hemolysis, and increasing erythropoiesis and iron reserves [47].

Iron metabolism is also mediated by oxygen availability. Under an oxidative stress-induced condition (e.g., high-intensity exercise), the increased reactive nitrogen and oxygen species (RNOS) production causes a reduction in iron due to the affinity of iron for H_2O_2, which stimulates the formation of free radicals [48,49]. Inflammation and hypoxic exposure promote RNOS production, which regulates the expression of hepcidin [50]. Besides, the upregulation of pro-inflammatory cytokines under an inflammatory or hypoxic condition also enables the iron/H_2O_2-based formation of hydroxyl radicals, inducing ferritin degradation and iron release in erythrocytes [51,52]. Thus, the circulating concentrations of pro-inflammatory cytokines such as interleukin (IL)-6 may play a regulative role in iron metabolism [53,54], and as a consequence in hepcidin synthesis [55].

Therefore, regular physical activity has been proposed as a confounding variable that mediates the iron–hepcidin balance in humans [3,4,56]. However, the effects of a single session of exercise on the circulating expression of hepcidin have been scarcely analyzed before 2010 [28,57]. In those pioneer studies, an increase in urine concentrations of hepcidin at 3 h to 24 h after an exhausting exercise bout [28,57] suggest that circulating hepcidin and iron expressions could be modulated by acute bouts of exercise. Since chronic exercise bouts can promote an upregulation of hepcidin concentrations, compromising iron reserves and decreasing dietary iron absorption [19], this review aims to explore the potential regulative role of a single session of exercise on the serum hepcidin levels as a mediator of the iron absorption–degradation rate in humans.

2. Materials and Methods

Two researchers utilized the Dialnet, Elsevier, Medline, Pubmed, Scielo, and SPORTDiscus databases to search for articles published between 2010 and 1 August 2017. The strategy employed was hepcidin (Concept 1) AND "exercise" OR "sport" OR "physical activity" (Concept 2). The following exclusion criteria were used to ensure the purpose of the present review:

- Date of publication: before 2010.
- Language: publication in other language than English or Spanish.
- Type of manuscript: others than experimental studies, such as editorials, letters to the editor, congress or meetings abstracts, reviews, or meta-analyses.
- Type of study: other studies than those performed in an adult population (>18 years old) in which serum hepcidin had been analyzed in response to an acute exercise bout, such as in vitro or in vivo studies in animals, studies in children or an adolescent population, or studies in which serum hepcidin was either not measured or reported in response to an acute exercise bout.

The flow diagram of the inclusion/exclusion process of the systematic review is illustrated in Figure 1. A total of 313 studies were obtained from the initial search. Initially, articles published in a language other than Spanish or English, before 2010, non-experimental studies (duplicates, letters, proceedings of congresses, and reviews or meta-analyses) or duplicated articles (*n* = 140) were excluded. Then, the full-text examination of the 82 potentially eligible studies retrieved 21 articles that satisfied the inclusion/exclusion criteria. A brief description of the studies included in the current review is presented in Table 1, where the pre-exercise versus post-exercise differences of the circulating concentration of hepcidin are reported for each study.

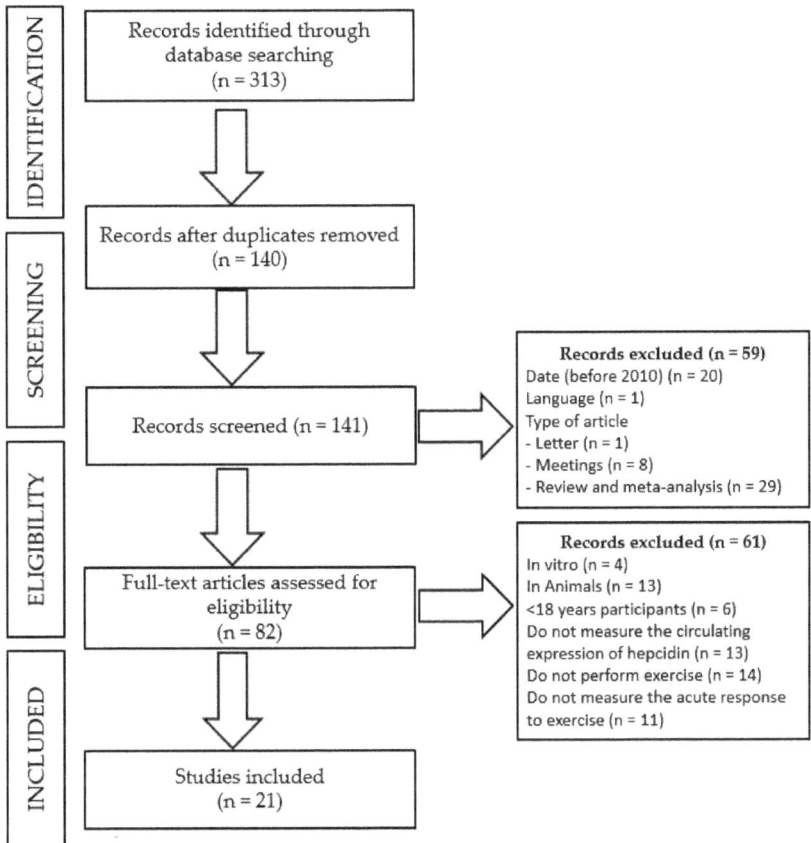

Figure 1. Flow diagram of the inclusion/exclusion process of the systematic review.

From the articles included, the following information was obtained: authors, date of publication, sample size, population characteristics, exercise protocol, pre-exercise conditions, and time-points at which circulating levels of hepcidin were measured.

3. Results

3.1. Population Characteristics

A total of 321 participants were recruited in the 21 studies included in the present review (Table 1). Notably, the majority of the participants were males ($n = 272$) compared to females ($n = 50$), and the fitness stratification revealed the inclusion of athletes ($n = 224$), physically active ($n = 38$) participants, and sedentary participants ($n = 10$). Although the athlete population included judokas ($n = 11$), the vast majority of them performed endurance modalities ($n = 222$). Among the endurance athletes, 162 participants reported having a moderate–high level of training (VO_{2peak}, from 60.1 ± 1.4 to 69.8 ± 5.7 mL·kg^{-1}·min^{-1}), while 60 individuals took part in international competitions (walkers, $n = 24$; rowers, $n = 36$).

Table 1. Summary of the studies investigating the effect of a single session of exercise on serum hepcidin levels.

Author	Population	n	Exercise Protocol	Experimental Conditions	TP	Main Outcomes — Pre vs. Post Comparison	EC Differences
Sim et al. [35]	Trained males (66 ± 2 mL·kg⁻¹·min⁻¹ VO₂peak)	10	Endurance exercise (Running and Cycling) EP1: 60 min at 65% VO₂peak EP2: 8 × (3 min at 85% VO₂peak & 1.5 min at 60% VO₂peak)	EC1: EP1 running EC2: EP1 cycling EC3: EP2 running EC4: EP2 cycling	Pre & 3 h PE	* EC1: −1.6 vs. −2.4 nmol·L⁻¹ * EC2: −1.1 vs. −2.0 nmol·L⁻¹ * EC3: −1.5 vs. −2.5 nmol·L⁻¹ * EC4: −1.2 vs. −2.6 nmol·L⁻¹	ANOVA time but no EC or interaction effect
Badenhorst et al. [36]	Male endurance athletes (63 ± 6 mL·kg⁻¹·min⁻¹ VO₂peak)	10	Endurance exercise (Running) 8 × (3 min at 85% VO₂peak & 1.5 min at 60% VO₂peak)	EC1: Recovery in hypoxia (FiO₂ ~0.1513) EC1: Recovery in normoxia (FiO₂ ~0.2093)	Pre, 3 h & 24 h PE	Pre vs. 3 h PE * EC1: 3.2 ± 1.9 vs. 5.4 ± 3.2 nM * EC2: 3.2 ± 1.2 vs. 7.4 ± 4.0 nM	ANOVA time and interaction effect. EC1 > EC2 at 3 h PE
Badenhorst et al. [39]	Male endurance athletes (63 ± 4 mL·kg⁻¹·min⁻¹ VO₂peak)	11	Endurance exercise (Running) 8 × (3 min at 85% VO₂peak & 1.5 min at 60% VO₂peak)	EC1: Early recovery (0.5 & 2 h) CHO (1.2 g·kg⁻¹) intake EC2: Late recovery (2 & 4 h PE) CHO (1.2 g·kg⁻¹) intake	Pre, 3 h, 5 h PE.	Pre vs. 3 h PE * EC1: 6.5 ± 9.6 vs. 9.7 ± 3.5 nM * EC2: 4.9 ± 2.4 vs. 7.5 ± 3.6 nM Pre vs. 5 h PE * EC1: 6.5 ± 9.6 vs. 9.7 ± 3.8 nM * EC2: 4.9 ± 2.4 vs. 7.1 ± 3.5 nM	ANOVA time, but no EC or interaction effect
Sim et al. [44]	Male endurance athletes (63 ± 4 mL·kg⁻¹·min⁻¹ VO₂peak)	11	Endurance exercise (Running) 8 × 3 min at 85% VO₂peak & 1.5 min at 60% VO₂peak	EC1: 24 h LCHO (3 g·kg·day⁻¹) EC2: 24 h HCHO (10 g·kg·day⁻¹)	Pre & 3 h PE	* EC1: (Pre vs. 3 h PE): 4.2 ± 3.6 vs. 6.4 ± 5.1 nM * EC2 (Pre vs. 3 h PE): 2.2 ± 1.1 vs. 4.1 ± 3.2 nM	ANOVA time and EC, but no interaction effect. * EC1 > EC2 at pre-exercise NS, EC1 vs. EC2 at 3 h PE
Badenhorst et al. [61]	Male endurance athletes (64 ± 5 mL·kg⁻¹·min⁻¹ VO₂peak)	12	Endurance exercise (Running) Two sessions of 45 min at 65% VO₂peak (day 1 -D1- and day 7 -D7-)	EC1: LCHO diet (3 g·kg·day⁻¹) EC2: HCHO diet (8 g·kg·day⁻¹)	Pre & 3 h PE	EC1 (Pre vs. 3 h PE): * D1: 2.0 ± 1.9 vs. 7.6 ± 6.0 nM * D7: 1.8 ± 1.2 vs. 6.5 ± 4.7 nM EC2 (Pre vs. 3 h PE): * D1: 1.9 ± 1.2 vs. 6.4 ± 3.9 nM * D7: 1.8 ± 0.7 vs. 5.4 ± 3.4 nM	ANOVA time, but no EC or interaction effect
Sim et al. [62]	Male endurance athletes (60 ± 1 mL·kg⁻¹·min⁻¹ VO₂peak)	11	Endurance exercise (Running) 90 min at 75% VO₂peak	EC1: CHO drink (6%) during exercise EC2: H₂O during exercise	Pre, 3 h, 24 h PE	Pre vs. 3 h PE: * EC1: −3.0 vs. −7.5 nm·l⁻¹ * EC2: −3.0 vs. −9.0 nm·l⁻¹	ANOVA time but no EC or interaction effect
Newlin et al. [63]	PA females (52 ± 4 mL·kg⁻¹·min⁻¹ VO₂peak)	11	Endurance exercise (Running) 65% VO₂peak	EC1: 60 min EC2: 120 min	Pre, 0 h, 3 h, 6 h, 9 h & 24 h PE	* EC1 (Pre vs. 3 h PE): −0.7 vs. −1.9 nmol·L⁻¹ * EC2 (Pre vs. 3 h PE): −1.1 vs. −4.5 nmol·L⁻¹	ANOVA time and EC, but no interaction effect * EC2 > EC1 at 3 h PE
Peeling et al. [64]	Endurance athletes (60 ± 7 mL·kg⁻¹·min⁻¹ VO₂peak).	♂38 ♀54	Endurance exercise (5 Running sessions) S1: 8 × 3 min at 85% VO₂peak S2: 5 × 4 min at 90% VO₂peak S3: 90 min at 75% VO₂peak S4: 40 min at 75% VO₂peak S5: 40 min at 65% VO₂peak	Baseline SF: SF1 (n = 12): SF ≤ 30 μg·L⁻¹ SF2 (n = 8): SF = 30–50 μg·L⁻¹ SF3 (n = 14): SF = 50–100 μg·L⁻¹ SF4 (n = 20): SF ≥ 100 μg·L⁻¹	Pre & 3 h	SF1: −0.8 vs. −1.2 nM SF2: −2.1 vs. −4.5 nM SF3: −2.2 vs. −5.3 nM SF4: −3.5 vs. −8.0 nM	ANOVA effect (Pre and 3 h PE) particularly SF1 compared with SF2, SF3, and SF4. Baseline SF and 3 h PE hepcidin correlation (r = 0.52).

Table 1. *Cont.*

Author	Population	n	Exercise Protocol	Experimental Conditions	TP	Main Outcomes Pre vs. Post Comparison	EC Differences
Burden et al. [65]	ID endurance athletes without anemia (64 ± 6 mL·kg^{-1}·min^{-1} VO$_{2peak}$)	♂6 ♀9	Endurance exercise (Running) Incremental test at day 1 (D1), day 2 (D2) and week 4 (W4)	EC1: Iron (500 mg) EC2: Placebo	Pre, 0 h, and 3 h PE	EC1 (Pre vs. 3 h PE) * D2: −110 vs. −210 ng·mL^{-1} * W4: −70 vs. −210 ng·mL^{-1} NS increase in EC2.	D1: ANOVA time effect D2: ANOVA time and EC effect (EC1 > EC2) W4: ANOVA time and EC effect (EC1 > EC2 at 3 h post-exercise).
Dahlquist et al. [66]	Male trained cyclists (67 ± 4 mL·kg^{-1}·min^{-1} VO$_{2peak}$)	10	Endurance exercise (Running) 8×3 min at 85% & 1.5 min at 60% VO$_{2peak}$	EC1: PE CHO (75 g), Pro (25 g), vit.D (5000 IU) & vit.K(100 mcg). EC2: PE CHO (75 g), Pro (25 g) EC3: Placebo PE	Pre, 0 h, and 3 h PE	Pre vs. 0 h PE * EC1: 14.2 ± 14.9 vs. 17.8 ± 19.8 nmol·L^{-1} * EC2: 9.9 ± 8.9 vs. 11.8 ± 10.2 nmol·L^{-1} * EC3: 10.4 ± 14.6 vs. 10.1 ± 7.7 nmol·L^{-1} Pre vs. 3 h PE * EC1: 14.2 ± 14.9 vs. 25.4 ± 11.9 nmol·L^{-1} * EC2: 9.9 ± 8.9 vs. 22.3 ± 13.4 nmol·L^{-1} * EC3: 10.4 ± 14.6 vs. 22.6 ± 15.6 nmol·L^{-1}	ANOVA time (in EC1 & EC2), but no EC effect or interaction
Díaz et al. [67]	Trained males (70 ± 6 mL·kg^{-1}·min^{-1} VO$_{2peak}$)	10	Endurance exercise (Running) 90 min at 75% VO$_{2peak}$ in before (D1) & after the 4 W intervention (W4).	EC1: Vit.C (500 mg) & vit.E (400 IU). EC2: Placebo	Pre, 0 h, 3 h, 6 h, and 10 h PE	Pre vs. 3 h PE (D1 & W4) * EC1: −11 vs. −26 ng·mL^{-1} EC2: NR Pre vs. 6 h PE (D1 & W4) * EC1: −11 vs. −21 ng·mL^{-1} EC2: NR	ANOVA time but no EC effect.
Sim et al. [68]	PA females who ingested oral contraceptives (53 ± 2 mL·kg^{-1}·min^{-1} VO$_{2peak}$)	10	Endurance exercise (Running) 40 min at 75% VO$_{2peak}$	EC1: D2 to D4 of the menstrual cycle EC2: D12 to D14 of the menstrual cycle	Pre and 3 h PE	* EC1: −1.9 vs. −4.4 ng·mL^{-1} * EC2: −3.6 vs. −4.5 ng·mL^{-1}	ANOVA time, but no EC or interaction effect.
Peeling et al. [69]	Male race-walker athletes (64.9 ± 5.9 mL·kg^{-1}·min^{-1} VO$_{2peak}$)	24	Endurance exercise (Running) 25 km race-walk at 75% VO$_{2peak}$	EC1: All walkers EC2: lower 50th percentile EC3: higher 50th percentile	Pre and 3 h PE	* EC1: 1.1 ± 1.0 vs. 8.6 ± 5.3 nM * EC2: 0.8 ± 0.5 vs. 6.0 ± 3.6 nM * EC3: 1.5 ± 1.2 vs. 11.3 ± 5.4 nM	EC differences at baseline. Correlation of hepcidin at 3 h with SF ($r = 0.69$) and serum iron ($r = 0.62$).
Govus et al. [70]	Endurance athletes (males 61 ± 6.3 and females 55.0 ± 5.9 mL·kg^{-1}·min^{-1} VO$_{2max}$)	♂7 ♀6	Endurance exercise (Running) 5×4 min of 90% VO$_{2peak}$ & 1.5 min of passive recovery	EC1: hypoxia (F$_i$O$_2$ ~0.1450) EC2: normoxia (F$_i$O$_2$ ~0.2093)	Pre, 0 h, and 3 h PE	Pre vs. 3 h PE * EC1: 3.32 vs. 4.17 nmol·L^{-1} * EC2: 2.85 vs. 4.44 nmol·L^{-1}	ANOVA time, but no EC or interaction effect.

Table 1. Cont.

Author	Population	n	Exercise Protocol	Experimental Conditions	TP	Main Outcomes	
						Pre vs. Post Comparison	EC Differences
Govus et al. [1]	Endurance athletes (65.6 ± 8.1 mL·kg⁻¹·min⁻¹ VO$_{2max}$)	♂6 ♀4	Endurance exercise (Running) 6 × 1000 m at 90% VO$_{2peak}$ & 1.5 min of passive recovery	EC1: hypoxia (F$_i$O$_2$ ~0.155) EC2: normoxia (600 m) EC3: 11 days of LHTL EC4: Iron (105 mg) plus Vit.C (1000 mg) during 1 week before the trials in participants with baseline SF < 100 μg·L⁻¹ (EG1, n = 5), no placebo was provided for those with SF ≥ 100 μg·L⁻¹ (EG2, n = 5).	Pre and 3 h PE	* EC1: aumento (NR) * EC2: aumento (NR) * EC3: Pre 4.0 vs. 2.0 nmol·L⁻¹	Baseline differences between EG1 and EG2 were observed. ANOVA time but not EC1, EC2, EC4 or interaction effect. ANOVA time and EC3 effect
Antosiewicz et al. [2]	Trained males (judokas) ^{A} and sedentary males ^{B} (NR VO$_{2peak}$)	11 ^{A} 10 ^{B}	Endurance exercise (Cycling) 3 × 30 s all-out sprint. (4.5 min recovery)	Population comparison: Trained (A) vs. Sedentary population (B).	Pre, 1 h, 24 h, and 5 D	Pre vs. 1 h PE * A: 64.7 ± 14.5 vs. 83.3 ± 23.3 ng·L⁻¹ * B: 32.0 ± 5.5 vs. 43.7 ± 9.9 ng·L⁻¹	NR ANOVA differences A > B at baseline and 1 h PE
Tomczyk et al. [3]	PA males (50.1 ± 8.9 mL·kg⁻¹·min⁻¹ VO$_{2peak}$)	17	Endurance exercise (Cycling) Incremental test before (D1) & after 3 days (D3) intervention	EC1: Glucose (4 g·kg⁻¹) EC2: Fructose (4 g·kg⁻¹) EC3: Placebo	Pre & 1 h PE	EC1: −61.3 vs. −60.0 ng·mL⁻¹ EC2: −61.5 vs. −57.5 ng·mL⁻¹ EC3: −56.0 vs. −63.5 ng·mL⁻¹	NR ANOVA EC effect
Kasprowicz et al. [4]	Trained males (NR VO$_{2peak}$ not specified)	6	Endurance exercise (Running) 100 km ultramarathon		Pre, 25 km, 50 km, 75 km, 0 h, and 14 h PE	Pre: −43 ng·L⁻¹ 25 km: −45 ng·L⁻¹ 50 km: −45 ng·L⁻¹ 75 km: −43 ng·L⁻¹ 0 h PE or 100 km: −44.5 ng·L⁻¹ 14 h PE: −48 ng·L⁻¹	
Skarpanska-Stejnborn et al. [5]	Male rowing athletes (NS VO$_{2peak}$)	20	Endurance exercise (Rowing) 2000 m maximum test		Pre, 0 h, and 1D PE	Pre: −0.25 ng·mL⁻¹ * 0 h PE: −1.7 ng·mL⁻¹ # 1D PE: −0.25 ng·mL⁻¹	
Skarpanska-Stejnborn et al. [6]	Male rowing athletes (NS VO$_{2peak}$)	16	Endurance exercise (Rowing) 2000 m maximum test before (D1) and after 6 weeks (W6)	EC1: Cranberry extract (648 mg·day⁻¹) (n = 9) EC2: Placebo (n = 7)	Pre, 0 h, and 1D PE	D1: NS W6 (Pre vs. 0 h Post): * EC1: −0.12 vs. −0.32 ng·dL⁻¹ EC2: −0.11 vs. −0.15 ng·dL⁻¹	No ANOVA time or EC effect EC1: ANOVA time effect
Robson-Ansley et al. [7]	Trained males (58 ± 4 mL·kg⁻¹·min⁻¹ VO$_{2max}$)	9	Endurance exercise (Running) 120 min at 60% VO$_{2peak}$ & 5 km time trial	EC1: CHO drink (6%) during exercise EC2: H$_2$O during exercise	Pre, 0 h, and 24 h PE	Pre vs. 0 h PE * EC1: −20 vs. −34 pg·mL⁻¹ * EC2: −15 vs. −30 pg·mL⁻¹	ANOVA time but no EC or interaction effect Plasma hepcidin and IL-6 correlation at 0 h PE: EC1 (R^2 = 0.13), EC2 (R^2 = 0.65).

Anemia = hemoglobin > 12.0 g·L⁻¹; ANOVA = analysis of variance; CHO = carbohydrate; D = day; EC = experimental condition; EG = experimental group; EP = exercise protocol; F$_i$O$_2$ = fraction of inspired oxygen; H = men; HCHO = high CHO diet; ID = iron deficiency (serum ferritin < 30–40 μg·L⁻¹); LCHO = low CHO diet; LHTL = live high, train low; min = minute; NR = not reported; PA = physically active; PE = post-exercise; S = exercise session; SF = serum ferritin; TP = time-points of which serum hepcidin levels was measured; VO$_{2peak}$ = peak oxygen consumption; W = week. ~estimated from the figures provided by authors; * significant differences compared to pre-exercise levels; # significant differences compared to 0 h post-exercise.

3.2. Measurements of Serum Hepcidin Levels

The majority of the studies included in the present review, 15 out of the 21 studies, assessed the circulating expression of hepcidin at 3 h post-exercise [23,58–71]. Moreover, the circulating fraction of serum hepcidin levels was evaluated immediately [63,64,70], as well as at 1 h [72,73], 5 h [59], 6 h [63,71], 9 h [63], 10 h [64], 14 h [74], 24 h [62,72,75,76], and five days after the exercise bout [72].

3.3. Serum Hepcidin Levels in Response to Exercise

An upregulation of the circulating expression of hepcidin was observed in 20 of the 21 studies analyzed [23,58–73,75–77]. Regarding the different time-points utilized, hepcidin increased immediately post-exercise in four out of five studies [66,75–77]; while after 1 h [72,73], 3 h [23,58–71], and 5 h [59], all of the studies reported a significant increase compared to baseline levels.

In addition, Diaz et al. [67] found an elevated hepcidin expression at 6 h post-exercise, while Newlin et al. [63] reported no significant increase. However, during the late recovery period post-exercise (>6 h), hepcidin concentration was not altered in any of the time-points analyzed at 9 h [63], 10 h [67], 14 h [74], 24 h [62,72,75,76], and five days after the exercise bout [72].

3.3.1. Effect of Exercise Type on Serum Hepcidin Levels

In all of the 21 studies included, the circulating hepcidin expression was measured in response to endurance exercise. Running was the endurance exercise utilized in the majority of the studies (16 out of 19) [23,58–68,70,71,74,77], while cycling [23,72,73], rowing [75,76], and athletic walking were used as well [61]. Continuous and intervallic endurance exercise strategies were carried out, and all of the studies reported a significant upregulation of serum hepcidin, except Kasprovicz et al. [74], where an ultramarathon did not modify hepcidin concentrations in blood during or after the race. No human studies assessed hepcidin expression after a resistance exercise session.

3.3.2. Effect of Exercise Intensity on Serum Hepcidin Levels

After an incremental exercise up to exhaustion, plasma hepcidin levels were upregulated in physically active males at 1 h post-exercise [73], while in national and international athletes, this effect was observed at 3 h post-exercise, but only in the group that was injected with iron [65]. In response to supramaximal intensity, three consecutive 30 s all-out sprints (Wingate test, 4.5 min recovery) reported a hepcidin elevation at 1 h post-exercise in untrained males and judokas [72]. Moreover, Skarpanska-Stejnborn et al. [75,76] examined the response of hepcidin to a 2000 m rowing race in elite rowers. Both studies found a significant increase in circulating hepcidin immediately post-exercise; however, that effect was attenuated after the administration of a cranberry extract [76].

Submaximal intensity also increased hepcidin levels. A single session of 40 min to 120 min of endurance exercise performed at 60% [77], 65% [23,61,63,64], or 75% VO_{2peak} [62,64,67–69] upregulated the expression of hepcidin. On the other hand, Kasprovicz et al. [74] did not find an elevation of hepcidin levels at 25 km, 50 km, 75 km, and 100 km of an ultramarathon race.

In addition to continuous exercise, different intensities of intervallic endurance exercise were evaluated. The most extended protocol utilized was eight series of 3 min running at 85% VO_{2peak} followed by 1.5 min at 60% VO_{2peak}, which reported a significant increase in hepcidin levels from 3 h to 5 h post-exercise [23,58–60,64,66]. Similarly, four more intervallic protocols were undergone [64,70–72]. In Peeling et al. [64] and Govus et al. [70], five series of 4 min each of running at 90% VO_{2peak} were performed, Govus et al. [71] analyzed six series of 1000 m at 90% VO_{2peak}, while in the previously mentioned study from Antosiewicz et al. [72], three consecutive Wingate tests were carried out. These four studies reported a significant upregulation of hepcidin concentration in blood from 1 h to 3 h post-exercise [64,70–72].

Finally, only two studies compared the effects of different exercise intensities on hepcidin expression [23,64]. In Peeling et al. [64], according to pre-exercise levels of iron, five running sessions were evaluated: (1) eight series of 3 min at 85% VO_{2peak}; (2) five series of 4 min at 90% VO_{2peak}; (3) 90 min at 75% VO_{2peak}; (4) 40 min at 75% VO_{2peak}; and (5) 40 min at 65% VO_{2peak}. In this study, the ferritin levels in blood determined the circulating concentrations of hepcidin post-exercise. While in Sim et al. [23], two sessions of cycling and running of 40 min at 65% or 85% VO_{2peak} were compared, and no differences were observed between groups or modalities.

3.3.3. Effect of Exercise Duration on Serum Hepcidin Levels

The duration of a single session of exercise on the serum hepcidin levels was also examined. Peeling et al. [64] did not find significant differences in the circulating levels of hepcidin of endurance athletes after a running session composed of 40 min or 90 min at 75% VO_{2peak}. Meanwhile, Newlin et al. [63] observed higher hepcidin levels in physically active females after 120 min of running at 65% VO_{2max} compared to 60 min at the same intensity. Similarly, an increase in hepcidin levels was observed after 40 min [64,68], 45 min [61], 60 min [23,63], 90 min [62,64,67], and 120 min [63,77] of endurance exercise performed at 60% to 75% VO_{2peax}. However, Kasprovicz et al. [74] did not report any significant alteration of hepcidin levels during or after a 100 km ultramarathon race (~10 h long).

3.3.4. Effect of Diet and Supplementation on the Response of Serum Hepcidin Levels to Exercise

In 10 of the 19 studies, the serum hepcidin levels were investigated in response to a diet or supplementation administration. Carbohydrates (CHO) ingestion was manipulated in seven studies [59–62,66,73,77]. During the 24 h before the exercise session, Badenhorst et al. [60] observed that a low CHO diet (3 g of CHO/kg of body mass) stimulated a higher response of serum hepcidin compared to a high CHO diet (10 g of CHO/kg of bm). However, later studies did not find significant differences on serum hepcidin levels after the ingestion of either 3 g, 4 g, or 8 g of CHO/kg of body mass [53,63]. The ingestion of CHO during exercise (6% CHO beverage) [62,77] or 2 h to 4 h post-exercise (1.2 g of CHO/kg of bm) [59] were not effective strategies to alter serum hepcidin in response to endurance exercise. Equally, CHO with protein supplementation alone or in combination with vitamins D and K did not modify the expression of serum hepcidin [66].

The effect of iron [65], vitamins C and E [66], and cranberry extract supplementation [76] on the response of serum hepcidin to endurance exercise were also investigated. As expected, iron injection treatment over seven weeks (500 mg·day^{-1} of intravenous iron) increased the circulating expression of hepcidin compared to a placebo [65]. Besides, cranberry extract (648 mg·day^{-1}) supplementation over six weeks caused an attenuation of hepcidin increase in response to an incremental test [76]. In contrast, four weeks supplementation with vitamin C (500 mg·day^{-1}) and E (400 international units·day^{-1}) did not alter the circulating expression of hepcidin post-exercise.

3.3.5. Effect of Hypoxia on the Response of Circulating Hepcidin to Exercise

In two different experimental designs, Govus et al. [70,71] did not find significant differences in serum hepcidin levels after intervallic endurance exercise (five series of 4 min or six series of 1000 min at 90%, respectively) performed in severe acute hypoxia (fraction of inspired oxygen, F_IO_2 ~0.145 and ~0.155, respectively) compared to normoxic conditions. In fact, in Govus et al. [71], prior exposure to a hypoxia condition (11 days) did not alter the exercise-induced response of serum hepcidin.

In contrast, Badenhorst et al. [58] observed that acute hypoxia exposure (F_IO_2 ~0.1513) during passive recovery after eight series of 3 min running at 85% VO_{2peak} followed by 1.5 min at 60% VO_{2peak} produced an attenuated response of serum hepcidin at 3 h post-exercise compared to normoxic conditions (F_IO_2 ~0.2093).

4. Discussion

4.1. Effect of Exercise Type, Intensity, and Duration on the Circulating Expression of Hepcidin

Although hemolysis has been traditionally associated with the mechanical impact produced in some types of exercise (e.g., running) [78], other exercise modes (e.g., swimming, cycling, or rowing) have also been shown to promote the lysis of erythrocytes [22]. Thus, the amount of exercise-induced red blood cells determines the rupture of these cells, in a process that allows iron to be released. Since elevated concentrations of free iron stimulate the hepatic production and the release of hepcidin, several studies have investigated the effects of different exercise types on circulating hepcidin expression. Endurance exercise upregulates the circulating fraction of hepcidin after running [23,58–68,74,77], cycling [23,72,73], rowing [75,76], or walking [69]. However, only one study compared two endurance exercise types, running and cycling, in response to moderate and high-intensity exercise protocols [23]. The study did not observe significant differences between any of the experimental groups, supporting the theory that that exercise-induced hepcidin upregulation may occur in response to hemolysis not promoted by mechanical impact.

In contrast, evidence is scarce regarding the effects of resistance exercise on hepcidin concentrations. In rodents, compared to endurance, resistance training has been presented as a better strategy for improving blood hemoglobin concentration in iron-deficient rats, potentially due to an increased heme synthesis [79,80]. Remarkably, this type of exercise seems to promote an elevation of iron absorption caused by an increase of recycled iron [81]. Nevertheless, despite the promising results of resistance exercise in iron metabolism [82], the effects of this exercise type—whether alone or in combination with endurance exercise—on hepcidin concentrations remains to be elucidated in humans.

In general, endurance exercise induced an increase on serum hepcidin levels during the early recovery phase post-exercise (~3 h). The present review supports that pattern of response, since an upregulation of hepcidin was found in the 13 studies in which hepcidin was evaluated at 3 h post-exercise [23,58–71]. Nonetheless, several studies reported increases in hepcidin concentrations before and after 3 h post-exercise; in fact, an upregulation of hepcidin levels was found in close proximity to the end of the exercise session (≤1 h) [64,72,73,75–77], as well as during the late recovery phase post-exercise (5–6 h) [59,67]. These studies suggest that the response of serum hepcidin levels to exercise may occur immediately post-exercise, peaking at ~3 h and returning to baseline levels at ~6 h post-exercise.

Intensity is another variable that modifies the magnitude of the adaptations promoted by exercise [83,84]. In this regard, continuous and intervallic endurance exercise sessions were performed at different intensities to determine the response of hepcidin to exercise. Sim et al. [23] compared two sessions of 40 min at 65% or 85% VO_{2peak} of both cycling and running, and reported a significant increase in circulating hepcidin at 3 h post-exercise. However, no intensity effect was found in either of the two endurance exercise modalities [23]. Likewise, in response to different exercise intensities, from 60% to 90% of VO_{2peak}, a similar elevation of circulating hepcidin concentration was reported [23,58–61,63–67,69–73,75–77]. Thus, moderate-to-high-intensity endurance exercise stimulates an analogous hepcidin response, suggesting that intensity may not be a major determinant of hepcidin response to endurance exercise. Nevertheless, it remains unknown whether lower intensities (<60 VO_{2peak}) may provoke an upregulation of serum hepcidin levels.

On the other hand, the duration of the endurance exercise session has been proposed to play a role in exercise-induced hepcidin. Newlin et al. [63] compared the duration of two endurance exercise sessions, 120 min versus 60 min, at the same intensity—65% VO_{2max}—in physically active women (52.1 ± 3.9 mL·kg^{-1}·min^{-1} VO_{2peak}). After the 120 min session, participants reported an elevation of hepcidin concentrations, while no differences between groups were observed for iron or ferritin status [63]. In contrast, Peeling et al. [64] did not find such an exercise duration-response of the circulating levels of hepcidin, when 40 min versus 90 min of endurance exercise at 75% VO_{2peak} were compared in athletes, who were previously divided according to their baseline levels of serum ferritin. Since 120 min of endurance exercise at 65% VO_{2max} may be an exhausting task for a physically active population compared to 90 min at 75% VO_{2peak} in athletes, fatigue-dependent mechanisms (e.g., reduced muscle glycogen availability) may explain the divergent response of circulating hepcidin in both studies. Nevertheless, in Kasprowicz et al. [74], hepcidin expression was not significantly modified during or after a 100-km ultramarathon run (~10 h), which seems to discard the fatigue-dependent mechanisms of hepcidin release. Therefore, exercise-induced hepcidin may not respond in a duration-dependent manner; in fact, the baseline status of some factors (e.g., ferritin) may play a critical role.

4.2. Effect of Diet and Supplementation on the Response of Circulating Hepcidin to Exercise

The influence of diet or supplementation strategies on the exercise-induced hepcidin expression have also been investigated [59,62,65–67,73,76,77].

In rodents, iron retention is decreased by lactose, sucrose, glucose, and starch ingestion [85], while fructose increased iron deposition, potentially due to a chelation-related mechanism. In humans, the influence of CHO on iron absorption and as a modifier of iron storage has been evaluated as well [59–62,66,73,77]. In contrast to animal studies, the pre-exercise manipulation of CHO in diet [52,53,63] or as a supplement during [62,77] or post-exercise [59] did not significantly alter the hepcidin expression in response to endurance exercise. Notably, Tomczyk et al. [73] compared three days of supplementation (4 $g \cdot kg^{-1} \cdot day^{-1}$) of glucose and fructose on an incremental test, and no increase in hepcidin levels were observed in any of the groups. Thus, the role of CHO in iron absorption and deposition may not be mediated by hepcidin in humans.

Furthermore, several vitamins have been administered as potential modulators of serum hepcidin. At baseline, vitamin D was shown to reduce serum hepcidin expression by ~30% in a healthy population [86] and in patients with chronic renal diseases [87], while vitamin K may also act in decreasing inflammatory markers and its deleterious effects [66,88]. However, only one study analyzed the effects of these two vitamins on the exercise-induced concentrations of hepcidin. In highly-trained cyclists (67.4 $\pm$ 4.4 $mL \cdot kg^{-1} \cdot min^{-1}$ VO_{2max}), Dahlquist et al. [66] observed a similar increase in hepcidin levels after a single session of intervallic endurance exercise prior to CHO and protein supplementation alone or in combination with vitamins D and K. Also, the antioxidant effects of vitamin C and E were evaluated, and non-significant differences in the hepcidin response to exercise after 28 days of supplementation with vitamin C (5 $mg \cdot day^{-1}$) and E (400 $IU \cdot day^{-1}$) were reported [67]. Consequently, the anti-toxicity and antioxidant capacity of these vitamins (C, D, E, and K) may not interfere with serum hepcidin levels rising post-exercise.

In contrast, cranberry flavonoids may mediate in the hepcidin response to exercise. Skarpanska-Stejnborn et al. [76] found that six weeks of cranberry extract supplementation (648 $mg \cdot day^{-1}$) abrogated the increased expression of circulating hepcidin at 3 h after an extenuating 2000 m rowing test. Flavonoids are an abundant nutraceutical compound of cranberries that have been shown to promote oxidative [89], antioxidant, and anti-inflammatory effects [90,91]. Thus, despite the lack of effects reported by vitamin C and E supplementation [67], hepcidin production may be regulated by a decreased oxidative stress [48], caused by the administration of cranberry flavonoids [66]. Nonetheless, further studies are required to delineate how polyphenols may regulate hepcidin and iron metabolism in response to exercise.

Finally, since hepcidin and iron storage work in a controlled feedback system [46,47], it is expected that a diet or a supplement rich in iron may produce an upregulation of the post-exercise levels of hepcidin as an attempt to ensure iron homeostasis. Accordingly, in iron-deficient athletes, the intravenous injection of iron (500 $mg \cdot day^{-1}$ over seven weeks) stimulated an increased response of serum hepcidin and ferritin expressions post-exercise compared to a placebo, an effect that was preserved at four weeks post-treatment [65]. Previously, iron supplementation has been used as strategy to improve ventilatory thresholds, VO_{2max}, and energetic efficiency in iron-deficient athletes [92,93]; still, the effect of iron supplementation on performance has been questioned [94]. In this regard, the Burden et al. [65] study seems to suggest that in iron-deficient athletes, iron supplementation (500 mg·day^{-1}) provokes a transitory elevation of this mineral, despite the absence of a direct improvement in performance [65,95]. Of note, moderate doses of iron supplementation (24 mg·day^{-1}) have also been reported as effectively increasing serum hepcidin in iron deficient-athletes [96]. Thus, these findings indicate that ferritin deficiency determines the response of hepcidin to endurance exercise, and accordingly, iron supplementation may activate a counter-regulative mechanism by which hepcidin is released into circulation after a single session of endurance exercise.

4.3. A Mechanistic Approach to Exercise-Induced Hepcidin Expression

4.3.1. Iron Status

The increase of the serum hepcidin in response to exercise has been commonly attributed to an increased inflammatory status [50]. In iron-deficient rodents, lipopolysaccharide treatment produced a reduction on the mRNA expression of hepatic HAMP, IL-6, and TNF-α, suggesting that an iron deficit may blunt hepcidin expression in response to inflammatory inducers [97]. In humans, the anemia of inflammation patients showed greater circulating hepcidin concentrations at baseline, as compared to their healthy iron-deficient homologues [98,99]. In fact, under an elevated inflammatory state, non-anemic individuals reported higher hepcidin levels compared with an anemic population [100]. In regards to exercise, Peeling et al. [64] found that hepcidin did not respond to exercise in those athletes with pre-exercise levels of serum ferritin < 30 µg·L^{-1}, but in contrast, an upregulation of hepcidin concentrations post-exercise was observed in those individuals who reported higher levels of ferritin at baseline [64]. Supporting this idea, in iron-deficient athletes (serum ferritin < 30–40 µg·L^{-1} and hemoglobin > 12.0 g·L^{-1}), iron supplementation facilitates the post-exercise elevation of hepcidin in blood [65]. Therefore, these studies, together with those in which iron supplementation have induced a greater increase in hepcidin response to exercise compared to placebo, indicate that despite the relevant role of inflammation as a hepcidin activator, the pre-exercise iron status may be a master regulator of this exercise-induced liver-derived hormone. Hence, when a pathological or non-pathological iron deficit occurs, exercise-induced hepcidin is blunted, at least in part. Consequently, since the magnitude of response of hepcidin to exercise seems to be dependent on ferritin levels and subsequently to iron stores, the normalization of these parameters is essential in order to further explore the effects of exercise in the regulation of the iron-hepcidin relationship.

4.3.2. Inflammation

Although iron deficit appears to determine post-exercise hepcidin expression, an increase in the inflammatory status also mediates the exercise-induced upregulation of hepcidin in non-iron deficient populations [50,57].

In hepatocyte cells, systemic inflammation diseases or infections facilitate the activation of hepcidin via the IL-6/STAT3 signaling pathway [50,101]. The Jak/STAT signaling pathway is stimulated by several cytokines (e.g., IL-6 or IL-15) in different cell types that mainly promote pro-inflammatory and anti-inflammatory effects [53]. In rodents, cyclosporine A administrated after an exhausting endurance exercise session produced a decrease in plasma IL-6 and the transcriptional expression of IL-6 inhibitory signaling (SOCS3 and IL-6 receptor alpha) and hepcidin in hepatocytes, immediately and 2 h post-exercise, respectively [102]. However, in the study, the mRNA and protein expression of IL-6, the protein expression of hepcidin, and the iron status were not reported [92], which confounds the role of pro-inflammatory factors as mediators of exercise-induced hepcidin. Adding an extra layer of complexity, cyclosporine A produces diverse effects depending on the cell type [103,104]. While in macrophages, cyclosporine A administration stimulates a downregulation of IL-6 protein, it does not stimulate mRNA expression [103]; in human skeletal muscle, cyclosporine A promotes an upregulation of the IL-6 expression, and a decrease of the TNF-α expression [105], thus questioning the role of IL-6 as a pro-inflammatory activator of hepcidin expression.

In the past decade, IL-6 was identified as a myokine that is increased in response to exercise, depending on glucose availability, and the intensity and duration of the exercise bout [106–108]. IL-6 has been shown to exert several endocrine effects when it is released by skeletal muscle in response to exercise; among them, IL-6 promotes anti-tumorigenic [99,109] and anti-inflammatory effects [110,111]. In humans, the acute elevation of the circulating expression of IL-6 is associated with increased IL-1rα and IL-10 expressions [111], and reduced TNF-α production [110]. These studies suggest a critical role for skeletal muscle-derived IL-6 in leukocyte trafficking, promoting anti-inflammatory effects. Thus, the elevation of the circulating fraction of IL-6 in response to exercise may not reflect a pro-inflammatory function of this cytokine. In fact, the transcriptional upregulation of IL-6 inhibitory signals (SOCS3 and IL-6rα) in hepatocyte cells, observed by Banzet et al. [102], may be interpreted as a counteracting mechanism by which in response to an elevation of muscle-derived IL-6 in blood, these cells acutely reduce IL-6 uptake, thereby allowing the anti-inflammatory effects of this myokine.

Nevertheless, although the post-exercise elevation of the circulating fraction of IL-6 may have an anti-inflammatory function, the chronic increase of this cytokine is known to be an inflammatory marker found in different populations [112,113]. The coexisting pro-inflammatory and anti-inflammatory roles have been observed in other myokines. IL-15 has been shown to exert pro-inflammatory effects when this cytokine is chronically elevated at baseline [114]; however, in response to a single session of exercise, serum IL-15 is upregulated [115,116], and instead of showing a pro-inflammatory function, this myokine exerts oxidative effects in adipose tissue [117]. In fact, in physically active individuals, the baseline concentration of IL-15 and its cognate alpha receptor were decreased in a population with inflammatory-related diseases [118], potentially suggesting an anti-inflammatory effect of IL-15 in response to chronic exercise bouts.

Consequently, instead of the post-exercise increase, the chronic elevation of IL-6 at baseline may be interpreted as a pro-inflammatory signal that may activate the inflammatory-induced expression of hepcidin observed in vitro and in vivo [46,119]. Supporting this idea, only one study has reported a correlation between circulating IL-6 and hepcidin levels immediately post-exercise [77], while the majority of the studies did not find such a relationship [23,59–64,66,68,69,72,75] or showed contrasting results between these two factors [58,64,65,67,73,74,76]. Therefore, pre-exercise iron status and IL-6 levels may be responsible for the association reported by Robson-Ansley et al. [77] immediately post-exercise. Thus, in addition to the iron status, pre-exercise IL-6 concentrations need to be monitored in order to understand the hepcidin response to exercise.

4.3.3. Hypoxia

Endurance athletes are routinely exposed to hypoxic environments in order to improve performance (VO_{2max}) due to the increase in red blood cell population induced by this condition [120,121]. Intriguingly, hypoxia is another regulator of hepcidin synthesis [50]. Cell culture studies have found that the activation of the hypoxia-induced factors (HIF-1α and HIF-2α) suppress hepcidin activity, and increase the bioavailability of iron-stimulating erythropoiesis [122]. Moreover, in rodents, an increased erythropoiesis stress has shown to stimulate the expression of erythroferrone (ERFE), a hormone that suppresses serum hepcidin, facilitating iron mobilization and absorption [123]. In humans, prolonged exposure to a reduced fraction of inspired oxygen has been shown to attenuate hepcidin expression [124], and thus increase ferroportin and DMT1 expressions [125].

This reduction in hepcidin may be solely attributed to the iron requirements of erythropoietin (EPO) stimulation in the bone marrow to promote erythrocytes production [125–128]. Hence, the regulative role of hypoxia-inducible factors in hepcidin synthesis has been questioned, since EPO is a key activator of HIF-1α and HIF-2α [129]. Nevertheless, the hypoxia-inducible factor may be stimulated by different signaling mechanisms [130], and potentially have an EPO-independent effect on hepcidin production [126,131]. HIF-1α and HIF-2α are considered sensors of iron and oxygen status; thus, when the availability of iron or oxygen is reduced, for instance in response to high-intensity exercise, these two factors are upregulated [21]. In addition, ERFE may also play a critical role in hepcidin metabolism [123]; however, human studies are required to evaluate this idea.

In this context, Badenhorst et al. [58] analyzed the effect of exposure to a severe acute hypoxia (F_IO_2 ~0.1513, simulated altitude of ~2900 m) compared to normoxia (F_IO_2 ~0.2093) during the recovery period of an intervallic endurance exercise session (eight series of 3 min of running at 85% VO_{2peak} followed by 1.5 min at 60% VO_{2peak}). The study found a decreased in serum hepcidin levels at 3 h post-exercise, which supports the suppressing effects of hypoxia in the synthesis of hepcidin. In contrast, Govus et al. [70] observed that exposure to severe acute hypoxia (F_IO_2 ~0.1450, simulated altitude of ~3000 m) during intervallic endurance exercise (five series of 4 min of running at 90% VO_{2peak}) increased serum hepcidin levels at 3 h post-exercise, similar to the normoxic condition. A potential explanation for these apparently opposing studies may reside in the exposure time to the hypoxic gas mixture. While in Govus et al. [70], participants were only exposed to hypoxia during the exercise session (~31 min), in Badenhorst et al. [58], participants were exposed during 3 h post-exercise.

Live high–train low (LHTL) is a recurrent strategy among athletes to improve their endurance performance [132]. To assess the effect of this strategy on hepcidin metabolism, Govus et al. [71] analyzed serum hepcidin responses to an intervallic endurance session (six series of 1000 m of running at 90% VO_{2peak}) in hypoxia (F_IO_2 ~0.155) or normoxic conditions (600 m of altitude), before and after 11 days of LHTL. Supporting the previous work performed by this research group [70], the exposure to either hypoxia or normoxia during exercise produced a similar increase in serum hepcidin at 3 h post-exercise in trained runners [71]. Despite the lack of an acute response, Govus et al. [71] found that the LHTL strategy increased serum hepcidin levels at baseline, but not in response to exercise. This suppression of serum hepcidin levels may be interpreted as a mechanism to facilitate dietary or recycled (hemolysis) iron in order to maintain the erythropoietic demands promoted by hypoxia exposure [125]. Interestingly, in Govus et al. [71], pre-exercise serum ferritin levels seem to influence the hepcidin response to exercise after LHTL, which supports that the magnitude of response of serum hepcidin to exercise performed in either normoxia [56,57] or hypoxia, Govus et al. [71] is dependent on pre-exercise ferritin levels.

Therefore, exercise-induced disturbances in oxygen availability or the upregulation of hypoxia-inducible factors may attenuate hepcidin synthesis at baseline, while in response to exercise, the normalization of serum ferritin is required in order to examine the effect of hypoxia in human hepcidin metabolism.

4.3.4. Oral Contraceptives

Iron deficiency is five to seven times more prevalent in female than in male athletes [6,7], at least in part as a consequence of elevated iron losses due to menstruation [133]. Besides, differences in sex hormones may also explain the gender difference in iron deficit, since estrogen hormones have shown to stimulate hepcidin synthesis [134], while testosterone promotes an inhibition of hepcidin [135,136].

In this regard, in an attempt to regulate menstrual bleeding, some female athletes use contraceptive pills, despite them containing estradiol, a sex hormone belonging to the subgroup of estrogens, which may affect the expression of hepcidin. In this regard, Sim et al. [68] assessed the effect of contraceptive pills administration on the hepcidin response in a group of physically active women after 40 min of endurance exercise at 70% VO_{2peak}, during days 2–4 and 12–14 of the menstrual cycle. A significant increase in serum hepcidin was found 3 h post-exercise in the two periods of the menstrual cycle measured, and no interaction of contraceptive pill was reported. Although this study did not reveal significant differences, the circulating concentrations of sex hormones deserve further attention as a potential hepcidin synthesis modulator.

5. Conclusions

Iron deficiency is a frequent event in the career of athletes, and it may cause deleterious effects on endurance performance, reducing oxygen availability, and exercise economy. Hepcidin has been presented as a crucial regulator of the iron absorption–degradation rate, which may be mediated by exercise. The current review revels that a single session of 30 min to 120 min of endurance exercise (intervallic or continuous) at moderate or high intensity (60% to 90% of VO_{2peak}) facilitates the upregulation of the circulating expression of hepcidin between 0 h and 6 h post-exercise, peaking after 3 h of the end of the exercise session.

The magnitude of response of hepcidin to exercise seems to be dependent on the pre-exercise status of iron (ferritin levels) and the circulating expression of pro-inflammatory cytokines (prominently IL-6). Moreover, oxygen disturbances and the upregulation of hypoxia-inducible factors during or post-exercise may also regulate the expression of hepcidin. Lastly, iron and cranberry flavonoid supplementation have been found to modulate the post-exercise circulating expression of hepcidin, while vitamins C, D, E, or K, and CHO supplementation, did not alter the expression of hepcidin. Further studies are required to explore the effect of different exercise types (resistance exercise), intensities (<60 VO_{2peak}), and volumes (chronic exercise bouts) on the circulating fraction of hepcidin.

Author Contributions: R.D. and F.M.-O. conceived and designed the review; A.F.-M. and M.G.-P. selected the articles included; A.J.S.-O., A.F.-M., M.G.-P. and A.P.-L. analyzed the articles included and prepared figures and tables; R.D., A.J.S.-O., F.M.-O., A.L.-S. and A.P.-L. drafted the manuscript; A.F.-M. and M.G.-P. revised the manuscript; R.D., A.J.S.-O., F.M.-O., A.F.-M., M.G.-P., A.L.-S. and A.P.-L. approved the final version of the manuscript.

Conflicts of Interest: The authors declare no conflict of interest.

References

1. Umbreit, J. Iron deficiency: A concise review. *Am. J. Hematol.* **2005**, *78*, 225–331. [CrossRef] [PubMed]
2. De Benois, B.; McLean, E.; Egli, I.; Cogswell, M. *Worldwide Prevalence of Anaemia 1993–2005. WHO Database on Anaemia*; World Health Organization: Geneve, Switzerland, 2008.
3. Gropper, S.S.; Blessing, D.; Dunham, K.; Barksdale, M. Iron status of female collegiate athletes involved in different sports. *Biol. Trace Elem. Res.* **2006**, *109*, 1–14. [CrossRef]
4. Woolf, K.; St Thomas, M.M.; Hahn, N.; Vaughan, L.A.; Carlson, A.G.; Hinton, P. Iron status in highly active and sedentary young women. *Int. J. Sport Nutr. Exerc. Metab.* **2009**, *1*, 519–535. [CrossRef]
5. Zoller, H.; Vogel, W. Iron supplementation in athletes-first do no harm. *Nutrition* **2004**, *20*, 615–619. [CrossRef] [PubMed]
6. Sinclair, L.M.; Hinton, P.S. Prevalence of iron deficiency with and without anemia in recreationally active men and women. *J. Am. Diet. Assoc.* **2005**, *105*, 975–978. [CrossRef] [PubMed]
7. DellaValle, D.M.; Haas, J.D. Impact of iron depletion without anemia on performance in trained endurance athletes at the beginning of a training season: A study of female collegiate rowers. *Int. J. Sport Nutr. Exerc. Metab.* **2011**, *21*, 501–506. [CrossRef] [PubMed]
8. Lukaski, H.C. Vitamin and mineral status: Effects on physical performance. *Nutrition* **2004**, *20*, 632–644. [CrossRef] [PubMed]
9. Hinton, P.S. Iron and the endurance athlete. *Appl. Physiol. Nutr. Metab.* **2014**, *39*, 1012–1018. [CrossRef] [PubMed]
10. DellaValle, D.M. Iron supplementation for female athletes: Effects on iron status and performance outcomes. *Curr. Sports Med. Rep.* **2013**, *12*, 234–239. [CrossRef] [PubMed]
11. DellaValle, D.M.; Haas, J.D. Iron supplementation improves energetic efficiency in iron-depleted female rowers. *Med. Sci. Sports Exerc.* **2014**, *46*, 1204–1215. [CrossRef] [PubMed]
12. Garvican, L.A.; Lobigs, L.; Telford, R.; Fallon, K.; Gore, C.J. Haemoglobin mass in an anaemic female endurance runner before and after iron supplementation. *Int. J. Sports Physiol. Perform.* **2011**, *6*, 137–140. [CrossRef] [PubMed]
13. Latunde-Dada, G.O. Iron metabolism in athletes—Achieving a gold standard. *Eur. J. Haematol.* **2013**, *90*, 10–15. [CrossRef] [PubMed]
14. Brownlie, T.T.; Utermohlen, V.; Hinton, P.S.; Giordano, C.; Haas, J.D. Marginal iron deficiency without anemia impairs aerobic adaptation among previously untrained women. *Am. J. Clin. Nutr.* **2002**, *75*, 734–742. [CrossRef] [PubMed]

15. Brownlie, T.T.; Utermohlen, V.; Hinton, P.S.; Haas, J.D. Tissue iron deficiency without anemia impairs adaptation in endurance capacity after aerobic training in previously untrained women. *Am. J. Clin. Nutr.* **2004**, *79*, 437–443. [CrossRef] [PubMed]

16. Valko, M.; Jomova, K.; Rhodes, C.; Kuča, K.; Musílek, K. Redox- and non-redoxmetal-induced formation of free radicals and their role in human disease. *Arch. Toxicol.* **2016**, *90*, 1–37. [CrossRef] [PubMed]

17. Domínguez, R.; Garnacho-Castaño, M.V.; Maté-Muñoz, J.L. Effect of hepcidin on iron metabolism in athletes. *Nutr. Hosp.* **2014**, *30*, 1218–1231. [PubMed]

18. Food and Nutrition Board. *Dietary Reference Intakes for Vitamin A, Vitamin K, Arsenic, Boron, Chromium, Copper, Iodine, Iron, Manganese, Molybdenum, Nickel, Silicon, Vanadium, and Zinc*; National Academy Press: Washington, DC, USA, 2001; pp. 290–393.

19. Peeling, P.; Dawson, B.; Goodman, C.; Landers, G.; Trinder, D. Athletic induced iron deficiency: New insights into the role of inflammation, cytokines and hormones. *Eur. J. Appl. Physiol.* **2008**, *103*, 381–391. [CrossRef] [PubMed]

20. Reeder, B.; Wilson, M. The effects of pH on the mechanism of hydrogen peroxide and lipid hydroperoxide consumption by myoglobin: A role for the protonated ferryl species. *Free Radic. Biol. Med.* **2001**, *30*, 1311–1318. [CrossRef]

21. Yusof, A.; Leithauser, R.M.; Roth, H.J.; Finkernagel, H.; Wilson, M.T.; Beneke, R. Exercise-induced hemolysis is caused by protein modification and most evident during the early phase of an ultraendurance race. *J. Appl. Physiol.* **2007**, *102*, 582–586. [CrossRef] [PubMed]

22. Telford, R.D.; Sly, G.J.; Hahn, A.G.; Cunningham, R.B.; Bryant, C.; Smith, J.A. Footstrike is the major cause of hemolysis during running. *J. Appl. Physiol.* **2003**, *94*, 38–42. [CrossRef] [PubMed]

23. Sim, M.; Dawson, B.; Landers, G.; Swinkels, D.W.; Tjasma, H.; Trinder, D.; Peeling, P. Effect of exercise modality and intensity on postexercise interleukin-6 and hepcidina levels. *Int. J. Sports Nutr. Exerc. Metab.* **2013**, *23*, 178–186. [CrossRef]

24. Pattini, A.; Schena, F.; Guidi, G.C. Serum ferritin and serum iron after cross-country and roller sky endurance races. *Eur. J. Appl. Physiol. Occpat. Phyisiol.* **1990**, *61*, 55–60. [CrossRef]

25. Babic, Z.; Papa, B.; Sikirika-Bosnjakovic, M.; Prkacin, I.; Misigoj-Durakovic, M.; Katicic, M. Occult gastrointestinal bleeding in rugby players. *J. Sports Med. Phys. Fit.* **2011**, *41*, 399–402.

26. Lampre, J.W.; Slavin, J.L.; Apple, F.S. Iron status of active women and effect of running a marathon on bowel function and gastrointestinal blood-loss. *Int. J. Sport Med.* **1991**, *12*, 173–179. [CrossRef] [PubMed]

27. Lopes, T.R.; Kirsztajn, G.M. Renal analysis in 75 km ultra-marathon participants. *Acta Paul. Enferm.* **2009**, *22*, 487–489. [CrossRef]

28. Roecker, L.; Meier-Buttermilch, R.; Bretchel, L.; Nemeth, E.; Ganz, T. Iron-regulatory protein hepcidin is increased in female athletes after a marathon. *Eur. J. Appl. Physiol.* **2005**, *95*, 569–571. [CrossRef] [PubMed]

29. Troadec, M.B.; Lainé, F.; Daniel, V.; Rochcongar, P.; Ropert, M.; Cabillic, F.; Perrin, M.; Morcet, J.; Loréal, O.; Olbina, G.; et al. Daily regulation of serum and urinary hepcidin is not influenced by submaximal cycling exercise in humans with normal iron metabolism. *Eur. J. Appl. Physiol.* **2010**, *106*, 435–444. [CrossRef] [PubMed]

30. Le Blanc, S.; Garrick, M.D.; Arredondo, M. Heme carrier protein 1 transports heme and is involved in heme-Fe metabolism. *Am. J. Physiol. Cell Physiol.* **2012**, *302*, 1780–1785. [CrossRef] [PubMed]

31. McKie, A.T.; Barrow, D.; Latunde-Dada, G.O.; Rolfs, A.; Sager, G.; Mudaly, E.; Mudaly, M.; Richardson, C.; Barlow, D.; Bomford, A.; et al. An iron-regulated ferric reductase associated with the absorption of dietary iron. *Science* **2001**, *291*, 1755–1759. [CrossRef] [PubMed]

32. Gunshin, H.; Mackenzie, B.; Berger, U.V.; Gunshin, Y.; Romero, M.F.; Boron, W.F.; Nussberger, S.; Gollan, J.L.; Hediger, M.A. Cloning and characterization of a mammalian proton-coupled metal-ion transporter. *Nature* **1997**, *388*, 482–488. [CrossRef] [PubMed]

33. Donker, A.E.; Raymakers, R.A.P.; Vlasveld, L.T.; van Barneveld, T.; Terink, R.; Dors, N.; Brons, P.P.; Knoers, N.V.; Swinkels, D.W. Practice guidelines for the diagnosis and management of microcytic anemias due to genetic disorders of iron metabolism or heme synthesis. *Blood* **2014**, *123*, 3873–3886. [CrossRef] [PubMed]

34. Munro, H.N.; Linder, M.C. Ferritin: Structure, biosynthesis, and role in iron metabolism. *Physiol. Rev.* **1978**, *58*, 317–396. [CrossRef] [PubMed]

35. Donovan, A.; Brownlie, A.; Zhou, Y.; Shepard, J.; Pratt, S.J.; Moynihan, J.; Paw, B.H.; Drejer, A.; Barut, B.; Zapata, A.; et al. Positional cloning of zebrafish ferroportin 1 identifies a conserved vertebrate iron exporter. *Nature* **2000**, *403*, 776–781. [CrossRef] [PubMed]

36. Yeh, K.Y.; Yeh, M.; Glass, J. Interactions between ferroportin and hephaestin in rat enterocytes are reduced after iron ingestion. *Gastroenterology* **2011**, *141*, 292–299. [CrossRef] [PubMed]

37. Cherukuri, S.; Potla, R.; Sarkar, J.; Nurko, S.; Harris, Z.L.; Fox, P.L. Unexpected role of ceruloplasmin in intestinal iron absorption. *Cell Metab.* **2005**, *2*, 309–319. [CrossRef] [PubMed]

38. Ganz, T. Systemic iron homeostasis. *Physiol. Rev.* **2013**, *93*, 1721–1741. [CrossRef] [PubMed]

39. Ganz, T. Hepcidin and iron metabolism, 10 years later. *Blood* **2012**, *117*, 4425–4433. [CrossRef] [PubMed]

40. Krause, A.; Neitz, S.; Magert, H.J.; Schulz, A.; Forssmann, W.G.; Schulz-Knappe, P.; Adermann, K. LEAP-1, a novel highly disulfide-bonded human peptide, exhibits antimicrobial activity. *FEBS Lett.* **2000**, *480*, 147–150. [CrossRef]

41. Park, C.H.; Valore, E.V.; Waring, A.J.; Ganz, T. Hepcidin, a urinary antimicrobial peptide synthesized in the liver. *J. Biol. Chem.* **2001**, *276*, 7806–7810. [CrossRef] [PubMed]

42. Brasse-Lagnel, C.; Karim, Z.; Letteron, P.; Bekri, S.; Bado, A.; Beaumont, C. Intestinal DMT1 cotransporter is down-regulated by hepcidin via proteasome internalization and degradation. *Gastroenterology* **2011**, *140*, 1261–1271. [CrossRef] [PubMed]

43. Barrios, Y.; Espinoza, M.; Barón, M.A. Pro-hepcidin, its relationship with iron metabolism and inflammation indicators in hemodialyzed patients, with or without recombinant erythropoietin treatment. *Nutr. Hosp.* **2010**, *25*, 555–560. [PubMed]

44. Kroot, J.C.; Tjalsma, H.; Fleming, R.; Swinkels, D.W. Hepcidin in human iron disorders: Diagnostic implications. *Clin. Chem.* **2011**, *57*, 1650–1669. [CrossRef] [PubMed]

45. Nicolas, G.; Bennoun, M.; Devaux, I.; Beaumont, C.; Grandchamp, B.; Kahn, A.; Vaulont, S. Lack of hepcidin gene expression and severe tissue iron overload in upstream stimulatory factor 2 (USF2) knockout mice. *Proc. Natl. Acad. Sci. USA* **2001**, *98*, 8780–8785. [CrossRef] [PubMed]

46. Nemeth, E.; Rivera, S.; Gabayan, V.; Keller, C.; Taudorf, S.; Pedersen, B.K.; Ganz, T. IL-6 mediates hypoferremia of inflammation by inducing the synthesis of the iron regulatory hormone hepcidin. *J. Clin. Investig.* **2004**, *113*, 1271–1276. [CrossRef] [PubMed]

47. Jonker, F.A.; Calis, J.C.; Phiri, K.; Kraaijenhagen, R.J.; Brabin, B.J.; Faragher, B.; Wiegerink, E.T.; Tjalsma, H.; Swinkels, D.W.; van Hensbroek, M.B. Low hepcidin levels in severely anemic Malawian children with high incidence of infectious diseases and bone marrow iron deficiency. *PLoS ONE* **2013**, *8*, e78964. [CrossRef] [PubMed]

48. Kruszewski, M. Labile iron pool: The main determinant of cellular response to oxidative stress. *Mutat. Res.* **2003**, *531*, 81–92. [CrossRef] [PubMed]

49. Bresgen, N.; Eckl, P. Oxidative stress and the homeodynamics of iron metabolism. *Biomolecules* **2015**, *5*, 808–847. [CrossRef] [PubMed]

50. Nicolas, G.; Chauvet, C.; Viatte, L.; Danan, J.L.; Bigard, X.; Beaumont, C.; Kahn, A.; Vaulont, S. The gene encoding the iron regulatory peptide hepcidin is regulated by anaemia, hypoxia and inflammation. *J. Clin. Investig.* **2002**, *110*, 1037–1044. [CrossRef] [PubMed]

51. Antosiewicz, J.; Ziolkowski, W.; Kaczor, J.J.; Herman-Antosiewicz, A. Tumor necrosis factor-alpha-induced reactive oxygen species formation is mediated by JNK1-dependent ferritin degradation. *Radic. Biol. Med.* **2007**, *43*, 265–270. [CrossRef] [PubMed]

52. Borkowska, A.; Sielicka-Dudzin, A.; Herman-Antosiewicz, A.; Halon, M.; Wozniak, M.; Antosiewicz, J. P66Shc mediated ferritin degradation—A novel mechanism of ROS formation. *Free Radic. Biol. Med.* **2011**, *51*, 658–663. [CrossRef] [PubMed]

53. Villarino, A.V.; Huang, E.; Hunter, C.A. Understanding the pro- and anti-inflammatory properties of IL-27. *J. Immunol.* **2004**, *173*, 715–720. [CrossRef] [PubMed]

54. Wallberg, L.; Mattsson, C.M.; Enqvist, J.K.; Ekblom, B. Plasma IL-6 concentration during ultra-endurance exercise. *Eur. J. Appl. Physiol.* **2011**, *111*, 1081–1088. [CrossRef] [PubMed]

55. Nemeth, E.; Ganz, T. The role of hepcidin in iron metabolism. *Acta Haematol.* **2009**, *122*, 78–86. [CrossRef] [PubMed]

56. Mainous, A.G.; Diaz, V.A. Relation of serum ferritin level to cardiovascular fitness among young men. *Am. J. Cardiol.* **2009**, *103*, 115–118. [CrossRef] [PubMed]

57. Peeling, P.; Dawson, B.; Goodman, C.; Landers, G.; Wiegerinck, E.T.; Swinkels, D.W.; Trinder, D. Effects of exercise on hepcidin response and iron metabolism during recovery. *Int. J. Sport Nutr. Exerc. Metab.* **2009**, *19*, 583–597. [CrossRef] [PubMed]

58. Badenhorst, C.E.; Dawson, W.; Goodman, C.; Sim, M.; Cox, G.R.; Gore, C.J.; Tjalsma, H.; Swinkels, D.W.; Peeling, P. Influence of post-exercise hypoxic exposure on hepcidina response in athletes. *Eur. J. Appl. Physiol.* **2014**, *114*, 951–959. [CrossRef] [PubMed]

59. Badenhorst, C.E.; Dawson, B.; Cox, G.R.; Laarakkers, C.M.; Swinkels, D.W.; Peeling, P. Timing of post-exercise carbohydrate ingestion: Influence on IL-6 and hepcidin responses. *Eur. J. Appl. Physiol.* **2015**, *115*, 2215–2222. [CrossRef] [PubMed]

60. Badenhorst, C.E.; Dawson, B.; Cox, G.R.; Laarakkers, C.M.; Swinkels, D.W.; Peeling, P. Acute dietary carbohydrate manipulation and the subsequent inflammatory and hepcidin responses to exercise. *Eur. J. Appl. Physiol.* **2015**, *115*, 2521–2530. [CrossRef] [PubMed]

61. Badenhorst, C.E.; Dawson, B.; Cox, G.R.; Sim, M.; Laarakkers, C.M.; Swinkels, D.W.; Peeling, P. Seven days of high carbohydrate ingestion does not attenuate post-exercise IL-6 and hepcidin levels. *Eur. J. Appl. Physiol.* **2016**, *116*, 1715–1724. [CrossRef] [PubMed]

62. Sim, M.; Dawson, B.; Landers, G.; Swinkels, D.W.; Tjalsma, H.; Trinder, D.; Peeling, P. The effects of carbohydrate ingestion during endurance running on post-exercise inflammation and hepcidina levels. *Eur. J. Appl. Physiol.* **2012**, *12*, 1889–1898.

63. Newlin, M.K.; Williams, S.; McNamara, T.; Tjalsma, H.; Swinkels, D.W.; Haymes, E.M. The effects of acute exercise bouts on hepcidina in women. *Int. J. Sports Nutr. Exerc. Metab.* **2012**, *22*, 79–89. [CrossRef]

64. Peeling, P.; Sim, M.; Badenhorst, C.E.; Dawson, B.; Govus, A.D.; Abbiss, C.R.; Swinkels, D.W.; Trinder, D. Iron status and the acute post-exercise hepcidin response in athletes. *PLoS ONE* **2014**, *9*, e93002. [CrossRef] [PubMed]

65. Burden, R.J.; Pollock, N.; Whyte, G.P.; Richards, T.; Moore, B.; Busbridge, M.; Srai, S.K.; Otto, J.; Pedlar, C.R. Effect of intravenous iron on aerobic capacity and iron metabolism in elite athletes. *Med. Sci. Sports Exerc.* **2015**, *47*, 1399–1407. [CrossRef] [PubMed]

66. Dahlquist, D.T.; Stellingwerff, T.; Dieter, B.P.; McKenzie, D.C.; Koehle, M.S. Effects of macro- and micronutrients on exercise induced hepcidin response in highly trained endurance athletes. *Appl. Physiol. Nutr. Metab.* **2017**, *42*, 1036–1043. [CrossRef] [PubMed]

67. Díaz, V.; Peinado, A.B.; Barba-Moreno, L.; Altamura, S.; Butragueño, J.; González-Gross, M.; Alteheld, B.; Stehle, P.; Zapico, A.G.; Muckenthaler, M.U.; et al. Elevated hepcidin serum level in response to inflammatory and iron signals in exercising athletes is independent of moderate supplementation with vitamin C and E. *Physiol. Rep.* **2015**, *3*, e12475. [CrossRef] [PubMed]

68. Sim, M.; Dawson, B.; Landers, G.; Swinkels, D.W.; Tjasma, H.; Yeap, B.B.; Trinder, D.; Peeling, P. Oral contraception does not alter typical post-exercise interleukin-6 and hepcidin levels in females. *J. Sci. Med. Sport* **2015**, *18*, 8–12. [CrossRef] [PubMed]

69. Peeling, P.; McKay, A.K.A.; Pyne, D.B.; Guelfi, K.J.; McCormick, R.H.; Laarakkers, C.M.; Swinkels, D.W.; Garvican-Lewis, L.A.; Ross, M.L.R.; Sharma, A.P.; et al. Factors influencing the post-exercise hepcidin-25 response in elite Athletes. *Eur. J. Appl. Physiol.* **2017**, *117*, 1233–1239. [CrossRef] [PubMed]

70. Govus, A.D.; Abbiss, C.R.; Garvican-rvica, L.A.; Swinkels, D.W.; Laarakkers, C.M.; Gore, C.J.; Peeling, P. Acute hypoxic exercise does not alter post-exercise iron metabolism in moderately trained endurance athletes. *Eur. J. Appl. Physiol.* **2014**, *114*, 2183–2191. [CrossRef] [PubMed]

71. Govus, A.D.; Peeling, P.; Abbiss, C.R.; Lawler, N.G.; Swinkels, D.W.; Laarakkers, C.M.; Thompson, K.G.; Peiffer, J.J.; Gore, C.J.; Garvican-Lewis, L.A. Live high, train low-influence on resting and post-exercise hepcidin levels. *Scand. J. Med. Sci. Sports* **2017**, *27*, 704–713. [CrossRef] [PubMed]

72. Antosiewicz, J.; Kaczor, J.J.; Kasprowicz, K.; Laskowski, R.; Kujach, S.; Luszczyk, M.; Radziminski, L.; Ziemann, E. Repeated "all out" interval exercise causes an increase in serum hepcidin concentration in both trained and untrained men. *Cell Immunol.* **2013**, *283*, 12–17. [CrossRef] [PubMed]

73. Tomczyk, M.; Kortas, J.; Flis, D.; Skrobot, W.; Camilleri, R.; Antosiewicz, J. Simple sugar supplementation abrogates exercise-induced increase in hepcidin in young men. *J. Int. Soc. Sports Nutr.* **2017**, *14*, 10. [CrossRef] [PubMed]

74. Kasprovicz, K.; Ziemann, E.; Ratkowski, W.; Laskowski, R.; Kaczor, J.J.; Dadci, R.; Antosiewicz, J. Running a 100-km-ultra-marathon induces an inflammatory response but does not raise the level of the plasma iron-regulatory protein hepcidina. *J. Sports Med. Phys. Fit.* **2013**, *53*, 533–537.

75. Skarpanska-Stejnborn, A.; Basta, P.; Trzeciak, J.; Szczesniak-Pilaczynska, L. Effect of intense physical exercise on hepcidin levels and selected parameters of iron metabolism in rowing athletes. *Eur. J. Appl. Physiol.* **2015**, *115*, 345–351. [CrossRef] [PubMed]

76. Skarpańska-Stejnborn, A.; Basta, P.; Trzeciak, J.; Michalska, A.; Kafkas, M.E.; Woitas-Ślubowska, D. Effects of cranberry (Vaccinum macrocarpon) supplementation on iron status and inflammatory markers in rowers. *J. Int. Soc. Sports Nutr.* **2017**, *14*, 7. [CrossRef] [PubMed]

77. Robson-Ansley, P.; Walsh, Q.; Sala, D. The effect of carbohydrate ingestion on plasma interleukin-6, hepcidina and iron concentrations following prolonged exercise. *Cytokine* **2011**, *53*, 196–200. [CrossRef] [PubMed]

78. Schmidt, W.; Prommer, N. Impact of alterations in total hemoglobin mass on VO_{2max}. *Exerc. Sport Sci. Rev.* **2010**, *38*, 68–75. [CrossRef] [PubMed]

79. Fujii, T.; Asai, T.; Matsuo, T.; Okamura, K. Effect of resistance exercise on iron status in moderately iron-deficient rats. *Biol. Trace Elem. Res.* **2011**, *144*, 983–991. [CrossRef] [PubMed]

80. Matsuo, T.; Suzuki, H.; Suzuki, M. Resistance exercise increses the capacity of heme biosynthesis more than aerobic exercise in rats. *J. Clin. Biochem. Nutr.* **2000**, *29*, 19–27. [CrossRef]

81. Fujii, T.; Matsuo, T.; Okamura, K. Effects of resistance exercise on iron absorption and balance in iron-deficient rats. *Biol. Trace Elem. Res.* **2014**, *161*, 101–106. [CrossRef] [PubMed]

82. Deruisseau, K.C.; Roberts, L.M.; Kushnick, R.M.; Evans, A.M.; Austin, K.; Haymes, E.M. Iron status of young males and females performing weight-training exercise. *Med. Sci. Sports Exerc.* **2004**, *36*, 241–248. [CrossRef] [PubMed]

83. Helgerud, J.; Høydal, K.; Wang, E.; Karlsen, T.; Berg, P.; Bjerkaas, M.; Simonsen, T.; Helgesen, C.; Hjorth, N.; Bach, R.; et al. Aerobic high-intensity intervals improve VO_{2max} more than moderate training. *Med. Sci. Sports Exerc.* **2007**, *39*, 665–671. [CrossRef] [PubMed]

84. Domínguez, R.; Garnacho-Castaño, M.V.; Maté-Muñoz, J.L. Methodology to determine the aerobic-anaerobic transition in functional evaluation. *Arch. Med. Deporte* **2015**, *32*, 387–392.

85. Amine, E.K.; Hegsed, D.M. Effect of diet on iron absorption in rion-deficient rats. *J. Nutr.* **1971**, *101*, 927–936. [CrossRef] [PubMed]

86. Bacchetta, J.; Zaritsky, J.J.; Sea, J.L.; Chun, R.F.; Lisse, T.S.; Zavala, K.; Nayak, A.; Wesseling-Perry, K.; Westerman, M.; Hollis, B.W.; et al. Suppression of iron-regulatory hepcidin by vitamin D. *J. Am. Soc. Nephrol.* **2014**, *25*, 564–572. [CrossRef] [PubMed]

87. Zughaier, S.M.; Alvarez, J.A.; Sloan, J.H.; Konrad, R.J.; Tangpricha, V. The role of vitamin D in regulating the iron-hepcidin-ferroportin axis in monocytes. *J. Clin. Transl. Endocrinol.* **2014**, *1*, 19–25. [CrossRef] [PubMed]

88. Ohsaki, Y.; Shirakawa, H.; Hiwatashi, K.; Furukawa, Y.; Mizutani, T.; Komai, M. Vitamin K suppresses lipopolysaccharide-induced inflammation in the rat. *Biosci. Biotechnol. Biochem.* **2006**, *70*, 926–932. [CrossRef] [PubMed]

89. Anhê, F.F.; Roy, D.; Pilon, G.; Dudonné, S.; Matamoros, S.; Varin, T.V.; Garofalo, C.; Moine, Q.; Desjardins, Y.; Levy, E.; et al. A polyphenol-rich cranberry extract protects from diet-induced obesity, insulin resistance and intestinal inflammation in association with increased *Akkermansia* spp. population in the gut microbiota of mice. *Gut* **2015**, *64*, 872–883. [CrossRef] [PubMed]

90. Pappas, E.; Schaich, K.M. Phytochemicals of cranberries and cranberry products: Characterization, potential health effects, and processing stability. *Crit. Rev. Food Sci. Nutr.* **2009**, *49*, 741–781. [CrossRef] [PubMed]

91. Denis, M.C.; Desjardins, Y.; Furtos, A.; Marcil, V.; Dudonné, S.; Montoudis, A.; Garofalo, C.; Delvin, E.; Marette, A.; Levy, E. Prevention of oxidative stress, inflammation and mitochondrial dysfunction in the intestine by different cranberry phenolic fractions. *Clin. Sci.* **2015**, *128*, 197–212. [CrossRef] [PubMed]

92. Hinton, P.S.; Sinclair, L.M. Iron supplementation maintains ventilatory threshold and improves energetic efficiency in iron-deficient nonanaemic athletes. *Eur. J. Clin. Nutr.* **2007**, *61*, 30–39. [CrossRef] [PubMed]

93. Garvican, L.A.; Saunders, P.U.; Cardoso, T.; Macdougall, I.C.; Lobigs, L.M.; Fazakerley, R.; Fallon, K.E.; Anderson, B.; Anson, J.M.; Thompson, K.G.; et al. Intravenous iron supplementation in distance runners with low or suboptimal ferritin. *Med. Sci. Sports Exerc.* **2014**, *46*, 376–385. [CrossRef] [PubMed]

94. Blee, T.; Goodman, C.; Dawson, B.; Stapff, A. The effect of intramuscular iron injections of serum ferritin levels and physical performance in elite netballers. *J. Sci. Med. Sport* **1999**, *2*, 311–321. [CrossRef]

95. Pedlar, C.R.; Whyte, G.P.; Burden, R.J.; Moore, B.; Horgan, G.; Pollock, N. A case study of an iron-deficient female Olympic 15,000 m runner. *Int. J. Sports Physiol. Perform.* **2013**, *8*, 696–698. [CrossRef]
96. Ishibashi, A.; Maeda, N.; Kamei, A.; Goto, K. Iron supplementation during three consecutive days of endurance training augmented hepcidin levels. *Nutrients* **2017**, *9*, 809. [CrossRef] [PubMed]
97. Darshan, D.; Frazer, D.M.; Wilkins, S.J.; Anderson, G.J. Severe iron deficiency blunts the response of the iron regulatory gene Hamp and pro-inflammatory cytokines to lipopolysaccharide. *Haematologica* **2010**, *95*, 1660–1667. [CrossRef] [PubMed]
98. Nemeth, E.; Valore, E.V.; Territo, M.; Schiller, G.; Lichtenstein, A.; Ganz, T. Hepcidin, a putative mediator of anemia of inflammation, is a type II acutephase protein. *Blood* **2003**, *101*, 2461–2463. [CrossRef] [PubMed]
99. Van Santen, S.; van Dongen-Lases, E.C.; de Vegt, F.; van Riel, P.L.; van Ede, A.E.; Swinkels, D.W. Hepcidin and hemoglobin content parameters in the diagnosis of iron deficiency in rheumatoid arthritis patients with anemia. *Arthritis Rheum.* **2011**, *63*, 3672–3680. [CrossRef] [PubMed]
100. Jaeggi, T.; Moretti, D.; Kvalsvig, J.; Holding, P.A.; Tjalsma, H.; Kortman, G.A.; Jooste, I.; Mwangi, A.; Zimmermann, M.B. Iron status and systemic inflammation, but not gut inflammation, strongly predict gender specific concentrations of serum hepcidin in infants in rural Kenya. *PLoS ONE* **2013**, *8*, e57513. [CrossRef] [PubMed]
101. Ganz, T.; Nemeth, E. Hepcidin and iron homeostasis. *Biochim. Biophys. Acta* **2012**, *1823*, 1434–1443. [CrossRef] [PubMed]
102. Banzet, S.; Sanchez, H.; Chapot, R.; Bigard, X.; Vaulont, S.; Koulmann, N. Interleukin-6 contributes to hepcidin mRNA increase in response to exercise. *Cytokine* **2012**, *58*, 158–161. [CrossRef] [PubMed]
103. Garcia, J.E.; López, A.M.; de Cabo, M.R.; Rodríguez, F.M.; Losada, J.P.; Sarmiento, R.G.; López, A.J.; Arellano, J.L. Cyclosporin A decreases human machrophage interleukin-6 synthesis at post-transcriptional level. *Mediat. Inflamm.* **1999**, *8*, 253–259. [CrossRef] [PubMed]
104. Williamson, M.S.; Miller, E.K.; Plemons, J.; Rees, T.; Iacopino, A.M. Cyclosporine A upregulates interleukin-6 gene expression in human gingiva: Possible mechanism for gingival overgrowth. *J. Periodontol.* **1994**, *65*, 895–903. [CrossRef] [PubMed]
105. Keller, C.; Hellsten, Y.; Steensberg, A.; Pedersen, B.K. Differential regulation of IL-6 and TNF-alpha via calcineurin in human skeletal muscle cells. *Cytokine* **2006**, *36*, 141–147. [CrossRef] [PubMed]
106. Keller, C.; Steensberg, A.; Pilegaard, H.; Osada, T.; Saltin, B.; Pedersen, B.K.; Neufer, P.D. Transcriptional activation of the IL-6 gene in human contracting skeletal muscle: Influence of muscle glycogen content. *FASEB J.* **2001**, *15*, 2748–2750. [CrossRef] [PubMed]
107. Pedersen, B.K.; Febbraio, M.A. Muscle as an endocrine organ: Focus on muscle-derived interleukin-6. *Physiol. Rev.* **2008**, *88*, 1379–1406. [CrossRef] [PubMed]
108. Pedersen, B.K. The diseasome of physical inactivity—And the role of myokines in muscle-fat cross talk. *J. Physiol.* **2009**, *587*, 5559–5568. [CrossRef] [PubMed]
109. Pedersen, L.; Idorn, M.; Olofsson, G.H.; Lauenborg, B.; Nookaew, I.; Hansen, R.H.; Johannesen, H.H.; Becker, J.C.; Pedersen, K.S.; Dethlefsen, C.; et al. Voluntary running suppresses tumor growth through epinephrine- and IL-6-Dependent NK cell mobilization and redistribution. *Cell Metab.* **2016**, *23*, 554–562. [CrossRef] [PubMed]
110. Starkie, R.; Ostrowski, S.R.; Jauffred, S.; Febbraio, M.; Pedersen, B.K. Exercise and IL-6 infusion inhibit endotoxin-induced TNF-alpha production in humans. *FASEB J.* **2003**, *17*, 884–886. [CrossRef] [PubMed]
111. Steensberg, A.; Fischer, C.P.; Keller, C.; Moller, K.; Pedersen, B.K. IL-6 enhances plasma IL-1ra, IL-10, and cortisol in humans. *Am. J. Physiol. Endocrinol. Metab.* **2003**, *285*, 433–437. [CrossRef] [PubMed]
112. Dandona, P.; Aljada, A.; Bandyopadhyay, A. Inflammation: The link between insulin resistance, obesity and diabetes. *Trends Immunol.* **2004**, *25*, 4–7. [CrossRef] [PubMed]
113. Duncan, B.B.; Schmidt, M.I.; Pankow, J.S.; Ballantyne, C.M.; Couper, D.; Vigo, A.; Hoogeveen, R.; Folsom, A.R.; Heiss, G.; Atherosclerosis Risk in Communities Study. Low-grade systemic inflammation and the development of type 2 diabetes: The atherosclerosis risk in communities study. *Diabetes* **2003**, *52*, 1799–1805. [CrossRef] [PubMed]
114. Budagian, V.; Bulanova, E.; Paus, R.; Bulfone-Paus, S. IL-1/IL-15 receptor biology: A guided tour through an expanding universe. *Cytokine Growth Factor Rev.* **2006**, *17*, 259–280. [CrossRef] [PubMed]

115. Tamura, Y.; Watanabe, K.; Kantani, T.; Hayashi, J.; Ishida, N.; Kaneki, M. Upregulation of circulating IL-15 by treadmill running in healthy individuals: Is IL-15 an endocrine mediator of the beneficial effects of endurance exercise. *Endocrin. J.* **2011**, *58*, 211–215. [CrossRef]

116. Pérez-López, A.; McKendry, J.; Martin-Rincón, M.; Morales-Alamo, D.; Pérez-Köhler, B.; Valadés, D.; Buján, J.; Calbet, J.A.L.; Breen, L. Skeletal muscle IL-15/IL-15Rα and myofibrillar protein synthesis after resistance exercise. *Scand. J. Med. Sci. Sports* **2017**, *28*, 116–125. [CrossRef] [PubMed]

117. Quinn, L.S.; Strait-Bodey, L.; Anderson, B.G.; Argiles, J.M.; Havel, P.J. Interleukin-15 stimulates adiponectin secretion by 3T3-L1 adipocytes: Evidence for a skeletal muscle-to-fat signaling pathway. *Cell Biol. Int.* **2005**, *29*, 449–457. [CrossRef] [PubMed]

118. Pérez-López, A.; Valadés, D.; Vázquez Martínez, C.; de Cos Blanco, A.I.; Buján, J.; Garcia-Honduvilla, N. Serum IL-15 and IL-15Rα levels are decreased in lean and obese physically active humans. *Scand. J. Med. Sci. Sports* **2017**. [CrossRef] [PubMed]

119. Kemna, E.; Pickkers, P.; Nemeth, E.; van der Hoeven, H.; Swinkels, D. Time-course analysis of hepcidin, serum iron, and plasma cytokine levels in humans injected with LPS. *Blood* **2005**, *106*, 1864–1866. [CrossRef] [PubMed]

120. Christoulas, K.; Karamouzis, M.; Mandroukas, K. "Living high-training low" vs. "living high-training high": Erythropoietic responses and performance of adolescent cross-country skiers. *J. Sport Med. Phys. Fit.* **2011**, *51*, 74–81.

121. Son, H.J.; Kim, H.J.; Kim, J.H.; Ohno, H.; Kim, C.K. Erythropoietin, 2,3 DPG, oxygen transport capacity, and altitude training in adolescent Alpine skiers. *Aviat. Space Envirn. Med.* **2012**, *83*, 50–53. [CrossRef]

122. Peyssonnaux, C.; Zinkernagel, A.S.; Schuepbach, R.A.; Rankin, E.; Vaulont, S.; Haase, V.H.; Nizet, V.; Johnson, R.S. Regulation of iron homeostasis by the hypoxia-inducible transcription factors(HIFs). *J. Clin. Investig.* **2007**, *117*, 1926–1932. [CrossRef] [PubMed]

123. Kautz, L.; Jung, G.; Valore, E.V.; Rivella, S.; Nemeth, E.; Ganz, T. Identification of erythroferrone as an erythroid regulator of iron metabolism. *Nat. Genet.* **2014**, *46*, 678–684. [CrossRef] [PubMed]

124. Talbot, N.P.; Lakhal, S.; Smith, T.G.; Privat, C.; Nickol, A.H.; Rivera-Ch, M.; León-Velarde, F.; Dorrington, K.L.; Mole, D.R.; Robbins, P.A. Regulation of hepcidin expression at high altitude. *Blood* **2012**, *119*, 857–860. [CrossRef] [PubMed]

125. Goetze, O.; Schmitt, J.; Spliethoff, K.; Theurl, I.; Weiss, G.; Swinkels, D.W.; Tjalsma, H.; Maggiorini, M.; Krayenbuhl, P.; Rau, M.; et al. Adaptation of iron transport and metabolism to acute highaltitude hypoxia in mountaineers. *Hepatology* **2013**, *58*, 2153–2162. [CrossRef] [PubMed]

126. Lui, Q.; Davidoff, O.; Niss, K.; Haase, V.H. Hypoxia-inducible factor regulates hepcidin via erythropoietin-induced erythropoiesis. *J. Clin. Investig.* **2012**, *122*, 4635–4644.

127. Robach, P.; Cairo, G.; Gelfi, C.; Bernuzzi, F.; Pilegaard, H.; Viganò, A.; Santambrogio, P.; Cerretelli, P.; Calbet, J.A.; Moutereau, S.; et al. Strong iron demand during hypoxia-induced erythropoiesis is associated with down-regulation of iron-related proteins and myoglobin in human skeletal muscle. *Blood* **2007**, *109*, 4724–4731. [CrossRef] [PubMed]

128. Robach, P.; Recalcati, S.; Girelli, D.; Gelfi, C.; Aachmann-Andersen, N.J.; Thomsen, J.J.; Norgaard, A.M.; Alberghini, A.; Campostrini, N.; Castagna, A.; et al. Alterations of systemic and muscle iron metabolism in human subjects treated with low dose recombinant erythropoietin. *Blood* **2009**, *113*, 6707–6715. [CrossRef] [PubMed]

129. Volke, M.; Gale, D.P.; Maegdefrau, U.; Schley, G.; Klanke, B.; Bosserhoff, A.K.; Maxwell, P.H.; Eckardt, K.U.; Warnecke, C. Evidence for a lack of a direct transcriptional suppression of the iron regulatory peptide hepcidin by hypoxia-inducible factors. *PLoS ONE* **2009**, *4*, e7875. [CrossRef] [PubMed]

130. Choudhry, H.; Harris, A.L. Advances in Hypoxia-inducible factor biology. *Cell Metab.* **2017**, *27*, 281–298. [CrossRef] [PubMed]

131. Piperno, A.; Galimberti, S.; Mariani, R.; Pelucchi, S.; Ravasi, G. Modulation of hepcidin production during hypoxia-induced erythropoiesis in humans in vivo: Data from the HIGHCARE project. *Blood* **2011**, *117*, 2953–2959. [CrossRef] [PubMed]

132. Hauser, A.; Troesch, S.; Saugy, J.J.; Schmitt, L.; Cejuela-Anta, R.; Faiss, R.; Steiner, T.; Robinson, N.; Millet, G.P.; Wehrlin, J.P. Individual hemoglobin mass response to normobaric and hypobaric "live high-train low": A one-year crossover study. *J. Appl. Physiol.* **2017**, *123*, 387–393. [CrossRef] [PubMed]

133. Harvey, L.J.; Armah, C.N.; Dainty, J.R.; Foxall, R.J.; John Lewis, D.; Langford, N.J.; Fairweather-Tait, S.J. Impact of menstrual blood loss and diet on iron deficiency among women in the UK. *Br. J. Nutr.* **2005**, *94*, 557–564. [CrossRef] [PubMed]

134. Ikeda, Y.; Tajima, S.; Izawa-Ishizawa, Y.; Kihira, Y.; Ishizawa, K.; Tomita, S.; Tsuchiya, K.; Tamaki, T. Estrogen regulates hepcidin expression via GPR30-BMP6-dependent signaling in hepatocytes. *PLoS ONE* **2012**, *7*, e40465. [CrossRef] [PubMed]

135. Guo, W.; Bachman, E.; Li, M.; Roy, C.N.; Blusztajn, J.; Wong, S.; Chan, S.Y.; Serra, C.; Jasuja, R.; Travison, T.G.; et al. Testosterone administration inhibits hepcidin transcription and is associated with increased iron incorporation into red blood cells. *Aging Cell* **2013**, *12*, 280–291. [CrossRef] [PubMed]

136. Fernández-Díaz, P.; Domínguez, R. Effects of testosterone supplementation on endurance performance. *Rev. Andal. Med. Deporte* **2016**, *9*, 131–137. [CrossRef]

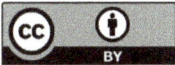

nutrients

MDPI

Review

Approaches for Reducing the Risk of Early-Life Iron Deficiency-Induced Brain Dysfunction in Children

Sarah E. Cusick [1,3], Michael K. Georgieff [2,3] and Raghavendra Rao [2,3,]

[1] Division of Global Pediatrics, Department of Pediatrics, and Center for Neurobehavioral Development, University of Minnesota, Minneapolis, MN 55455, USA; scusick@umn.edu

[2] Division of Neonatology, Department of Pediatrics, Institute of Child Development, and Center for Neurobehavioral Development, University of Minnesota, Minneapolis, MN 55455, USA; georg001@umn.edu

[3] Center for Neurobehavioral Development, University of Minnesota, 717 Delaware Street SE, Suite 333, Minneapolis, MN 55414, USA

* Correspondence: raghurao@umn.edu; Tel.: +1-612-625-3260

Received: 19 January 2018; Accepted: 14 February 2018; Published: 17 February 2018

Abstract: Iron deficiency is the most common micronutrient deficiency in the world. Women of reproductive age and young children are particularly vulnerable. Iron deficiency in late prenatal and early postnatal periods can lead to long-term neurobehavioral deficits, despite iron treatment. This may occur because screening and treatment of iron deficiency in children is currently focused on detection of anemia and not neurodevelopment. Anemia is the end-stage state of iron deficiency. The brain becomes iron deficient before the onset of anemia due to prioritization of the available iron to the red blood cells (RBCs) over other organs. Brain iron deficiency, independent of anemia, is responsible for the adverse neurological effects. Early diagnosis and treatment of impending brain dysfunction in the pre-anemic stage is necessary to prevent neurological deficits. The currently available hematological indices are not sensitive biomarkers of brain iron deficiency and dysfunction. Studies in non-human primate models suggest that serum proteomic and metabolomic analyses may be superior for this purpose. Maternal iron supplementation, delayed clamping or milking of the umbilical cord, and early iron supplementation improve the iron status of at-risk infants. Whether these strategies prevent iron deficiency-induced brain dysfunction has yet to be determined. The potential for oxidant stress, altered gastrointestinal microbiome and other adverse effects associated with iron supplementation cautions against indiscriminate iron supplementation of children in malaria-endemic regions and iron-sufficient populations.

Keywords: iron; iron deficiency; iron supplementation; infants; children; neurodevelopment; brain dysfunction

1. Introduction

Iron is essential for the normal development and function of all tissues in the body. Iron-containing heme proteins (Hemoglobin [Hgb] and cytochromes) participate in tissue oxygen delivery and energy metabolism. In the brain, iron and iron-containing enzymes are necessary for neuronal and glial energy metabolism, myelin synthesis and neurotransmission [1]. From a public health point of view, iron deficiency is the most common micronutrient deficiency in the world [2]. Women of childbearing age and preschool age children are particularly vulnerable. In addition to being the most common cause of anemia, iron deficiency during the late prenatal and early postnatal periods is a risk factor for long-term neurodevelopmental abnormalities [1,3,4]. Thus, early detection and prompt treatment of iron deficiency is of public health significance. Conversely, excess iron supplementation is associated with growth failure, altered gastrointestinal microbiome and other adverse effects in children, suggesting the need for a balanced approach. In the following sections, we review the causes and adverse neurological consequences of iron deficiency in infants and children, the current screening and treatment recommendations, and recent advances in diagnosis and treatment strategies for preventing iron-deficiency-induced adverse neurological effects.

2. Children At-Risk of Iron Deficiency

Children are at risk of iron deficiency at three time points: in the late prenatal and neonatal period; between 6 and 24 months of age; and at adolescence. The former two time periods (first 1000 days; hereafter called early-life iron deficiency) coincide with the period of rapid brain growth and development and can negatively impact neurodevelopment. The common causes of iron deficiency in the fetal and neonatal period are maternal iron-deficiency anemia, preterm birth, and gestational complications such as maternal diabetes mellitus, intrauterine growth restriction, maternal smoking, maternal obesity and inflammation. Consumption of a diet that is low in iron and/or contains iron binders and chronic gastrointestinal blood loss due to cow milk intolerance or hookworm infestation are the common causes of iron deficiency in the post-neonatal period. Iron deficiency during adolescence is common in female athletes due to a combination of insufficient dietary iron intake, menstrual blood losses and exercise-induced hepcidin upregulation [5]. In contrast to early-life iron deficiency, the neurological effects of iron deficiency at adolescence and beyond are reversible with iron supplementation [6], likely because the brain is fully developed by this age.

3. Early-Life Iron Deficiency and Brain Dysfunction

3.1. Inter-Organ Prioritization of Iron in Early-Life Iron Deficiency

The majority (60–70%) of the total body iron is in the red blood cells (RBCs) as Hgb; the rest is in tissues and storage form [7]. During negative iron balance in early life, available iron is prioritized to the RBCs over all other organs, including the brain [8–11]. This risk is greatest in the late fetal through infancy periods when the iron needs of growth competes with those of erythropoiesis. Studies in infant humans [8,12], monkeys [13], lambs [9,14] and rats [15] demonstrate that brain iron is reduced prior to the appearance of anemia. Similar prioritization (RBC before brain) also occurs during recovery from iron deficiency. The Hgb is normalized before the brain becomes iron replete in anemic infant rats and monkeys during treatment [13,15]. The slower recovery of brain iron is of concern, because iron transport across the blood–brain barrier is developmentally regulated [16] and delaying iron treatment misses out this window of opportunity, leaving the brain iron deficient [17]. Residual brain iron deficiency is likely responsible for the persistent neurological deficits in children with a history of early-life iron deficiency [3,4].

3.2. Neurological Sequelae of Early-Life Iron Deficiency

An in-depth review of the neurological effects of early-life iron deficiency is beyond the scope of this review. Excellent reviews are available elsewhere [1,18]. Briefly, late prenatal and neonatal iron deficiency is associated with altered temperament [19], abnormal recognition memory [20,21], and mental and psychomotor deficits in full-term infants [22], and abnormal neurological reflexes [23] and auditory brain-stem response in preterm infants [24]. An association between fetal iron deficiency and schizophrenia has been reported [25]. Postnatally, iron deficiency between 6 and 24 months of age is associated with lower IQ, slower processing speed, deficits in attention, motor, cognitive and behavioral functions, and disrupted sleep–wake rhythm [26]. While early treatment improves motor performance, behavioral deficits often persist into adulthood [27].

3.3. Biology of Abnormal Neurodevelopment in Early-Life Iron Deficiency

Rodent and non-human primate models demonstrate that early-life iron deficiency anemia causes impaired cerebral energy metabolism [15,28], hypomyelination, altered monoamine metabolism [29], abnormal synaptic architecture, and suppression of growth factor expression [15,30–34]. The hippocampus, striatum and cerebellum are targeted. Similar effects are seen with non-anemic hippocampus-specific iron deficiency, suggesting that brain tissue iron deficiency is primarily responsible for the adverse effects. The animal studies also highlight the importance of timing iron treatment for reversing the adverse neurological effects. Whereas early iron treatment corrects brain iron deficiency and restores brain metabolism and function [35], late treatment after the onset of anemia fails to produce similar beneficial effects [36], even when higher than the standard iron doses are used [36,37]. Thus, early detection and treatment is important for ensuring the normal neurodevelopment of children at risk of early-life iron deficiency.

4. Screening and Treatment Strategies

4.1. Current Recommendation

The American Academy of Pediatrics currently endorses universal screening for anemia at 12 months of age through the determination of Hgb and an assessment of risk factors for iron deficiency [38]. If anemia (Hgb < 110 g/L) is present, then additional screening for iron deficiency by measuring serum ferritin and C-reactive protein (CRP) levels (to rule out false elevation in serum ferritin due to inflammation) or reticulocyte Hgb concentration is recommended [38]. This strategy is unlikely to ensure neuroprotection. As mentioned above, anemia is the end-stage state of iron deficiency due to the prioritization of iron to the RBCs over other organs [8,14,39,40]. The brain is already iron deficient by the time anemia is diagnosed. Animal studies show that it is brain-tissue iron deficiency, independent of anemia, that is responsible for the neurological deficits [17,41]. Screening for anemia also fails to detect non-anemic iron deficiency, which is 3-fold more common than iron deficiency anemia even in the United States [42], and a risk factor for neurological impairments [43]. Furthermore, the laboratory tests used for screening (Hgb, ferritin and reticulocyte Hgb) are biomarkers of hematological changes. Our recent study in non-human primates demonstrates that these hematological and iron panel biomarkers are not sensitive for detecting brain iron deficiency and cerebral metabolic dysfunction in the pre-anemic period [44]. Finally, starting iron treatment after the onset of anemia does not correct the adverse neurological effects, even when an extended duration of iron therapy is used [45].

4.2. Potential Biomarkers of Brain Dysfunction in Early-Life Iron Deficiency

We have previously reported that a cord blood ferritin < 35 µg/L predicts brain iron deficiency and dysfunction as indexed by impaired recognition memory at birth, and lower psychomotor development at 1 year of age in full-term infants with iron deficiency due to maternal gestational diabetes [20]. A cord blood ferritin concentration ≤75 µg/L correlates with slower auditory brainstem-evoked responses that are suggestive of reduced auditory tract myelination in the newborn period [24,46]. A cord blood zinc protoporphyrin/heme (ZnPP/H) ratio > 118 µM/M predicts worse recognition memory at 2 months [21]. Unfortunately, a similar association between a serum iron panel index and brain iron deficiency and dysfunction beyond the newborn period has yet to be determined. Reticulocyte Hgb content is the strongest predictor of iron deficiency and response to iron supplementation in children [47,48]. Unpublished studies in neonatal rats from our lab suggest that reticulocyte Hgb is a sensitive peripheral biomarker of impending brain iron deficiency. Validation in human infants is necessary before reticulocyte Hgb could be recommended as a screening tool. Our studies in non-human primate models of infantile iron deficiency suggest that proteomic and metabolomic analysis of biofluids (serum and cerebrospinal fluid) may provide sensitive biomarkers of impending brain metabolic dysfunction in the pre-anemic period [44]. It is important to note, however, that while all of these biomarkers appear to be sensitive for detecting early-life iron deficiency-induced brain dysfunction, currently there is no evidence that instituting iron supplementation based on these biomarkers will prevent or reverse the adverse neurological effects.

5. Prevention of Early-Life Iron Deficiency-Induced Brain Dysfunction

Given the difficulties with early detection of brain dysfunction and the ineffectiveness of iron treatment started after the onset of anemia in reversing the neurological deficits, strategies aimed at prevention of early-life iron deficiency are of the utmost importance and potentially should begin with ensuring adequate iron accretion by the fetus. Currently, routine iron supplementation via diet (e.g., iron-fortified cereal) or medicinal iron is recommended for full-term breastfed infants from 4 months of age [38]. In children aged 4–24 months, daily iron supplementation improves hematological status [42,49]. Mental and psychomotor performances are not affected. This lack of beneficial effect on neurodevelopment with iron supplementation has been used as an argument for continuing with the current screening recommendation [50]. However, it is also possible that waiting until 4 months of age to begin iron supplementation may have been too late for preventing brain iron deficiency and associated adverse effects in those at risk of early-life iron deficiency (e.g., those born with low iron stores). Consistent with this possibility, previous studies have demonstrated that iron supplementation using an iron-containing formula within a month of birth improves psychomotor development of at-risk infants [51,52]. Since low iron endowment at birth predisposes to iron deficiency in early-infancy [53], measures that enhance iron stores before and/or soon after birth are likely to be beneficial.

5.1. Ensuring Early-Life Iron Sufficiency

5.1.1. Maternal Iron Supplementation

Maternal iron supplementation during pregnancy is a cost-effective method of ensuring iron sufficiency in the mother–infant dyad. The Institute of Medicine recommends that women consume 27 mg/day of iron during pregnancy [54]. However, most women in low- and middle-income countries need additional iron to prevent iron deficiency and maintain adequate stores. Typically, 30–60 mg of elemental iron per day is recommended, with up to 120 mg of elemental iron daily for those with anemia [55,56]. A meta-analysis of 44 trials involving more than 40,000 women in 2015 showed that daily oral iron supplementation during pregnancy reduces maternal anemia by 70%, iron-deficiency anemia by 67%, and iron deficiency by 57% at term gestation [56]. Women receiving iron were more likely to have higher Hgb at delivery and in the postpartum period, and less likely to have low birth weight and preterm infants, compared with those not receiving iron supplementation [56]. An additional theoretical benefit of maternal iron supplementation is better mother–infant interaction due to an improved iron status of the mother. However, compliance with iron supplementation may be poor due to a lack of education and side effects associated with enteral supplementation. In a prospective study in north-east India, the incidence of maternal anemia during pregnancy was 90% due to a combination of the consumption of an iron-poor diet, the habit of drinking large quantities of black tea (which binds to iron in the intestinal lumen and prevents its absorption) with meals, and poor compliance with recommended iron supplementation [57]. There is also a potential for adverse effects with excessive iron supplementation during pregnancy. The above-mentioned meta-analysis found that mothers on iron supplementation were more likely to have Hgb concentration of 130 g/L, a value associated with maternal and fetal adverse effects [56]. Thus, there is a need for considering methods beyond maternal iron supplementation for enhancing offspring's iron stores. Two examples of such a strategy are delayed clamping or milking of the umbilical cord and early iron supplementation.

5.1.2. Delayed Clamping or Milking of the Umbilical Cord

Delaying clamping of the umbilical cord for 30–45 s after birth is an effective method of increasing Hgb concentration and iron stores in healthy full-term infants. Whereas the improvement in Hgb is limited to the first 24–48 h after birth, the beneficial effects on iron stores last at least until 6 months of age [58]. A similar beneficial effect on iron stores is also seen with immediate clamping of a long segment of the umbilical cord followed by milking it towards the infant [59]. This strategy is useful in situations where delayed clamping of the umbilical cord is not feasible (for example, when there is a need for resuscitation of the infant at birth). The beneficial effects on iron stores were present in infants of both anemic mothers and non-anemic mothers [59], suggesting that the procedure could be undertaken universally in areas where maternal gestational iron deficiency is common. An association between delayed cord clamping and improved scores in fine motor and social domains at 4 years of age in boys has been reported [60].

5.1.3. Initiation of Supplementation Earlier than the Recommended Period

Beginning iron supplementation earlier than the recommended 4 months of age may be beneficial in infants at risk of early-life iron deficiency. In full-term breastfed infants, 7–7.5 mg per day of elemental iron from 1 to 6 months of age leads to higher Hgb and improved iron status at 6 months of age, and better visual acuity and psychomotor development at 13 months of age [52,61]. In areas where iron deficiency is prevalent, starting iron supplementation even earlier may be beneficial. Unpublished data suggest that iron supplementation in a dose of 2 mg/kg daily started on the second day after birth and continued until 6 months improves iron stores and motor development at 6 months of age in breastfed full-term infants in regions with high prevalence of iron deficiency (Bora, personal communication). Whether such supplementation leads to better long-term neurodevelopment has yet to be determined.

6. Potential Risk with Universal Iron Supplementation in Children

Public policy approaches to address common and potentially dangerous nutrient deficiencies include fortification and universal supplementation. Folate supplementation of grains and iodide supplementation of salt represent two such successful campaigns that have resulted in subsequent reductions in morbidity from neural tube defects and hypothyroidism/goiter. The decision to universally supplement or fortify with a nutrient takes into consideration the risks and benefits of the nutrient. While no apparent harm has occurred through folate and iodide supplementation, the case for universal supplementation of iron is more difficult because of emerging evidence of the potential toxicities of iron. Two populations at risk of this complication are discussed below.

6.1. Iron Supplementation of Children in Malaria-Endemic Areas

In many of the same regions where iron deficiency is most prevalent, malaria is also endemic. The potential danger of giving iron to children living in malaria-endemic regions was brought to the world's attention by a large, randomized, placebo-controlled trial of prophylactic iron supplementation for young children living on malaria-endemic Pemba Island, Tanzania [62]. This trial was the first large-scale study to test the former recommendation of the World Health Organization (WHO) for daily, universal iron supplementation of children living in areas where the prevalence of anemia was 40% or greater. The Pemba study was stopped early due to an observed increased risk of hospitalizations and deaths among children who received iron. The results of a sub study of the larger study, which included more specific iron-status measures such as ZnPP, as well as more immediate access to prompt malaria diagnosis and treatment, demonstrated that children who were anemic or who had an elevated ZnPP (reflective of iron deficiency) had a significantly lower rate of serious adverse events compared with iron-deficient children who did not receive iron.

With more than 30,000 children enrolled, the Pemba trial was a landmark study, and its results shook the global nutrition world, changing the policy and practice of giving iron to the tens of millions of children around the world who live in malaria-endemic areas. The most recent of three Cochrane reviews on the topic that were conducted after the Pemba study found (as did the other two reviews) no harmful effect of iron in malaria-endemic area when iron is given in conjunction with malaria management services [63], subsequent studies continued to underscore the potentially dangerous interaction of iron with malaria and other infections. One study of iron-containing multiple micronutrient supplementation reported an increased risk of malaria episodes in iron-deficient

Tanzanian children [64], and another study of iron-containing micronutrient powder supplementation reported an increased risk of diarrhea and respiratory illness among Pakistani children [65]. A large birth cohort study in a malaria-endemic area of Tanzania in which no iron was given found an increased risk of all-cause mortality among children who remained iron-replete in the first four years of life compared with children who developed iron-deficiency [66]. More than a decade later, the best way to help young children living in malaria-endemic areas to safely maintain a healthy iron status in order to protect brain development thus remains unclear, although significant research has helped elucidate the pathophysiology of the interaction between iron and malaria, clarifying several potential intervention strategies.

A meta-analysis of more than 55 randomized controlled trials of iron supplementation in children reported that the Hgb response to iron is diminished in malaria-endemic areas [67]. This finding is in line with malaria itself as an important cause of anemia among children in endemic regions and the diminished iron absorption that accompanies malaria infection. There are more than 200 million cases of uncomplicated malaria among children in sub-Saharan Africa each year alone. Young children in malaria-endemic areas have multiple, recurring malaria infections throughout childhood, likely leading to varying levels of chronic inflammation. The inflammatory response that accompanies malaria and other infections leads to increased production of the hepatic protein hepcidin, which cause the degradation of ferroportin, the iron efflux protein that permits dietary iron to be released from intestinal cells into the circulation and iron that would be recycled from senescent red blood cells to be released from macrophages [68]. Recent work suggests that hepcidin is lowest at the end of a malarial season in areas of seasonal transmission and best predicts the response to iron therapy, causing some to suggest timing the administration of iron to the end of the malaria season [69,70].

Low hepcidin also best predicted successful incorporation of dietary iron into red blood cells in an iron-stable isotope study in Gambian children [71,72]. This study also confirmed that dietary iron incorporation—an indirect measure of absorption—into red blood cells is diminished in children recovering from post-malarial anemia as compared with children recovering from iron-deficiency anemia alone. However, children recovering from malarial anemia had a greater Hgb gain than children recovering from iron-deficiency anemia, leading researchers to conclude that immediate iron needs in these children were initially met by iron trapped in reticuoendothelial stores during the inflammation of malaria, but then released for supporting Hgb synthesis following antimalarial treatment [71].

Delaying the start of iron therapy until after effective treatment of malaria and an accompanying reduction in inflammation and hepcidin thus may be another strategy to safely increase iron absorption and utilization. We recently reported that iron therapy begun 28 days after antimalarial treatment in children with iron deficiency and malaria was more than twice as well incorporated (16.5% vs. 7.9%) as iron therapy that was started concurrently with antimalarial treatment per the current WHO standard of care [73]. In accordance with the greater incorporation, hepcidin concentrations were also significantly lower in the delayed iron group as compared with the immediate iron group at day 28. At day 56, after all children had received the same length of iron therapy, Hgb and iron markers (ferritin, soluble transferrin receptor, ZnPP) were equivalent between the two groups.

An additional finding was that children in the delayed iron group had a significantly lower incidence of all-cause sick-child visits to the study clinic during the 56-day follow-up period [74]. The most common diagnosis was upper respiratory infection, followed by malaria. Although the mechanism behind the lower morbidity associated with delayed iron therapy is unclear, it follows that the greater percentage iron incorporation that we observed with delayed treatment would be accompanied by less unabsorbed iron in the intestinal lumen. In multiple studies of iron-fortified micronutrient powder, unabsorbed iron has been associated with a shift in the composition of the intestinal microbiome of young children living in malaria-endemic areas, shifting from predominant beneficial barrier strains (e.g., bifidobacteriaceae), to more pathogenic strains (e.g., enterobacteria), and leading to intestinal inflammation [75–77].

Recent work suggests that this shift to pathogenic strains may be mitigated by the addition of prebiotic galacto-oligosaccharides (GOS) to micronutrient formulations. In a randomized controlled trial in Kenyan infants, infants who received daily supplementation with multiple micronutrient powder fortified with 5 mg of iron and GOS had no increase in pathogenic bacteria and a lower incidence of respiratory infections compared to children who received iron-fortified power without GOS [78]. The increased incidence of respiratory tract infections with iron reported in this study [78], the Soofi study [65], and in our recent work [74] is in line with pre-clinical evidence demonstrating that the gut microbiome is an important modulator of immunity. Of note, associations between the gut microbiome and respiratory infections are described, with pathogenic shifts in the gut microbiome associated with an increased risk of a range of respiratory tract infections, including pneumococcal pneumonia [79].

Many questions remain after the Pemba study on how to optimize the iron status in children living in malaria-endemic areas. Recent in vitro evidence suggests that iron-deficient RBCs resist invasion of the malaria parasite [80,81], but iron deficiency cannot be a malaria-control strategy because of the risk it poses to the developing brain described above. Establishment of a safe and effective management strategy to address both iron deficiency and malaria when they coexist is thus a public health imperative.

6.2. Iron Supplementation of Iron-Sufficient Pediatric Populations

As noted previously, iron deficiency is the most common nutrient disorder worldwide. The estimated prevalence is 2 billion cases, a number that exceeds the rate of iodine deficiency for which universal supplementation policies have been implemented. However, given that the world population now exceeds 7 billion, more than 5 billion people are not iron deficient. The situation is further enhanced in developed countries. For example, in the United States, the prevalence of total body iron deficiency is 15% in toddlers, and 10–16% in women of reproductive age [82], which means that the majority population is iron sufficient. Thus, careful consideration must be given to the balance between potential risks and benefits. Studies clearly indicate that iron supplementation of iron-deficient individuals and populations improves iron status, and in some cases, neurodevelopment (see above). Conversely, little, if any, evidence suggests that iron supplementation of iron-sufficient populations improves hematologic or neurodevelopmental status.

Acute toxicity (poisoning) from iron overdose is well described and is characterized by acute liver failure. Small children are at highest risk through accidental ingestion of maternal iron supplements. Questions remain whether routine iron supplementation in therapeutic or preventative doses is a risk to the health of pregnant women and young children. The concerns revolve around the theoretical health risks of iron and the epidemiological and clinical trials in which iron supplementation was associated with adverse outcomes.

The main theoretical risks of iron supplementation in general, but particularly of iron-sufficient populations are the generation of reactive oxygen species, alteration of the intestinal microbiome toward a more "pathogenic" profile with or without an increase in diarrheal diseases, and an increased risk of non-gastrointestinal infections [83,84]. In contrast to the large preclinical and clinical research literature on the negative effects of early-life iron deficiency, the literature on the potential negative effects of iron supplementation of iron-sufficient populations is relatively limited. Further investigation of the topic seems imperative given the theoretical risks and the small amount of data in humans.

Typically, iron is protein-bound both in the serum, where it is attached to transferrin and other members of the total iron-binding protein family, and in the tissues to storage and chaperone molecules. Non-protein bound iron (NPBI) can mediate cellular DNA damage under prooxidant conditions. NPBI appears in the serum when the iron-binding capacity (TIBC) is overwhelmed, which can occur with a rapid release of iron during hemolysis or with rapid infusions of iron. Since enteral iron uptake is well regulated by the hepcidin system from a very early age, the chances of NPBI being present with enteral iron supplementation are low. Nevertheless, Brittenham et al. have recently demonstrated that in healthy women iron given at the standard treatment dose on an empty stomach can result in measurable NPBI in the serum, although no evidence of oxidative stress was observed [85].

Pediatric populations that would be at risk of NPBI and oxidative stress when given enteral iron include premature infants, because of their immature antioxidant systems and low serum transferrin concentrations and consequently, low TIBC. Studies of premature infants given up to 18 mg of iron/kg of body weight daily have failed to demonstrate increased oxidative stress [86]. Only one clinical trial in full-term infants suggests that enteral iron may be detrimental to a relevant health outcome such as neurodevelopment when given to an iron-sufficient population. In one arm of a trial of formula iron supplementation in Chile, Lozoff et al. gave an iron-fortified formula to iron-sufficient infants at 6 months of age and found poorer neurodevelopmental outcomes at 10 years of age, compared with infants given a low-iron formula [87]. Interestingly, the authors indicated that within this trial, it was only the infants who had higher than normal Hgb concentrations that demonstrated the negative neurodevelopmental effects with the iron-supplemented formula. Since the trial was targeted more toward providing iron-fortified formula to a population with a high rate of iron deficiency, supporting evidence regarding NPBI or oxidative stress markers was not available for this unanticipated finding. Nevertheless, this trial has been cited as evidence that enteral iron supplementation to iron-sufficient individuals may be problematic. Preclinical studies to support the notion have been scarce. Iron-sufficient rat pups given iron in doses between 2.5 mg/kg and 30 mg/kg body weight showed increased risk to memory performance as adults as a function of iron dose [88]. Again, no brain-tissue evidence of global or regional iron overload or oxidative stress was provided, making it difficult to assess the causative link between iron dosing and biologically plausible specific brain pathology.

The concern about enteral iron altering the intestinal microbiome to a more pathogenic state mentioned above in the context of malaria-endemic areas also extends to other areas. Prior to the recent advent of microbiome analyses, concerns of iron supplementation increasing the risk of diarrhea from siderophilic organisms such as *E. coli* and Salmonella had been raised. Yip et al. reported no increase in diarrheal disease in US breastfed infants supplemented with iron [89]. The concern about enteral iron supplementation in iron-sufficient individuals with intact hepcidin regulation of intestinal absorption is that an iron-sufficient individual absorbs less than 20% of enteral iron. The unabsorbed iron progresses downstream in the intestine to the colon and results in a high intraluminal iron concentration that fosters the growth of siderophilic bacteria. Lactobacillus, which is gut-protective, is not siderophilic and thrives in a low-iron environment compared with *E. coli*. A recent study in Africa, while performed in children at risk for iron deficiency, emphasized this shift in intestinal microbiota [90]. Other populations that may be at greater risk from this type of microbiome shift include premature infants with their higher risk of necrotizing enterocolitis. No studies have yet assessed whether unabsorbed enteral iron plays any role in this devastating disease. Similarly, whether the risk of non-diarrheal disease, such as upper respiratory tract infections mentioned above, is present in iron-sufficient populations supplemented with iron remains to be tested.

It is reasonable to postulate that the newborn infant is "set up" to require minimal exposure to enteral iron in the first months after birth when it is most vulnerable to infection and yet maintains iron sufficiency at the tissue level in order to maintain growth and development [91]. The appropriate weight for a gestational age full-term infant with no risk factors for iron deficiency during gestation [92] who undergoes "delayed" cord clamping, is breastfed and grows at the standard velocity on WHO curves has enough iron to meet its requirements until at least 4 months and likely 6 months of age. Thus, there appears to be little need for a large source of dietary iron in these otherwise iron-sufficient babies. Indeed, human milk provides very little iron and that iron is tightly bound by lactoferrin and thus not readily available for the pathophysiological processes described above [91].

7. Summary and Conclusions

Early-life iron deficiency is common and can negatively affect the brain development of children. Therefore, approaches aimed at reducing the risk of early-life iron deficiency and brain dysfunction are of public health importance. Ensuring maternal iron sufficiency during pregnancy, delayed clamping or milking of the umbilical cord, and promotion of breastfeeding are the most cost-effective approaches for ensuring that the infant begins postnatal life with sufficient iron stores. While current screening and treatment recommendations may suffice for iron-sufficient populations, biomarker-based early screening and treatment strategies may be necessary for those at risk of early-life iron deficiency. Routine iron supplementation is a cost-effective method of improving iron nutrition of at-risk children, but indiscriminant iron supplementation of children in malaria-endemic regions and iron-sufficient populations should be avoided.

Acknowledgments: The authors' studies cited in the manuscript are funded by grants HD-089989, HD-029421 and HD-074262 from the National Institutes of Health.

Author Contributions: Cusick participated in manuscript preparation and primarily wrote the section on iron supplementation in malaria-endemic regions. Georgieff participated in manuscript preparation and primarily wrote the section on iron supplementation in iron-sufficient populations. Rao conceived the idea for the review and was the lead author of the manuscript and its revision.

Conflicts of Interest: The authors declare no conflict of interest. The founding sponsors had no role in the writing of the manuscript.

References

1. Lozoff, B.; Georgieff, M.K. Iron deficiency and brain development. *Semin. Pediatr. Neurol.* **2006**, *13*, 158–165. [CrossRef] [PubMed]
2. World Health Organization. Iron Deficiency Anaemia. Assessment, Prevention, and Control. A Guide for Programme Managers. Available online: http://www.who.int/nutrition/publications/en/ida_assessment_prevention_control.pdf (accessed on 5 October 2017).
3. Lukowski, A.F.; Koss, M.; Burden, M.J.; Jonides, J.; Nelson, C.A.; Kaciroti, N.; Jimenez, E.; Lozoff, B. Iron deficiency in infancy and neurocognitive functioning at 19 years: Evidence of long-term deficits in executive function and recognition memory. *Nutr. Neurosci.* **2010**, *13*, 54–70. [CrossRef] [PubMed]
4. Chang, S.; Wang, L.; Wang, Y.; Brouwer, I.D.; Kok, F.J.; Lozoff, B.; Chen, C. Iron-deficiency anemia in infancy and social emotional development in preschool-aged Chinese children. *Pediatrics* **2011**, *127*, e927–e933. [CrossRef] [PubMed]
5. Peeling, P. Exercise as a mediator of hepcidin activity in athletes. *Eur. J. Appl. Physiol.* **2010**, *110*, 877–883. [CrossRef] [PubMed]
6. Murray-Kolb, L.E.; Beard, J.L. Iron treatment normalizes cognitive functioning in young women. *Am. J. Clin. Nutr.* **2007**, *85*, 778–787. [CrossRef] [PubMed]
7. Widdowson, E.M. Trace elements in foetal and early postnatal development. *Proc. Nutr. Soc.* **1974**, *33*, 275–284. [CrossRef] [PubMed]
8. Petry, C.D.; Eaton, M.A.; Wobken, J.D.; Mills, M.M.; Johnson, D.E.; Georgieff, M.K. Iron deficiency of liver, heart, and brain in newborn infants of diabetic mothers. *J. Pediatr.* **1992**, *121*, 109–114. [CrossRef]
9. Guiang, S.F., III; Georgieff, M.K.; Lambert, D.J.; Schmidt, R.L.; Widness, J.A. Intravenous iron supplementation effect on tissue iron and hemoproteins in chronically phlebotomized lambs. *Am. J. Physiol.* **1997**, *273*, R2124–R2131. [CrossRef] [PubMed]
10. Georgieff, M.K.; MIlls, M.M.; Gordon, K.; Wobken, J.D. Reduced neonatal liver iron concentrations after uteroplacental insufficiency. *J. Pediatr.* **1995**, *127*, 308–311. [CrossRef]
11. Dallman, P.R.; Siimes, M.A.; Manies, E.C. Brain iron: Persistent deficiency following short-term iron deprivation in the young rat. *Br. J. Haematol.* **1975**, *31*, 209–215. [CrossRef] [PubMed]
12. Georgieff, M.K.; Landon, M.B.; Mills, M.M.; Hedlund, B.E.; Faassen, A.E.; Schmidt, R.L.; Ophoven, J.J.; Widness, J.A. Abnormal iron distribution in infants of diabetic mothers: Spectrum and maternal antecedents. *J. Pediatr.* **1990**, *117*, 455–461. [CrossRef]

13. Geguchadze, R.N.; Coe, C.L.; Lubach, G.R.; Clardy, T.W.; Beard, J.L.; Connor, J.R. Csf proteomic analysis reveals persistent iron deficiency-induced alterations in non-human primate infants. *J. Neurochem.* **2008**, *105*, 127–136. [CrossRef] [PubMed]

14. Georgieff, M.K.; Schmidt, R.L.; Mills, M.M.; Radmer, W.J.; Widness, J.A. Fetal iron and cytochrome c status after intrauterine hypoxemia and erythropoietin administration. *Am. J. Physiol.* **1992**, *262*, R485–R491. [CrossRef] [PubMed]

15. Rao, R.; Tkac, I.; Townsend, E.L.; Gruetter, R.; Georgieff, M.K. Perinatal iron deficiency alters the neurochemical profile of the developing rat hippocampus. *J. Nutr.* **2003**, *133*, 3215–3221. [CrossRef] [PubMed]

16. Siddappa, A.J.; Rao, R.B.; Wobken, J.D.; Leibold, E.A.; Connor, J.R.; Georgieff, M.K. Developmental changes in the expression of iron regulatory proteins and iron transport proteins in the perinatal rat brain. *J. Neurosci. Res.* **2002**, *68*, 761–775. [CrossRef] [PubMed]

17. Fretham, S.J.; Carlson, E.S.; Wobken, J.; Tran, P.V.; Petryk, A.; Georgieff, M.K. Temporal manipulation of transferrin-receptor-1-dependent iron uptake identifies a sensitive period in mouse hippocampal neurodevelopment. *Hippocampus* **2012**, *22*, 1691–1702. [CrossRef] [PubMed]

18. Georgieff, M.K. Long-term brain and behavioral consequences of early iron deficiency. *Nutr. Rev.* **2011**, *69* (Suppl. 1), S43–S48. [CrossRef] [PubMed]

19. Wachs, T.D.; Pollitt, E.; Cueto, S.; Jacoby, E.; Creed-Kanashiro, H. Relation of neonatal iron status to individual variability in neonatal temperament. *Dev. Psychobiol.* **2005**, *46*, 141–153. [CrossRef] [PubMed]

20. Siddappa, A.M.; Georgieff, M.K.; Wewerka, S.; Worwa, C.; Nelson, C.A.; Deregnier, R.A. Iron deficiency alters auditory recognition memory in newborn infants of diabetic mothers. *Pediatr. Res.* **2004**, *55*, 1034–1041. [CrossRef] [PubMed]

21. Geng, F.; Mai, X.; Zhan, J.; Xu, L.; Zhao, Z.; Georgieff, M.; Shao, J.; Lozoff, B. Impact of fetal-neonatal iron deficiency on recognition memory at 2 months of age. *J. Pediatr.* **2015**, *167*, 1226–1232. [CrossRef] [PubMed]

22. Tamura, T.; Goldenberg, R.L.; Hou, J.; Johnston, K.E.; Cliver, S.P.; Ramey, S.L.; Nelson, K.G. Cord serum ferritin concentrations and mental and psychomotor development of children at five years of age. *J. Pediatr.* **2002**, *140*, 165–170. [CrossRef] [PubMed]

23. Armony-Sivan, R.; Eidelman, A.I.; Lanir, A.; Sredni, D.; Yehuda, S. Iron status and neurobehavioral development of premature infants. *J. Perinatol.* **2004**, *24*, 757–762. [CrossRef] [PubMed]

24. Amin, S.B.; Orlando, M.; Eddins, A.; MacDonald, M.; Monczynski, C.; Wang, H. In utero iron status and auditory neural maturation in premature infants as evaluated by auditory brainstem response. *J. Pediatr.* **2010**, *156*, 377–381. [CrossRef] [PubMed]

25. Insel, B.J.; Schaefer, C.A.; McKeague, I.W.; Susser, E.S.; Brown, A.S. Maternal iron deficiency and the risk of schizophrenia in offspring. *Arch. Gen. Psychiatry* **2008**, *65*, 1136–1144. [CrossRef] [PubMed]

26. Lozoff, B.; Beard, J.; Connor, J.; Barbara, F.; Georgieff, M.; Schallert, T. Long-lasting neural and behavioral effects of iron deficiency in infancy. *Nutr. Rev.* **2006**, *64*, S34–S91. [CrossRef] [PubMed]

27. Lozoff, B.; Smith, J.B.; Kaciroti, N.; Clark, K.M.; Guevara, S.; Jimenez, E. Functional significance of early-life iron deficiency: Outcomes at 25 years. *J. Pediatr.* **2013**, *163*, 1260–1266. [CrossRef] [PubMed]

28. Rao, R.; Ennis, K.; Oz, G.; Lubach, G.R.; Georgieff, M.K.; Coe, C.L. Metabolomic analysis of cerebrospinal fluid indicates iron deficiency compromises cerebral energy metabolism in the infant monkey. *Neurochem. Res.* **2013**, *38*, 573–580. [CrossRef] [PubMed]

29. Ward, K.L.; Tkac, I.; Jing, Y.; Felt, B.; Beard, J.; Connor, J.; Schallert, T.; Georgieff, M.K.; Rao, R. Gestational and lactational iron deficiency alters the developing striatal metabolome and associated behaviors in young rats. *J. Nutr.* **2007**, *137*, 1043–1049. [CrossRef] [PubMed]

30. Carlson, E.S.; Tkac, I.; Magid, R.; O'Connor, M.B.; Andrews, N.C.; Schallert, T.; Gunshin, H.; Georgieff, M.K.; Petryk, A. Iron is essential for neuron development and memory function in mouse hippocampus. *J. Nutr.* **2009**, *139*, 672–679. [CrossRef] [PubMed]

31. Brunette, K.E.; Tran, P.V.; Wobken, J.D.; Carlson, E.S.; Georgieff, M.K. Gestational and neonatal iron deficiency alters apical dendrite structure of ca1 pyramidal neurons in adult rat hippocampus. *Dev. Neurosci.* **2010**, *32*, 238–248. [CrossRef] [PubMed]

32. Tran, P.V.; Carlson, E.S.; Fretham, S.J.; Georgieff, M.K. Early-life iron deficiency anemia alters neurotrophic factor expression and hippocampal neuron differentiation in male rats. *J. Nutr.* **2008**, *138*, 2495–2501. [CrossRef] [PubMed]

33. Tran, P.V.; Fretham, S.J.; Wobken, J.; Miller, B.S.; Georgieff, M.K. Gestational-neonatal iron deficiency suppresses and iron treatment reactivates IGF signaling in developing rat hippocampus. *Am. J. Physiol. Endocrinol. Metab.* **2012**, *302*, E316–E324. [CrossRef] [PubMed]

34. Patton, S.M.; Coe, C.L.; Lubach, G.R.; Connor, J.R. Quantitative proteomic analyses of cerebrospinal fluid using iTRAQ in a primate model of iron deficiency anemia. *Dev. Neurosci.* **2012**, *34*, 354–365. [CrossRef] [PubMed]

35. Beard, J.L.; Unger, E.L.; Bianco, L.E.; Paul, T.; Rundle, S.E.; Jones, B.C. Early postnatal iron repletion overcomes lasting effects of gestational iron deficiency in rats. *J. Nutr.* **2007**, *137*, 1176–1182. [CrossRef] [PubMed]

36. Unger, E.L.; Hurst, A.R.; Georgieff, M.K.; Schallert, T.; Rao, R.; Connor, J.R.; Kaciroti, N.; Lozoff, B.; Felt, B. Behavior and monoamine deficits in prenatal and perinatal iron deficiency are not corrected by early postnatal moderate-iron or high-iron diets in rats. *J. Nutr.* **2012**, *142*, 2040–2049. [CrossRef] [PubMed]

37. Rao, R.; Tkac, I.; Unger, E.L.; Ennis, K.; Hurst, A.; Schallert, T.; Connor, J.; Felt, B.; Georgieff, M.K. Iron supplementation dose for perinatal iron deficiency differentially alters the neurochemistry of the frontal cortex and hippocampus in adult rats. *Pediatr. Res.* **2013**, *73*, 31–37. [CrossRef] [PubMed]

38. Baker, R.D.; Greer, F.R. Committee on Nutrition American Academy of Pediatrics. Diagnosis and prevention of iron deficiency and iron-deficiency anemia in infants and young children (0–3 years of age). *Pediatrics* **2010**, *126*, 1040–1050. [CrossRef] [PubMed]

39. Wallin, D.J.; Tkac, I.; Stucker, S.; Ennis, K.M.; Sola-Visner, M.; Rao, R.; Georgieff, M.K. Phlebotomy-induced anemia alters hippocampal neurochemistry in neonatal mice. *Pediatr. Res.* **2015**, *77*, 765–771. [CrossRef] [PubMed]

40. Zamora, T.G.; Guiang, S.F., III; Georgieff, M.K.; Widness, J.A. Iron is prioritized to red blood cells over the brain in phlebotomized anemic newborn lambs. *Pediatr. Res.* **2016**, *79*, 922–928. [CrossRef] [PubMed]

41. Carlson, E.S.; Fretham, S.J.; Unger, E.; O'Connor, M.; Petryk, A.; Schallert, T.; Rao, R.; Tkac, I.; Georgieff, M.K. Hippocampus specific iron deficiency alters competition and cooperation between developing memory systems. *J. Neurodev. Disord.* **2010**, *2*, 133–143. [CrossRef] [PubMed]

42. McDonagh, M.S.; Blazina, I.; Dana, T.; Cantor, A.; Bougatsos, C. Screening and routine supplementation for iron deficiency anemia: A systematic review. *Pediatrics* **2015**, *135*, 723–733. [CrossRef] [PubMed]

43. Lozoff, B.; Armony-Sivan, R.; Kaciroti, N.; Jing, Y.; Golub, M.; Jacobson, S.W. Eye-blinking rates are slower in infants with iron-deficiency anemia than in nonanemic iron-deficient or iron-sufficient infants. *J. Nutr.* **2010**, *140*, 1057–1061. [CrossRef] [PubMed]

44. Rao, R.; Ennis, K.; Lubach, G.R.; Lock, E.F.; Georgieff, M.K.; Coe, C.L. Metabolomic analysis of CSF indicates brain metabolic impairment precedes hematological indices of anemia in the iron-deficient infant monkey. *Nutr. Neurosci.* **2018**, *38*, 573–580. [CrossRef] [PubMed]

45. Lozoff, B.; Wolf, A.W.; Jimenez, E. Iron-deficiency anemia and infant development: Effects of extended oral iron therapy. *J. Pediatr.* **1996**, *129*, 382–389. [CrossRef]

46. Amin, S.B.; Orlando, M.; Wang, H. Latent iron deficiency in utero is associated with abnormal auditory neural myelination in ≥35 weeks gestational age infants. *J. Pediatr.* **2013**, *163*, 1267–1271. [CrossRef] [PubMed]

47. Brugnara, C.; Zurakowski, D.; DiCanzio, J.; Boyd, T.; Platt, O. Reticulocyte hemoglobin content to diagnose iron deficiency in children. *JAMA* **1999**, *281*, 2225–2230. [CrossRef] [PubMed]

48. Parodi, E.; Giraudo, M.T.; Ricceri, F.; Aurucci, M.L.; Mazzone, R.; Ramenghi, U. Absolute reticulocyte count and reticulocyte hemoglobin content as predictors of early response to exclusive oral iron in children with iron deficiency anemia. *Anemia* **2016**, *2016*, 7345835. [CrossRef] [PubMed]

49. Pasricha, S.R.; Hayes, E.; Kalumba, K.; Biggs, B.A. Effect of daily iron supplementation on health in children aged 4–23 months: A systematic review and meta-analysis of randomised controlled trials. *Lancet Glob. Health* **2013**, *1*, e77–e86. [CrossRef]

50. Siu, A.L.; Force, U.S.P.S.T. Screening for iron deficiency anemia in young children: Uspstf recommendation statement. *Pediatrics* **2015**, *136*, 746–752. [CrossRef] [PubMed]

51. Moffatt, M.E.; Longstaffe, S.; Besant, J.; Dureski, C. Prevention of iron deficiency and psychomotor decline in high-risk infants through use of iron-fortified infant formula: A randomized clinical trial. *J. Pediatr.* **1994**, *125*, 527–534. [CrossRef]

52. Friel, J.K.; Aziz, K.; Andrews, W.L.; Harding, S.V.; Courage, M.L.; Adams, R.J. A double-masked, randomized control trial of iron supplementation in early infancy in healthy term breast-fed infants. *J. Pediatr.* **2003**, *143*, 582–586. [CrossRef]
53. Ziegler, E.E.; Nelson, S.E.; Jeter, J.M. Iron stores of breastfed infants during the first year of life. *Nutrients* **2014**, *6*, 2023–2034. [CrossRef] [PubMed]
54. Institue of Medicine. Iron. In *Dietary Reference Intakes for Vitamin A, Vitamin K, Arsenic, Boron, Chromium, Copper, Iodine, Iron, Manganese, Molybdenum, Nickel, Silicon, Vanadium, and Zinc*; National Academy Press: Washington, DC, USA, 2001; pp. 290–393.
55. World Health Organization. *Daily Iron and Folic Acid Supplementation in Pregnant Women*; World Health Organization: Geneva, Switzerland, 2012.
56. Pena-Rosas, J.P.; De-Regil, L.M.; Garcia-Casal, M.N.; Dowswell, T. Daily oral iron supplementation during pregnancy. *Cochrane Database Syst. Rev.* **2015**, CD004736. [CrossRef] [PubMed]
57. Bora, R.; Sable, C.; Wolfson, J.; Boro, K.; Rao, R. Prevalence of anemia in pregnant women and its effect on neonatal outcomes in northeast India. *J. Matern. Fetal Neonatal Med.* **2014**, *27*, 887–891. [CrossRef] [PubMed]
58. McDonald, S.J.; Middleton, P.; Dowswell, T.; Morris, P.S. Effect of timing of umbilical cord clamping of term infants on maternal and neonatal outcomes. *Cochrane Database Syst. Rev.* **2013**, CD004074. [CrossRef] [PubMed]
59. Bora, R.; Akhtar, S.S.; Venkatasubramaniam, A.; Wolfson, J.; Rao, R. Effect of 40-cm segment umbilical cord milking on hemoglobin and serum ferritin at 6 months of age in full-term infants of anemic and non-anemic mothers. *J. Perinatol.* **2015**, *35*, 832–836. [CrossRef] [PubMed]
60. Andersson, O.; Lindquist, B.; Lindgren, M.; Stjernqvist, K.; Domellof, M.; Hellstrom-Westas, L. Effect of delayed cord clamping on neurodevelopment at 4 years of age: A randomized clinical trial. *JAMA Pediatr.* **2015**, *169*, 631–638. [CrossRef] [PubMed]
61. Ziegler, E.E.; Nelson, S.E.; Jeter, J.M. Iron supplementation of breastfed infants from an early age. *Am. J. Clin. Nutr.* **2009**, *89*, 525–532. [CrossRef] [PubMed]
62. Sazawal, S.; Black, R.E.; Ramsan, M.; Chwaya, H.M.; Stoltzfus, R.J.; Dutta, A.; Dhingra, U.; Kabole, I.; Deb, S.; Othman, M.K.; et al. Effects of routine prophylactic supplementation with iron and folic acid on admission to hospital and mortality in preschool children in a high malaria transmission setting: Community-based, randomised, placebo-controlled trial. *Lancet* **2006**, *367*, 133–143. [CrossRef]
63. Oral iron supplements for children in malaria-endemic areas. Available online: https://www.k4health.org/sites/default/files/okebe_2011.pdf (accessed on 16 February 2018).
64. Veenemans, J.; Milligan, P.; Prentice, A.M.; Schouten, L.R.; Inja, N.; van der Heijden, A.C.; de Boer, L.C.; Jansen, E.J.; Koopmans, A.E.; Enthoven, W.T.; et al. Effect of supplementation with zinc and other micronutrients on malaria in Tanzanian children: A randomised trial. *PLoS Med.* **2011**, *8*, e1001125. [CrossRef] [PubMed]
65. Soofi, S.; Cousens, S.; Iqbal, S.P.; Akhund, T.; Khan, J.; Ahmed, I.; Zaidi, A.K.; Bhutta, Z.A. Effect of provision of daily zinc and iron with several micronutrients on growth and morbidity among young children in Pakistan: A cluster-randomised trial. *Lancet* **2013**, *382*, 29–40. [CrossRef]
66. Gwamaka, M.; Kurtis, J.D.; Sorensen, B.E.; Holte, S.; Morrison, R.; Mutabingwa, T.K.; Fried, M.; Duffy, P.E. Iron deficiency protects against severe plasmodium falciparum malaria and death in young children. *Clin. Inf. Dis.* **2012**, *54*, 1137–1144. [CrossRef] [PubMed]
67. Gera, T.; Sachdev, H.P.; Nestel, P.; Sachdev, S.S. Effect of iron supplementation on haemoglobin response in children: Systematic review of randomised controlled trials. *J. Pediatr. Gastroenterol. Nutr.* **2007**, *44*, 468–486. [CrossRef] [PubMed]
68. Nemeth, E.; Valore, E.V.; Territo, M.; Schiller, G.; Lichtenstein, A.; Ganz, T. Hepcidin, a putative mediator of anemia of inflammation, is a type II acute-phase protein. *Blood* **2003**, *101*, 2461–2463. [CrossRef] [PubMed]
69. Atkinson, S.H.; Armitage, A.E.; Khandwala, S.; Mwangi, T.W.; Uyoga, S.; Bejon, P.A.; Williams, T.N.; Prentice, A.M.; Drakesmith, H. Combinatorial effects of malaria season, iron deficiency, and inflammation determine plasma hepcidin concentration in African children. *Blood* **2014**, *123*, 3221–3229. [CrossRef] [PubMed]
70. Pasricha, S.R.; Atkinson, S.H.; Armitage, A.E.; Khandwala, S.; Veenemans, J.; Cox, S.E.; Eddowes, L.A.; Hayes, T.; Doherty, C.P.; Demir, A.Y.; et al. Expression of the iron hormone hepcidin distinguishes different types of anemia in African children. *Sci. Transl. Med.* **2014**, *6*, 235re233. [CrossRef] [PubMed]

71. Doherty, C.P.; Cox, S.E.; Fulford, A.J.; Austin, S.; Hilmers, D.C.; Abrams, S.A.; Prentice, A.M. Iron incorporation and post-malaria Anaemia. *PLoS One* **2008**, *3*, e2133. [CrossRef] [PubMed]

72. Prentice, A.M.; Doherty, C.P.; Abrams, S.A.; Cox, S.E.; Atkinson, S.H.; Verhoef, H.; Armitage, A.E.; Drakesmith, H. Hepcidin is the major predictor of erythrocyte iron incorporation in anemic African children. *Blood* **2012**, *119*, 1922–1928. [CrossRef] [PubMed]

73. Cusick, S.E.; Opoka, R.O.; Abrams, S.A.; John, C.C.; Georgieff, M.K.; Mupere, E. Delaying iron therapy until 28 days after antimalarial treatment is associated with greater iron incorporation and equivalent hematologic recovery after 56 days in children: A randomized controlled trial. *J. Nutr.* **2016**, *146*, 1769–1774. [CrossRef] [PubMed]

74. Jaramillo, E.G.; Mupere, E.; Opoka, R.O.; Hodges, J.S.; Lund, T.C.; Georgieff, M.K.; John, C.C.; Cusick, S.E. Delaying the start of iron until 28 days after antimalarial treatment is associated with lower incidence of subsequent illness in children with malaria and iron deficiency. *PLoS ONE* **2017**, *12*, e0183977. [CrossRef] [PubMed]

75. Zimmermann, M.B.; Chassard, C.; Rohner, F.; N'Goran E, K.; Nindjin, C.; Dostal, A.; Utzinger, J.; Ghattas, H.; Lacroix, C.; Hurrell, R.F. The effects of iron fortification on the gut microbiota in African children: A randomized controlled trial in Cote d'ivoire. *Am. J. Clin. Nutr.* **2010**, *92*, 1406–1415. [CrossRef] [PubMed]

76. Jaeggi, T.; Kortman, G.A.; Moretti, D.; Chassard, C.; Holding, P.; Dostal, A.; Boekhorst, J.; Timmerman, H.M.; Swinkels, D.W.; Tjalsma, H.; et al. Iron fortification adversely affects the gut microbiome, increases pathogen abundance and induces intestinal inflammation in Kenyan infants. *Gut* **2015**, *64*, 731–742. [CrossRef] [PubMed]

77. Tang, M.; Frank, D.N.; Hendricks, A.E.; Ir, D.; Esamai, F.; Liechty, E.; Hambidge, K.M.; Krebs, N.F. Iron in micronutrient powder promotes an unfavorable gut microbiota in Kenyan infants. *Nutrients* **2017**, *9*. [CrossRef] [PubMed]

78. Paganini, D.; Uyoga, M.A.; Kortman, G.A.M.; Cercamondi, C.I.; Moretti, D.; Barth-Jaeggi, T.; Schwab, C.; Boekhorst, J.; Timmerman, H.M.; Lacroix, C.; et al. Prebiotic galacto-oligosaccharides mitigate the adverse effects of iron fortification on the gut microbiome: A randomised controlled study in Kenyan infants. *Gut* **2017**, *66*, 1956–1967. [CrossRef] [PubMed]

79. Schuijt, T.J.; Lankelma, J.M.; Scicluna, B.P.; de Sousa e Melo, F.; Roelofs, J.J.; de Boer, J.D.; Hoogendijk, A.J.; de Beer, R.; de Vos, A.; Belzer, C.; et al. The gut microbiota plays a protective role in the host defence against pneumococcal pneumonia. *Gut* **2016**, *65*, 575–583. [CrossRef] [PubMed]

80. Goheen, M.M.; Wegmuller, R.; Bah, A.; Darboe, B.; Danso, E.; Affara, M.; Gardner, D.; Patel, J.C.; Prentice, A.M.; Cerami, C. Anemia offers stronger protection than sickle cell trait against the erythrocytic stage of falciparum malaria and this protection is reversed by iron supplementation. *EBioMedicine* **2016**, *14*, 123–130. [CrossRef] [PubMed]

81. Clark, M.A.; Goheen, M.M.; Fulford, A.; Prentice, A.M.; Elnagheeb, M.A.; Patel, J.; Fisher, N.; Taylor, S.M.; Kasthuri, R.S.; Cerami, C. Host iron status and iron supplementation mediate susceptibility to erythrocytic stage plasmodium falciparum. *Nat. Commun.* **2014**, *5*, 4446. [CrossRef] [PubMed]

82. Gupta, P.M.; Hamner, H.C.; Suchdev, P.S.; Flores-Ayala, R.; Mei, Z. Iron status of toddlers, nonpregnant females, and pregnant females in the United States. *Am. J. Clin. Nutr.* **2017**, *106*, 1640S–1646S. [CrossRef] [PubMed]

83. Lonnerdal, B. Excess iron intake as a factor in growth, infections, and development of infants and young children. *Am. J. Clin. Nutr.* **2017**, *106*, 1681S–1687S. [CrossRef] [PubMed]

84. Krebs, N.F.; Domellof, M.; Ziegler, E. Balancing benefits and risks of iron fortification in resource-rich countries. *J. Pediatr.* **2015**, *167*, S20–S25. [CrossRef] [PubMed]

85. Brittenham, G.M.; Andersson, M.; Egli, I.; Foman, J.T.; Zeder, C.; Westerman, M.E.; Hurrell, R.F. Circulating non-transferrin-bound iron after oral administration of supplemental and fortification doses of iron to healthy women: A randomized study. *Am. J. Clin. Nutr.* **2014**, *100*, 813–820. [CrossRef] [PubMed]

86. Braekke, K.; Bechensteen, A.G.; Halvorsen, B.L.; Blomhoff, R.; Haaland, K.; Staff, A.C. Oxidative stress markers and antioxidant status after oral iron supplementation to very low birth weight infants. *J. Pediatr.* **2007**, *151*, 23–28. [CrossRef] [PubMed]

87. Lozoff, B.; Castillo, M.; Clark, K.M.; Smith, J.B. Iron-fortified vs. low-iron infant formula: Developmental outcome at 10 years. *Arch. Pediatr. Adolesc. Med.* **2012**, *166*, 208–215. [CrossRef] [PubMed]

88. Schroder, N.; Fredriksson, A.; Vianna, M.R.; Roesler, R.; Izquierdo, I.; Archer, T. Memory deficits in adult rats following postnatal iron administration. *Behav. Brain Res.* **2001**, *124*, 77–85. [CrossRef]

89. Scariati, P.D.; Grummer-Strawn, L.M.; Fein, S.B.; Yip, R. Risk of diarrhea related to iron content of infant formula: Lack of evidence to support the use of low-iron formula as a supplement for breastfed infants. *Pediatrics* **1997**, *99*, E2. [CrossRef] [PubMed]
90. Paganini, D.; Zimmermann, M.B. The effects of iron fortification and supplementation on the gut microbiome and diarrhea in infants and children: A review. *Am. J. Clin. Nutr.* **2017**, *106*, 1688S–1693S. [CrossRef] [PubMed]
91. Lonnerdal, B.; Georgieff, M.K.; Hernell, O. Developmental physiology of iron absorption, homeostasis, and metabolism in the healthy term infant. *J. Pediatr.* **2015**, *167*, S8–S14. [CrossRef] [PubMed]
92. Siddappa, A.M.; Rao, R.; Long, J.D.; Widness, J.A.; Georgieff, M.K. The assessment of newborn iron stores at birth: A review of the literature and standards for ferritin concentrations. *Neonatology* **2007**, *92*, 73–82. [CrossRef] [PubMed]

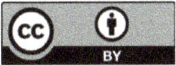

nutrients

MDPI

Article

Relative Bioavailability of Iron in Bangladeshi Traditional Meals Prepared with Iron-Fortified Lentil Dal

Rajib Podder [1], Diane M. DellaValle [2], Robert T. Tyler [3], Raymond P. Glahn [4], Elad Tako [4] and Albert Vandenberg [1,*]

1   Department of Plant Sciences, University of Saskatchewan, Saskatoon, SK S7N 5A8, Canada; rap039@mail.usask.ca
2   Department of Nutrition and Dietetics, Marywood University, 2300 Adams Avenue, Scranton, PA 18509, USA; ddellavalle@maryu.marywood.edu
3   Department of Food and Bioproduct Sciences, University of Saskatchewan, Saskatoon, SK S7N 5A8, Canada; bob.tyler@usask.ca
4   Robert W. Holley Center for Agriculture and Health, Agricultural Research Service, USDA, Ithaca, NY 14853, USA; rpg3@cornell.edu (R.P.G.); et79@cornell.edu (E.T.)
*   Correspondence: bert.vandenberg@usask.ca; Tel.: +1-306-221-2039 or +1-306-966-8786

Received: 15 January 2018; Accepted: 13 March 2018; Published: 15 March 2018

Abstract: Due to low Fe bioavailability and low consumption per meal, lentil must be fortified to contribute significant bioavailable Fe in the Bangladeshi diet. Moreover, since red lentil is dehulled prior to consumption, an opportunity exists at this point to fortify lentil with Fe. Thus, in the present study, lentil was Fe-fortified (using a fortificant Fe concentration of 2800 $\mu g\ g^{-1}$) and used in 30 traditional Bangladeshi meals with broad differences in concentrations of iron, phytic acid (PA), and relative Fe bioavailability (RFeB%). Fortification with NaFeEDTA increased the iron concentration in lentil from 60 to 439 $\mu g\ g^{-1}$ and resulted in a 79% increase in the amount of available Fe as estimated by Caco-2 cell ferritin formation. Phytic acid levels were reduced from 6.2 to 4.6 mg g^{-1} when fortified lentil was added, thereby reducing the PA:Fe molar ratio from 8.8 to 0.9. This effect was presumably due to dephytinization of fortified lentil during the fortification process. A significant ($p \leq 0.01$) Pearson correlation was observed between Fe concentration and RFeB% and between RFeB% and PA:Fe molar ratio in meals with fortified lentil, but not for the meal with unfortified lentil. In conclusion, fortified lentil can contribute significant bioavailable Fe to populations at risk of Fe deficiency.

Keywords: lentil; iron; fortification; bioavailability; Bangladesh

1. Introduction

Iron (Fe) deficiency is a public health problem and more than 30% of the world population (two billion) is anaemic, mainly due to Fe deficiency [1]. Fe deficiency is considered the major cause of anaemia, which mostly affects young children and pregnant and post-partum women [2]. In Bangladesh, anaemia is a public health concern and 40% of adolescents are anaemic [3]. In 2011, the national prevalence of anaemia in Bangladesh was 51% in children aged 6–59 months and 42% in non-pregnant women [4]. One of the major causes of Fe deficiency is low bioavailability of dietary Fe, especially in developing countries such as Bangladesh where diets are mostly cereal- and legume-based [5].

Among legumes, lentil is one of the oldest and most important cultivated crops. Lentil is consumed in both developed and developing countries around the world, and is a potential whole food source that can provide micronutrients such as Fe, zinc (Zn), and selenium (Se) [6]. In some developing countries, lentil is considered a staple food due to its nutritive value, especially as an inexpensive protein source compared to animal protein. Studies investigating ways to increase Fe content and bioavailability have focused mainly on biofortification strategies using marker-assisted breeding, improved agronomic practices, and removal of the seed coat from lentil seed [7–9]. However, Fe biofortification of food crops has several drawbacks, such as low bioavailability, limitations to increasing the total content in food crops, and insufficient consumption to show significant health benefits. The bioavailability of Fe from lentil is often compromised due to the presence of antinutritional factors (e.g., phytate, polyphenols, cotyledon cell wall) in the seed [10,11]. Fortification, on the other hand, often can overcome the inhibitors and provide significant bioavailable Fe [12] as long as the addition of Fe does not alter the appearance and taste of the target food product.

The main objective of any fortification program is to improve nutrient content and the nutritional quality of the added nutrients and thus help to eliminate or prevent deficiencies in the target population. Different strategies have been adopted to combat micronutrient deficiencies, such as biofortification, fortification, supplementation, dietary diversification, and nutrition education [13]. All of these strategies have limitations depending on sociocultural and economic factors as well as the age and gender of the target population. These may be overcome by food fortification, which has proven to be a cost-effective way to add micronutrients to processed food and improve the dietary quality of a target population without changing their food habits [14]. A systematic review of intervention of micronutrient fortified food and its impact on women and child health revealed that fortification with micronutrients, including Fe, significantly increased serum Fe concentrations with no significant adverse effect on hemoglobin levels [15].

Biofortification of lentil is not likely to have an impact on much of the Bangladeshi population as the consumption rate of pulses for the population of Bangladesh is 12 g/day/person [16], which is far below the desirable intake of 50 g/day/person that has been reported on the basis of previous studies and the current consumption pattern of the Bangladeshi population [17]. To address this shortfall, improving the nutritional quality of lentil by Fe fortification could provide a significant amount of the required daily Fe from a minimum amount of lentil dal, without having to increase the quantity of lentil in a given meal. To enable this approach, we previously developed a laboratory-scale protocol for fortifying de-hulled lentil seed (dal) using three Fe fortificants. NaFeEDTA was the most effective; at a fortificant Fe concentration of 1600 $\mu g \, g^{-1}$, NaFeEDTA provided 13–14 mg of additional Fe per 100 g of cooked lentil dal [18]. The United States Food and Drug Administration (FDA) published a food fortification policy featuring six principles for food fortification [19,20]. These are: "(1) the nutrient intake without fortification is below the desirable content for a significant portion of the population; (2) the food being fortified is consumed in quantities that would make a significant contribution to the population's intake of the nutrient; (3) the additional nutrient intake resulting from fortification is unlikely to create an imbalance of essential nutrients; (4) the nutrient added is stable under proper conditions of storage and use; (5) the nutrient is physiologically available from the food to which it is being added; and (6) there is reasonable assurance that it will not result in potentially toxic intakes." All of these principles have been considered with respect to lentil fortification.

We also investigated the sensory acceptability of fortified lentil dal with respect to appearance, odor, taste, texture, and overall acceptability by lentil consumers [21]. Fortification of lentil with NaFeEDTA minimally affected consumer perception of appearance, taste, texture, odour, and overall acceptability of cooked lentil compared to fortification with $FeSO_4 \cdot 7H_2O$ or $FeSO_4 \cdot H_2O$. Sensory acceptability was statistically similar to that of non-fortified lentil for almost all of the attributes.

The present study aimed to determine the concentration and relative bioavailability of Fe in different traditional Bangladeshi meal plan models featuring fortified and unfortified lentil dal. A Caco-2 cell bioassay was used to assess relative Fe bioavailability (RFeB%), expressed as a percentage of that of an unfortified control red lentil sample that was included in each run of the bioassay. This lentil sample had an Fe concentration of 50 $\mu g \, g^{-1}$. Ferritin formation by Caco-2 cell monolayers is a sensitive and accurate measurement tool for in vitro assessment of Fe bioavailability in food [22].

The concentration of phytic acid (PA), a known inhibitor of Fe bioavailability, also was determined in the meal plan models.

2. Materials and Methods

2.1. Preparation of Meal Models

A total of 30 meal combinations were prepared and assessed with respect to Fe concentration, RFeB%, and PA concentration (Table S1). Among these, models 1 to 11 and 15 to 25 featured either unfortified or fortified lentil dal, respectively, in different amounts (% by weight) along with other meal components. Three models (models 12 to 14) contained no lentil. The remaining five models (models 26 to 30) were prepared with only rice (model 26), vegetables (model 27), fish (model 28), unfortified cooked dal (model 29), or NaFeEDTA-fortified cooked dal (model 30). The fortified lentil had been treated with 2800 µg g^{-1} ppm NaFeEDTA, which in previous work comparing various fortificants and concentrations thereof, was determined to have the least effect on appearance and consumer acceptability measures such as taste and texture [18,21]. Lentil dal was prepared according to a traditional Bangladeshi recipe [23] where lentil, deionized water, canola oil, salt, turmeric powder and onion were used as ingredients in a 15:70:4:3:2:6 ratio, by weight. Along with the dal, rice (white, boiled and unenriched), vegetables (mixture of carrot, cauliflower, brinjal, potato, sweet potato, onion, salt, turmeric, garlic, oil, and water at a 10:10:8:10:5:2:1:1:1:12:40 ratio, by weight) and fish (fish fillets, salt, turmeric, and oil at a 90:2:3:5 ratio, by weight) were used in different ratios to prepare the meal models. All foods were cooked with 18 MΩ deionized water. Rice, fish, and vegetables were cooked in a traditional Bangladeshi fashion. Stainless steel cookware was used to prepare all meal components. Prepared dishes were cooled at room temperature for 2 h, frozen at −80 °C for 24 h, freeze-dried using a FreeZone 12 L Console Freeze Dry System with Stoppering Tray Dryers (Labconco, model 7759040, Prospect Avenue, Kansas City, MO, USA) for 72 h, and stored at room temperature [24]. A 10-g sample from each freeze-dried cooked dish (models 1 to 30) was finely ground and sent to the USDA-ARS Robert Holley Center for Agriculture and Health (Ithaca, NY, USA) to determine Fe concentration, phytic acid concentration, and RFeB%. From the 10-g sample, 0.5 g of each of the three repetitions was used in the Caco-2 cell bioassay to estimate the RFeB% [24,25].

2.2. Assessment of Fe Concentration, RFeB%, and PA Concentration

The concentrations of Fe for the 30 meal models were quantified with an inductively coupled argon-plasma emission spectrometer (iCAP 6500 series, Thermo Jarrell Ash Corp., Franklin, MA, USA) following the procedure of Glahn et al. (2017) [26]. Ferric chloride (FeCl$_3$) was used as the certified reference material in the iCAP analysis. Relative bioavailability of Fe for the 30 meal models was assessed using an established Caco-2 cell bioassay, where Caco-2 cell ferritin formation is used as the measure of cell Fe uptake and bioavailability [7,22,27]. The bioavailability assessment was conducted on three replicates for each cooked lentil sample. Ferritin values from the fortified lentil samples were compared with the control lentil (CDC Robin; Fe concentration of 50 µg g^{-1}) to calculate the RFeB%, using the following equation: Relative Fe bioavailability (RFeB %) = ((ng ferritin of the lentil sample/mg protein of the lentil sample)/(ng ferritin/mg protein of the control lentil)) × 100 [8]. The resulting index of relative Fe bioavailability (RFeB%) is used hereafter. Phytic acid content was measured as phosphorous released by phytase and alkaline phosphatase via a colorimetric assay kit (K-PHYT 12/12, Megazyme International, Wicklow, Ireland) [26].

2.3. Data Analysis

Data were analyzed statistically using SAS version 9.4 (SAS Institute Inc., Cary, NC, USA). One-way analysis of variance (ANOVA) was used to verify differences in Fe concentration, RFeB%, and PA concentration among different meal models. The outcomes for the three variables (Fe concentration, RFeB%, and PA concentration) represented the three replicates of each sample. Fisher's least significant difference (LSD) was calculated with the level of significance set at $p < 0.05$. Paired t-test analysis was used to assess differences in the five variables in the meal models featuring fortified vs. unfortified lentil. The associations among Fe concentration, RFeB%, and PA concentration were assessed using Pearson correlations at a $p < 0.05$ significance level [7]. Fe concentration, ferritin formation (ng ferritin/mg protein), RFeB%, PA, and PA:Fe molar ratio were compared to assess the effect of NaFeEDTA-fortified lentil (meal models 15 to 25) vs. unfortified lentil (meal models 1 to 11). A correlation analysis also was conducted for Fe concentration, PA concentration, and RFeB% to determine the relationships among these measures.

3. Results

3.1. Fe Concentration, RFeB%, and PA Concentration

The average Fe concentration, RFeB%, and PA concentration of 30 meal model samples prepared with unfortified and fortified lentil are shown in Figure 1 and in Table S2. Significant differences were observed for Fe concentration, RFeB%, and PA concentration. The Fe concentration of the 30 meal plan models ranged from 2.1 µg g^{-1} (model 26; 100% rice) to 439.2 µg g^{-1} (model 30; 100% NaFeEDTA fortified lentil) and the PA concentration ranged from 1.2 mg g^{-1} (model 26; 100% rice) to 6.2 mg g^{-1} (model 29; 100% unfortified dal). RFeB% ranged from 3.7% (model 27; 100% vegetable) to 48.6% (model 15; 50% rice + 50% NaFeEDTA-fortified lentil); the control lentil had an RFeB% value of 30.9%. The highest Fe concentration, PA concentration, and RFeB% were found for meal models 30, 29, and 15, respectively. Among the 11 meal models (models 1 to 11) where unfortified lentil was used as a meal component (usage ranged from 5–50%, by weight), the highest Fe and PA concentrations were found in model 1, whereas the highest RFeB% was observed in model 2 (Figure 1). In meal models 15 to 25, where fortified lentil was used, the highest Fe and PA concentrations and RFeB% were observed in meal model 15 (Figure 1).

The iron concentrations for model 29 (100% unfortified lentil; Fe concentration 60 µg g^{-1}) and model 30 (100% NaFeEDTA-fortified lentil; Fe concentration 439.2 µg g^{-1}) indicate that lentil was the main component providing Fe across all of the meal plans (Figure 1). This also is reflected in the six models (12, 13, 14, 26, 27, 28) that contained no lentil and had low Fe concentrations (Figure 1) compared to models containing either fortified or unfortified lentil. Fish, vegetables, and rice did not notably affect Fe concentration as these components contain low amounts of Fe. The vegetable curry contained a higher amount of Fe (19.4 µg g^{-1}) than did fish (11.4 µg g^{-1}) or rice (2.1 µg g^{-1}). The main component of meal models 2 to 14 and 16 to 25 was rice, ranging from 75 to 85%, by weight. Although the largest amounts of PA were found in unfortified lentil (6.2 mg g^{-1}) followed by fortified lentil dal (4.6 mg g^{-1}), the contribution of PA would have been mainly from rice, which comprised the major part of most meal models. For instance, meal models 9 and 23 had similar amounts of rice (85%) and lentil dal (15%), but the former contained unfortified dal and the latter, fortified dal. PA concentrations in meal models 9 and 23 were 2.4 and 1.7 mg g^{-1}, respectively, of which 1.02 mg g^{-1} was contributed by rice.

Among the six meal models (1, 5, 9, 15, 19, 23) in which rice and lentil were the only ingredients, increasing the amount of rice generally decreased the Fe concentration, PA concentration, and RFeB%. The meal model that included rice (50%), fish (25%), vegetables (25%), and no lentil (model 13) contained a very low amount of Fe (8.7 µg g^{-1}) but it was of higher relative bioavailability, which could be due to the low amount of PA in the meal. Models 4, 8, 18, and 22 contained similar amounts of vegetable (5%), but model 8 and 22 contained 10% more rice and 5% less fish and dal compared to models 4 and 18. This resulted in decreased Fe concentration, PA concentration, and RFeB%.

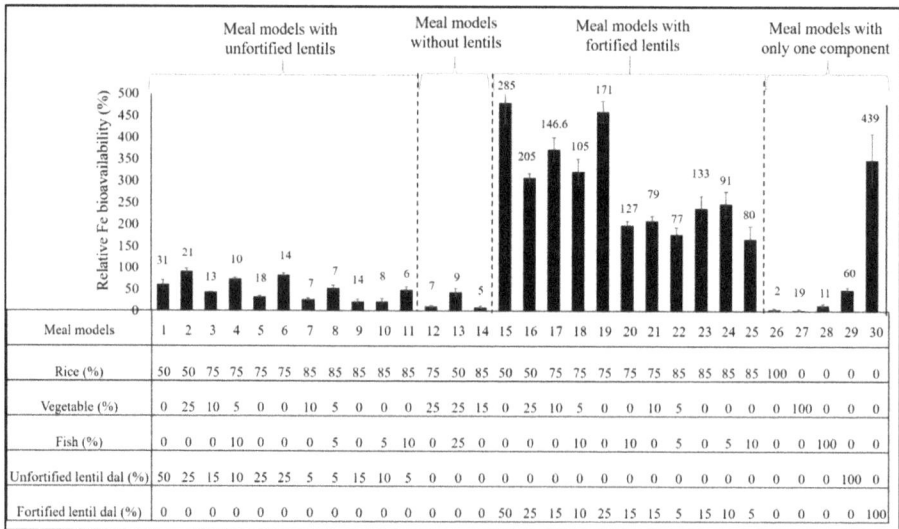

Figure 1. Relative iron bioavailability (RFeB%) and Fe concentration ($\mu g\ g^{-1}$, above each bar) of 30 traditional Bangladeshi meal plan models containing unfortified lentil (meal models 1–11), no lentil (meal models 12–14), fortified lentil (meal models 15–25) and single components (meal models 26–30), assessed using a Caco-2 cell bioassay.

3.2. Comparison between Meal Models Containing Unfortified vs. Fortified Lentil

A comparison of Fe concentration, ferritin formation (ng ferritin/mg protein), relative Fe bioavailability (% of control lentil), PA concentration, and PA:Fe molar ratio between meal model groups featuring unfortified lentil (models 1 to 11) vs. fortified lentil (meal models 15 to 25) revealed significant differences for all parameters considered. Specifically, the average Fe concentration was significantly ($p \leq 0.001$) higher in meal models with fortified lentil (136.2 $\mu g\ g^{-1}$) compared to those with unfortified lentil (13.5 $\mu g\ g^{-1}$). Ferritin formation (52.5 vs. 15.8 ng ferritin/mg protein) and RFeB% (290.0 vs. 51.2%) also were significantly ($p < 0.001$) higher in meal models with fortified lentil. PA concentration (2.1 vs. 2.4 mg g^{-1}, $p = 0.03$) and PA:Fe molar ratio (1.5 vs. 16.9) were significantly ($p \leq 0.001$) lower in meal models with fortified lentil.

3.3. Correlations between Measured Variables

Correlation coefficients between measured variables are presented in Table 1. Significant correlations were observed between Fe concentration and RFeB%, RFeB% and PA:Fe molar ratio, and Fe concentration and PA:Fe molar ratio when all meal models were considered. Significant correlations between Fe concentration and RFeB% as well as between RFeB% and PA:Fe molar ratio were observed for meal models with fortified lentil (models 15 to 25) but not unfortified lentil (models 1 to 11). Fe concentration and PA:Fe molar ratio had an inverse relationship for all meal models containing either unfortified or fortified lentil.

Table 1. Pearson correlation coefficients for iron (Fe) concentration vs. relative Fe bioavailability (RFeB%), bioavailability vs. phytic acid (PA):Fe molar ratio, and Fe concentration vs. PA:Fe molar ratio.

Meal Model	(Fe) vs. RFeB%	RFeB% vs. PA:Fe Molar Ratio	(Fe) vs. PA:Fe Molar Ratio
All (models 1 to 30)	0.832 **	−0.722 **	−0.627 **
(n = 30)	(<0.001)	(<0.001)	(<0.001)
Unfortified lentil (models 1 to 11)	−0.142	0.351	−0.628 *
(n = 11)	(0.685)	(0.299)	(0.0364)
Fortified lentil (model 15 to 25)	0.801 **	−0.763 **	−0.628 *
(n = 11)	(0.001)	(0.004)	(0.036)

** Correlation is significant at the 0.01 level (2-tailed); * Correlation is significant at the 0.05 level (2-tailed).

4. Discussion

Lentil fortification programs have been initiated with the aim of improving the Fe content in lentil because lentil serves as a major side dish in many countries, including Bangladesh. Due to poor absorption of intrinsic Fe from lentil, improvement in the Fe concentration in lentil dal and the increased absorption of Fe through fortification is a potential strategy to combat micronutrient malnutrition. In this study we assessed the bioavailability of Fe, using a Caco-2 cell bioassay, from a variety of traditional Bangladeshi meal models that contained either Fe-fortified or unfortified lentil.

In Bangladesh, the prevalence of anaemia in adolescent girls is ~30%, with iron deficiency considered the main cause [3]. Socioeconomic conditions also are reported to be a factor that, along with nutritional deficiency, influence dietary problems in rural Bangladeshi women, who consume lentil three (60%) or four (12%) times per week [28]. Lentil consumption is also increasing with the increasing price and reduced availability of animal protein. One study of the dietary habits of 384 rural women from northern Bangladesh revealed that 92% of respondents eat hotchpotch, a typical and traditional Bangladeshi dish with a pulse (usually lentil) and rice [28]. Thus, lentil fortification could be a potential approach to supplying a major part of the required amount of Fe to vulnerable people with Fe deficiency in Bangladesh.

Micronutrient bioavailability from fortified food depends on its absorption through the gastrointestinal tract for systemic utilization [29]. Bioavailability is the result of three major steps: digestibility (solubility of Fe in digesta), absorbability in the circulation system, and final processing and incorporation into a functional compartment of the body [30,31]. Different approaches, such as the chemical balance method, solubility or dialyzability, Caco-2 cell bioassay, hemoglobin repletion method, isotopic methods, and area under the curve for serum iron have been used to estimate non-heme iron absorption [32]. Other algorithms or combinations thereof have been used to assess Fe uptake based on Fe absorption from a single or complete meal [32]. In this study, a Caco-2 cell bioassay was used to measure Fe absorption. This model mimics conditions in the small intestine, and ferritin formation in the Caco-2 cell monolayers is considered as a marker for iron uptake [24]. Some limitations have been reported for the in vitro Caco-2 cell bioassay, for example, the in vitro model cannot fully mirror the human gut system that involves the effect of body Fe status and gut microflora on Fe uptake [24]. Considering these limitations, although this in vitro model is not a substitute for an in vivo model, it is a highly sensitive, cost-effective, and quick tool to measure Fe availability in foods [22,24]. Moreover, this model was found to be strongly correlated (R = 0.968, $p < 0.001$) with human Fe absorption studies [33], and with human and animal efficacy studies of Fe absorption from biofortified crops [34]. This model, therefore, can be considered to be thoroughly validated as a predictor of Fe absorption by humans. PA content was measured using a colorimetric assay kit, which is widely used as it gives accurate and reliable data, and saves cost and time [35]. Sometimes this kit gives a more accurate result than HPLC and quality controlling is easier than using HPLC if the person running the system is less experienced [36]. However, a limitation to the use of this kit is that it cannot measure *myo*-inositol in either its free or phytase/alkaline phosphatase released forms [35].

Iron absorption is influenced by both endogenous and exogenous factors [37]. The recipe used to prepare the various meal models used herein included different spices (turmeric, onion, garlic) and fat (canola oil). Bio-accessibility of Fe increased by 26.3% and 17.2% when 3.0 g of onion and 0.5 g of garlic, respectively, were cooked with 10 g of chickpea [38,39]. This could be due to the presence of sulfur-containing amino acids in *Allium* species that are reported to influence mineral status in animals. Moreover, spices also may contain phytic acid (inositol hexakisphosphate) and polyphenolic compounds (e.g., tannic acid and chlorogenic acid) [40]. The fortified and unfortified lentil used in the meal preparations are non-heme iron sources. Most polyphenols are located in the lentil seed coat, and the dehulled lentil used in this study would contain a low level of polyphenols, which would contribute to increased non-heme iron absorption in populations with limited Fe storage [41]. Turmeric is used extensively in countries of the Indian sub-continent, including Bangladesh. The most active constituent of turmeric is curcumin, a polyphenolic diketone. Curcumin forms a complex with solubilized Fe in aqueous solution with either Fe(II) or Fe(III) ion [42–44] and does not inhibit Fe absorption in young women [24]. Vegetables also contain significant amounts of vitamin A, carotenoids, and indigestible carbohydrates and the effect of these components on Fe absorption is unresolved [45]. Some vegetables used in this study to prepare vegetable curry, such as potato and sweet potato, contain a higher amount of Fe compared to the fish and the other vegetables used. This may explain the higher amount of Fe in vegetable (19.4 μg g^{-1}; meal model 27) than in fish (11.4 μg g^{-1}; meal model 28). A similar result also was found in another study conducted with traditional Bangladeshi meals [24].

Lentil consumption varies with age, gender, food habit, price, and availability of lentil in the market. The amount of vegetables in the meal models ranged from 5 to 25%, similar to traditional Bangladeshi meals. Fish comprised only 5 or 10% of the meals because the fish price in local markets is high and the consumption rate much lower than for other food items in the regular meal. Two meal models (models 3 and 17) are unique and represent hotchpotch, a ubiquitous meal for 1- to 5-year-olds and school-aged children in Bangladesh. In suburban areas of Bangladesh, "dal vaat" (rice and lentil or other pulses) is a common meal. Dried fish also is prevalent, and small amounts of dried fish with rice and lentil (models 6, 11, 20, and 25) also is a popular and widespread meal for local people in Bangladesh. The 30 meal models considered herein were designed with either unfortified or fortified lentil in varying amounts (5, 10, 15, 25, or 50%). Preliminary data (not shown) indicated that consumers prefer a thicker soup, which requires more lentil. This is favourable, as a higher amount of lentil dal in a meal will help to provide more of the required supply of Fe, and will increase the relative bioavailability.

The choice of NaFeEDTA-fortified lentil was based on the results of our two previous studies with respect to consumer acceptability [18,21]. Moreover, in the context of bioavailability, NaFeEDTA has proven to be more suitable than FeSO$_4$ as a fortificant in legume-based flours [46]. In cowpea flour, higher PA:Fe molar ratios (3.0:1 to 3.3:1) are related to low iron absorption [46]. PA chelates with positively charged multivalent cations such as Fe, Zn, Mg, and Ca, forming insoluble complexes that precipitate in the neutral pH condition of the small intestine, thus decreasing Fe absorption [47]. In models 29 (100% unfortified lentil) and 30 (100% NaFeEDTA-fortified lentil), the PA content was 6.2 and 4.6 mg g^{-1} and the RFeB% was 50.6 and 349.2%, respectively (Table S2). These differences could be attributed to: (i) the higher Fe concentration in the NaFeEDTA-fortified lentil; (ii) the lower PA content in the NaFeEDTA-fortified lentil; or (iii) the fortification process, as dephytinization can inactivate phytates to a large extent [47].

In this study, PA concentration was assessed using a PA (total P) test kit (Megazyme International, Ireland). However, the concentration of polyphenolic components also could differ between fortified and unfortified lentil dal due to the effect of the fortification process. The PA concentration in the unfortified lentil meal (model 29) was significantly higher than in the fortified lentil dal meal (model 30). Thus, the PA:Fe molar ratio also was reduced from 8.8 in meal model 29 to 0.9 in meal model 30

(Table S2). This could be due to dephytinization during the fortification process. A previous study reported that for Fe-fortified fonio porridge, dephytinization and fortification reduced the PA:Fe molar ratio from 24:1 to 0.3:1 [48]. Again, a significant inverse correlation was found between RFeB% and the PA:Fe molar ratio. A similar result with respect to RFeB% and PA:Fe molar ratio was observed for meal models prepared with dehulled lentil and whole lentil [24].

Although no recommendations are in place for lentil fortification, the World Health Organization (WHO) has recommended some Fe fortificants and appropriate doses for fortification of wheat flour in 13 countries [49]. The Food and Agriculture Organizations of the United Nations/World Health Organization recommended nutrient intakes (RNIs) of Fe (mg) for females and males 19–50 years of age are 29.4 and 13.7 mg, respectively, based on 10% bioavailability [14]. In this study, the amount of fortified lentil ranged from 5–50% in meal models 15 to 25. These meal models feature the fortified lentil as part of the meal, and not as a supplement. The meal model with fortified lentil only (model 30; 100% NaFeEDTA-fortified lentil) can provide ~43.9 mg of Fe from 100 g of cooked dal (dry basis). This means that 100 g (dry basis) of meal model 19, which contains 25% fortified lentil, would contain ~11 mg of Fe. This could provide a major portion of the recommended nutrient intakes (RNIs) of Fe for adult males and females aged 19–50 (mentioned in [14]). Because the tolerable upper intake level of Fe for adults is 45 mg/day [50], the meal model with fortified lentil only (50 g person^{-1}) is also safe for human consumption.

The study results showed that lentil was the major contributor of Fe and that the relative bioavailability of Fe increased when NaFeEDTA-fortified lentil was used in different meal models. Since different amounts of either fortified or unfortified lentil were used in different meal models, and the RNIs are advised on the basis of age, gender, pregnancy, and lactation period, recommendations for use of appropriate amounts of Fe-fortified lentil can be given for target populations. In this study, PA content was measured and considered to be the key inhibitor of Fe absorption. Since the PA concentration was significantly lower in the fortified lentil, it may be possible that levels of inhibitory polyphenols were also reduced in the fortified lentil, thereby increasing Fe absorption. However, it has been shown recently that not all polyphenols inhibit Fe absorption, and some have been identified as potential promoters of Fe uptake [51,52]. As we did not measure polyphenols in the meal models, our study cannot address this point.

5. Conclusions

Per capita global consumption of lentil is increasing rapidly. In some regions, however, the per capita consumption rate is actually decreasing due to higher demand. Fe-fortified lentil can provide a higher amount of Fe from a smaller amount of fortified lentil compared to unfortified lentil. This study demonstrated that lentil fortification is a promising and simple approach to help alleviate Fe deficiency, especially for countries in the developing world like Bangladesh, where most of the population consumes lentil in their daily meals.

Supplementary Materials: The following are available online at www.mdpi.com/2072-6643/10/3/354/s1. Table S1: Description of the 30 meal models, Table S2: Iron (Fe) concentration, relative Fe bioavailability (RFeB%), and phytic acid (PA) concentration (mean ± SD) and PA:Fe molar ratio of 30 meal plan models composed of varying percentages by volume of the amounts of rice, vegetable curry, fish and dal (lentil dish prepared with either fortified or unfortified lentil).

Acknowledgments: The authors would like to acknowledge financial assistance received from The Saskatchewan Ministry of Agriculture (Agriculture Development Fund) and Grand Challenges Canada. The authors are grateful for technical assistance provided by Barry Goetz, Crop Development Centre, University of Saskatchewan, and Mary Bodis, research support specialist and Yongpei (PeiPei) Chang, technician, Cornell University, USDA-ARS, Robert W. Holley Center, Ithaca, New York.

Author Contributions: Rajib Podder, Diane M. DellaValle, Raymond P. Glahn and Albert Vandenberg conceived and designed the study. Rajib Podder and Diane M. DellaValle analysed the study. Rajib Podder prepared the draft manuscript. All authors reviewed all documents critically and approved the final manuscript for submission to the journal.

Conflicts of Interest: The authors declare no conflict of interest.

References

1. WHO Micronutrient Defficiencies, Iron Defficiency Anaemia. Available online: http://www.who.int/nutrition/topics/ida/en/ (accessed on 25 February 2018).
2. De Benoist, B.; McLean, E.; Egll, I.; Cogswell, M. Worldwide Prevalence of Anaemia 1993–2005, WHO Global Database on Anaemia. Available online: http://whqlibdoc.who.int/publications/2008/9789241596657_eng.pdf?ua=1 (accessed on 15 November 2017).
3. Ahmed, F.; Khan, M.R.; Mohammad, A.; Rezaul, K.; Gail, W.; Harriet, T.; Ian, D.-H.; Dalmiya, N.; Banu, C.P.; Nahar, B. Long-term intermittent multiple micronutrient supplementation enhances hemoglobin and micronutrient status more than iron + folic acid supplementation in Bangladeshi rural adolescent girls with nutritional anemia. *J. Nutr.* **2010**, *140*, 1879–1886. [CrossRef] [PubMed]
4. National Institute for Population Research and Training. Bangladesh Demographic and Health Survey 2011. Available online: https://dhsprogram.com/pubs/pdf/fr265/fr265.pdf (accessed on 18 August 2017).
5. Zimmermann, M.B.; Chaouki, N.; Hurrell, R.F. Iron deficiency due to consumption of a habitual diet low in bioavailable iron: A longitudinal cohort study in Moroccan children. *Am. J. Clin. Nutr.* **2005**, *81*, 115–121. [CrossRef] [PubMed]
6. Thavarajah, D.; Thavarajah, P.; Wejesuriya, A.; Rutzke, M.; Glahn, R.P.; Combs, G.F.; Vandenberg, A. The potential of lentil (*Lens culinaris* L.) as a whole food for increased selenium, iron, and zinc intake: Preliminary results from a 3 year study. *Euphytica* **2011**, *180*, 123–128. [CrossRef]
7. DellaValle, D.M.; Thavarajah, D.; Thavarajah, P.; Vandenberg, A.; Glahn, R.P. Lentil (*Lens culinaris* L.) as a candidate crop for iron biofortification: Is there genetic potential for iron bioavailability? *Field Crops Res.* **2013**, *144*, 119–125. [CrossRef]
8. DellaValle, D.M.; Vandenberg, A.; Glahn, R.P. Seed Coat Removal Improves Iron Bioavailability in Cooked Lentils: Studies Using an in Vitro Digestion/Caco-2 Cell Culture Model. *J. Agric. Food Chem.* **2013**, *61*, 8084–8089. [CrossRef] [PubMed]
9. Khazaei, H.; Podder, R.; Caron, C.T.; Kundu, S.S.; Diapari, M.; Vandenberg, A.; Bett, K.E. Marker-Trait Association Analysis of Iron and Zinc Concentration in Lentil (*Lens culinaris* Medik.) Seeds. *Plant Genome* **2017**, *10*, 1–8. [CrossRef] [PubMed]
10. Grusak, M.A. Nutritional and health-beneficial quality. In *The Lentil: Botany, Production and Uses*; Erskine, W., Muehlbauer, F.J., Sarker, A., Sharma, B., Eds.; CABI International: Cambridge, MA, USA, 2009; pp. 368–390.
11. Glahn, R.P.; Tako, E.; Cichy, K.; Wiesinger, J. The cotyledon cell wall and intracellular matrix are factors that limit iron bioavailability of the common bean (Phaseolus vulgaris). *Food Funct.* **2016**, *7*, 3193–3200. [CrossRef] [PubMed]
12. Hurrell, R.F. Fortification: Overcoming Technical and Practical Barriers. *J. Nutr.* **2002**, *132*, 806S–812S. [CrossRef] [PubMed]
13. Northrop-Clewes, C.A. Food fortification. In *Nutrition in Infancy*; Humana Press: Totowa, NJ, USA, 2013; pp. 359–381.
14. Allen, L.; de Benoist, B.; Dary, O.; Hurrell, R. Guidelines on Food Fortification with Micronutrients. Available online: http://www.unscn.org/layout/modules/resources/files/fortification_eng.pdf (accessed on 21 April 2017).
15. Das, J.K.; Salam, R.A.; Kumar, R.; Bhutta, Z.A. fortification of food and its impact on woman and child health: A systematic review. *Syst. Rev.* **2013**, *2*, 1–24. [CrossRef] [PubMed]
16. Sarker, A.; Erskine, W.; Bakr, M.A.; Rahman, M.M.; Afzal, M.A.; Saxena, M.C. *Lentil Improvement in Bangladesh—A Success Story of Fruitful Partnership between the Bangladesh Agricultural Research Institute and International Center for Agricultural Research in the Dry Areas*; Asia-Pacific Association of Agricultural Research Institutions: Bangkok, Thailand, 2004.
17. FAO. Food-Based Dietary Guidelines—Bangladesh. Available online: http://www.fao.org/nutrition/education/fooddietaryguidelines/regions/countries/Bangladesh/en/ (accessed on 11 May 2017).
18. Podder, R.; Tar'an, B.; Tyler, R.T.; Carol, J.H.; DellaValle, D.M.; Vandenberg, A. Iron fortification of lentil (*Lens culinaris* Medik.) to address iron deficiency. *Nutrients* **2017**, *9*, 863. [CrossRef] [PubMed]
19. FDA. Guidance for Industry: Questions and Answers on FDA's Fortification Policy. Available online: https://www.fda.gov/food/guidanceregulation/guidancedocumentsregulatoryinformation/ucm470756.htm#A (accessed on 20 June 2017).

20. Dwyer, J.T.; Wiemer, K.L.; Dary, O.; Keen, C.L.; King, J.C.; Miller, K.B.; Philbert, M.A.; Tarasuk, V.; Taylor, C.L.; Gaine, P.C.; et al. Fortification and Health: Challenges and Opportunities. *Adv. Nutr. Int. Rev. J.* **2015**, *6*, 124–131. [CrossRef] [PubMed]

21. Podder, R.; Khan, S.M.; Tar'an, B.; Tyler, R.T.; Henry, C.J. Sensory acceptability of iron-fortified red lentil (*Lens culinaris* Medik.) dal. *J. Food Sci.* **2018**. [CrossRef] [PubMed]

22. Glahn, R.P.; Lee, O.A.; Yeung, A.; Goldman, M.I.; Miller, D.D. Caco-2 cell ferritin formation predicts nonradiolabeled food iron availability in an in vitro digestion/Caco-2 cell culture model. *J. Nutr.* **1998**, *128*, 1555–1561. [CrossRef] [PubMed]

23. Kohinoor, H.; Siddiqua, A.; Akhtar, S.; Hossain, M.G.; Podder, R.; Hossain, M.A. *Nutrition and Easy Cooking of Pulses*; Bangladesh Agricultural Research Institute: Gazipur, Bangladesh; Print Valley Printing Press: Gazipur, Bangladesh, 2010.

24. DellaValle, D.M.; Glahn, R.P. Differences in relative iron bioavailability in traditional Bangladeshi meal plans. *Food Nutr. Bull.* **2014**, *35*, 431–439. [CrossRef] [PubMed]

25. Glahn, R. The use of Caco-2 cells in defining nutrient bioavailability: Application to iron bioavailability of foods. *Des. Funct. Foods* **2009**, 340–361. [CrossRef]

26. Glahn, R.; Tako, E.; Hart, J.; Haas, J.; Mercy, L.; Beebe, S. Iron Bioavailability Studies of the First Generation of Iron-Biofortified Beans Released in Rwanda. *Nutrients* **2017**, *9*, 787. [CrossRef] [PubMed]

27. Tako, E.; Glahn, R.P. White beans provide more bioavailable iron than red beans Tako and Glahn. *Int. J. Vitam. Nutr. Res.* **2011**, *81*, 1–14.

28. Sheema, M.K.; Rahman, R.M.; Yasmin, Z.; Rahman, M.S.; Choudhary, M.Y.; Ali, M.F.R.; Javed, A. Food Habit and Nutritional Status of Rural Women in Bangladesh. *Am. J. Rural Dev.* **2016**, *4*, 114–119. [CrossRef]

29. Moretti, D.; Biebinger, R.; Bruins, M.J.; Hoeft, B.; Kraemer, K. Bioavailability of iron, zinc, folic acid, and vitamin A from fortified maize. *Ann. N. Y. Acad. Sci.* **2014**, *1312*, 54–65. [CrossRef] [PubMed]

30. Wienk, K.J.H.; Marx, J.J.M.; Beynen, A.C. The concept of iron bioavailability and its assessment. *Eur. J. Nutr.* **1999**, *38*, 51–75. [CrossRef] [PubMed]

31. Armah, S.M. *Models to Assess Food Iron Bioavailability*; Iowa State University: Ames, IA, USA, 2014.

32. Armah, M.S.; Carriquiry, A.; Sullivan, D.; Cook, J.D.; Reddy, M.B. A complete diet-based algorithm for predicting nonheme iron absorption in adults. *J. Nutr.* **2013**, *143*, 1136–1140. [CrossRef] [PubMed]

33. Yun, S.M.; Habicht, J.; Miller, D.; Glahn, R. An in vitro digestion/Caco-2 cell culture system accurately predicts the effects of ascorbic acid and polyphenolic compounds on iron bioavailability in humans. *J. Nutr.* **2004**, *134*, 2717–2721. [CrossRef] [PubMed]

34. Tako, E.; Bar, H.; Glahn, R.P. The combined application of the Caco-2 cell bioassay coupled with in vivo (Gallus gallus) feeding trial represents an effective approach to predicting fe bioavailability in humans. *Nutrients* **2016**, *8*, 732. [CrossRef] [PubMed]

35. Reason, D.A.; Watts, M.J.; Devez, V. *Quantification of Phytic Acid in Grains*; British Geological Survey: Nottingham, UK, 2015.

36. McKie, V.A.; McCleary, B.V. A novel and rapid colorimetric method for measuring total phosphorus and phytic acid in foods and animal feeds. *J. AOAC Int.* **2016**, *99*, 738–743. [CrossRef] [PubMed]

37. Hunt, J. Dietary and physiological factors that affect the absorption and bioavailability of iron. *J. Vitam. Nutr. Res.* **2005**, *75*, 375–384. [CrossRef] [PubMed]

38. Gautam, S.; Patel, K.; Srinivasan, K. Higher Bioaccessibility of Iron and Zinc from Food Grains in the Presence of Garlic and Onion. *J. Agric. Food Chem.* **2010**, *58*, 8426–8429. [CrossRef] [PubMed]

39. Greger, J.L.; Mulvaney, J. Absorption and tissue distribution of zinc, iron and copper by rats fed diets containing lactalbumin, soy and supplemental sulfur-containing amino acids. *J. Nutr.* **1985**, *115*, 200–210. [CrossRef] [PubMed]

40. Hunt, J.R. No TitleBioavailability of iron, zinc, and other trace minerals from vegetarian diets. *Am. J. Clin. Nutr.* **2003**, *78*, 633S–639S. [CrossRef] [PubMed]

41. Mennen, L.I.; Walker, R.; Bennetau-Pelissero, C.; Scalbert, A. Risks and safety of polyphenol consumption. *Am. J. Clin. Nutr.* **2005**, *81*, 326S–329S. [CrossRef]

42. Tuntipopipat, S.; Judprasong, K.; Zeder, C.; Wasantwisut, E.; Winichagoon, P.; Charoenkiatkul, S.; Hurrell, R.; Walczyk, T. Chili, but Not Turmeric, Inhibits Iron Absorption in Young Women from an Iron-Fortified Composite Meal. *J. Nutr.* **2006**, *136*, 2970–2974. [CrossRef] [PubMed]

43. Bernabé-Pineda, M.; Ramírez-Silva, M.T.; Romero-Romob, M.A.; González-Vergara, E.; Rojas-Hernández, A. Spectrophotometric and electrochemical determination of the formation constants of the complexes Curcumin–Fe(III)–water and Curcumin–Fe(II)–water. *Spectrochim. Acta Part A* **2004**, *60*, 1105–1113. [CrossRef]

44. Borsari, M.; Ferrari, E.; Grandi, R.; Monica, S. Curcuminoids as potential new iron-chelating agents: Spectroscopic, polarographic and potentiometric study on their Fe(III) complexing ability. *Inorg. Chim. Acta* **2002**, *328*, 61–68. [CrossRef]

45. Hurrell, R.; Egli, I. Iron bioavailability and dietary reference values. *Am. J. Clin. Nutr.* **2010**, *91*, 1461S–1467S. [CrossRef] [PubMed]

46. Abizari, A.R.; Moretti, D.; Schuth, S.; Zimmermann, M.B.; Armar-Klemesu, M.; Brouwer, I.D. Phytic Acid-to-Iron Molar Ratio Rather than Polyphenol Concentration Determines Iron Bioavailability in Whole-Cowpea Meal among Young Women. *J. Nutr.* **2012**, *142*, 1950–1955. [CrossRef] [PubMed]

47. Schlemmer, U.; Frølich, W.; Prieto, R.M.; Grases, F. Phytate in foods and significance for humans: Food sources, intake, processing, bioavailability, protective role and analysis. *Mol. Nutr. Food Res.* **2009**, *53*, S330–S375. [CrossRef] [PubMed]

48. Koréissi-Dembélé, Y.; Fanou-Fogny, N.; Moretti, D.; Schuth, S.; Dossa, R.A.M.; Egli, I.; Zimmermann, M.B.; Brouwer, I.D. Dephytinisation with Intrinsic Wheat Phytase and Iron Fortification Significantly Increase Iron Absorption from Fonio (Digitaria exilis) Meals in West African Women. *PLoS ONE* **2013**, *8*. [CrossRef] [PubMed]

49. Pachón, H.; Spohrer, R.; Mei, Z.; Serdula, M.K. Evidence of the effectiveness of flour fortification programs on iron status and anemia: A systematic review. *Nutr. Rev.* **2015**, *73*, 780–795. [CrossRef] [PubMed]

50. National Institutes of Health Iron-Dietary Supplement Fact Sheet. Available online: https://ods.od.nih.gov/pdf/factsheets/Iron-HealthProfessional.pdf (accessed on 11 August 2017).

51. Hart, J.J.; Tako, E.; Glahn, R.P. Characterization of Polyphenol Effects on Inhibition and Promotion of Iron Uptake by Caco-2 Cells. *J. Agric. Food Chem.* **2017**, *65*, 3285–3294. [CrossRef] [PubMed]

52. Hart, J.J.; Tako, E.; Kochian, L.V.; Glahn, R.P. Identification of Black Bean (*Phaseolus vulgaris* L.) Polyphenols That Inhibit and Promote Iron Uptake by Caco-2 Cells. *J. Agric. Food Chem.* **2015**, *63*, 5950–5956. [CrossRef] [PubMed]

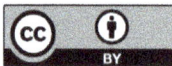

nutrients

MDPI

Article

Optimal Serum Ferritin Levels for Iron Deficiency Anemia during Oral Iron Therapy (OIT) in Japanese Hemodialysis Patients with Minor Inflammation and Benefit of Intravenous Iron Therapy for OIT-Nonresponders

Kazuya Takasawa [1,*], Chikako Takaeda [1], Takashi Wada [2] and Norishi Ueda [3,*]

1   Department of Internal Medicine, Division of Nephrology, Public Central Hospital of Matto Ishikawa, Ishikawa 9248588, Japan; takaeda@imcc-med.com
2   Department of Nephrology, Kanazawa University; Kanazawa, Ishikawa 9208641, Japan; twada@m-kanazawa.jp
3   Department of Pediatrics, Public Central Hospital of Matto Ishikawa, Ishikawa 9248588, Japan
*   Correspondence: kazuya@takasawa.org (K.T.); nueda@mattohp.com (N.U.);
    Tel.: +81-76-275-2222 (K.T. & N.U.)

Received: 10 February 2018; Accepted: 19 March 2018; Published: 29 March 2018

Abstract: Background: We determined optimal serum ferritin for oral iron therapy (OIT) in hemodialysis (HD) patients with iron deficiency anemia (IDA)/minor inflammation, and benefit of intravenous iron therapy (IIT) for OIT-nonresponders. **Methods:** Inclusion criteria were IDA (Hb <120 g/L, serum ferritin <227.4 pmol/L). Exclusion criteria were inflammation (C-reactive protein (CRP) $\geq$ 5 mg/L), bleeding, or cancer. IIT was withheld >3 months before the study. ΔHb $\geq$ 20 g/L above baseline or maintaining target Hb (tHB; 120–130 g/L) was considered responsive. Fifty-one patients received OIT (ferrous fumarate, 50 mg/day) for 3 months; this continued in OIT-responders but was switched to IIT (saccharated ferric oxide, 40 mg/week) in OIT-nonresponders for 4 months. All received continuous erythropoietin receptor activator (CERA). Hb, ferritin, hepcidin-25, and CERA dose were measured. **Results:** Demographics before OIT were similar between OIT-responders and OIT-nonresponders except low Hb and high triglycerides in OIT-nonresponders. Thirty-nine were OIT-responders with reduced CERA dose. Hb rose with a peak at 5 months. Ferritin and hepcidin-25 continuously increased. Hb positively correlated with ferritin in OIT-responders ($r = 0.913$, $p = 0.03$) till 5 months after OIT. The correlation equation estimated optimal ferritin of 30–40 ng/mL using tHb (120–130 g/L). Seven OIT-nonresponders were IIT-responders. **Conclusions:** Optimal serum ferritin for OIT is 67.4–89.9 pmol/L in HD patients with IDA/minor inflammation. IIT may be a second line of treatment for OIT-nonreponders.

Keywords: ferritin; hemodialysis; hepcidin-25; inflammation; iron deficiency anemia; oral iron therapy

---

1. Introduction

Iron deficiency anemia (IDA) is a common problem, which causes resistance to erythropoietin-stimulating agents (ESAs), is associated with patients on chronic hemodialysis (HD), and increases morbidity and mortality, whereas correction of anemia improves these events in HD patients [1]. IDA is generally defined by serum ferritin of <67.4 pmol/L and transferrin saturation (TSAT) <16%, while higher cutoffs of serum ferritin and TSAT are used to define IDA under inflammatory conditions such as chronic kidney disease (CKD) [2]. The Kidney Disease Improving Global Outcome (KDIGO) guidelines recommend that iron therapy should be initiated if CKD patients have serum ferritin

≤1123.5 pmol/L and TSAT ≤30% [3]. In Europe, it is recommended that serum levels of ferritin should be maintained at 898.8–1348.2 pmol/L for the management of IDA in HD patients [4]. However, the Japanese Society for Dialysis Therapy (JSDT) guidelines use more conservative criteria for IDA (serum ferritin <227.4 pmol/L and TSAT <20%) probably due to lower prevalence of inflammation in the Japanese HD patients [5]. In fact, prevalence of increased C-reactive protein (CRP) levels, a marker of inflammation, in HD patients was higher in Western countries than in Japan [6,7] and of catheter use for HD and obesity, which can increase inflammation, was lower in HD patients of Japan than those of Western countries [6].

Intravenous iron therapy (IIT) has been proposed to have superior benefit over oral iron therapy (OIT) for the management of IDA and efficient maintenance of target hemoglobin (tHb) in HD patients [8]. Recently, the majority of HD patients receiving IIT and ESAs have been shown to have hepatic iron overload evaluated by magnetic resonance imaging (MRI) [9,10]. A risk of hospitalization, cardiovascular events, infection, and mortality was significantly higher in HD patients receiving higher doses of IIT [11,12] and ESAs [13] than in those receiving lower doses [14]. Mortality was significantly higher in HD patients receiving an IV iron dose of >300 mg/month than in those receiving iron dose of <299 mg/month [11]. The MRI study suggested that the standard maximal amount of iron infused per month should be lowered to <250 mg/month in order to reduce a risk of iron overload and allow safer use of parenteral iron products [9]. These findings may call for a revision of clinical guidelines of the management of IDA in patients with chronic kidney disease (CKD), especially in HD patients, including the root and dose of iron supplementation.

Iron supplementation with avoidance of iron overload is crucial for the management of IDA in HD patients. For the purpose of appropriate management of IDA in CKD patients, rapid, accurate and noninvasive methods for monitoring iron stores in the body are mandatory, but unfortunately not available except the measurement of total body iron by MRI. Serum ferritin is a most commonly used and reliable biomarker of iron status in the absence of inflammation [2]. Serum levels of ferritin were positively correlated with liver iron content in HD patients [9,10]. High serum levels of ferritin reflected iron overload [10], resulting in iron toxicity and high mortality in CKD patients [15]. However, as acute reactants, serum ferritin and CRP are up-regulated by inflammation, which is frequently associated with CKD [2,16]. Thus, interpretation of data for serum ferritin should be with caution. Furthermore, both parameters were frequently increased in HD patients with functional IDA (FIDA) [17], accompanied by high inflammation, and HD patients with FIDA required higher dose of IIT than those without [18]. On the contrary, lower levels of CRP were predictive of a greater response to OIT in HD patients [19]. Taken together, these data suggest that therapeutic strategy for IDA should differ between HD patients with and without high inflammation.

Serum levels of ferritin were higher in HD patients treated with IIT than those with OIT [20], suggesting a possible risk of iron overload in HD patients receiving IIT compared to those receiving OIT. OIT is less toxic than IIT [8,21] and may reduce a risk of iron overload which leads to cardiovascular events, infection and mortality [22]. OIT has recently been shown to be as effective as IIT for the management of IDA in non-dialysis CKD [21] and HD patients [23–26] with relatively lower serum levels of ferritin and normal CRP. In the former study [21], IIT was associated with an increased risk of serious adverse events, including cardiovascular events and infectious disease. We have previously reported that OIT was beneficial for IDA in HD patients with minor inflammation and that ferritin and hepcidin-25 could be predictive of the OIT response [25]. However, it remains elusive what levels of serum ferritin are optimal for the management of IDA during iron supplementation in CKD patients to reduce a risk of iron overload-related adverse effects [2]. This prospective study was thus undertaken to determine the following, (1) what levels of serum ferritin are optimal for OIT in HD patients with IDA and minor inflammation receiving a continuous erythropoietin receptor activator (CERA)? And (2) whether IIT could be a second line of treatment for IDA in HD patients who are refractory to OIT.

2. Materials and Methods

Inclusion criteria of the study were adult HD patients ($\geq$18 years of age) and IDA (hemoglobin; Hb < 120 g/L and ferritin <227.4 pmol/L). Exclusion criteria were inflammation as defined by the presence of C-reactive protein (CRP) $\geq$ 5 mg/L, bleeding, cancer or poor adherence. Iron supplementation was withheld >3 months prior to the study.

At the initiation of the present study, there were 70 patients on maintenance HD in our hospital. Of these, 51 consecutive HD patients with IDA fulfilled the inclusion criteria and were enrolled in the study. This study was non-randomized and prospective study performed at our single center. All patients received oral ferrous fumarate (50 mg/day) for the first 3 months (Figure 1). The response to OIT was determined at 3 months after OIT since serum ferritin started to rise within this period (see in Section 3). At this time point, the patients were classified into two groups; OIT-responders and OIT-nonresponders. In OIT-responders, oral ferrous fumarate was continued for another 4 months. In OIT-nonresponders, OIT was switched to IIT (40 mg of saccharated ferric oxide), which was given 13 times during another 4 months. The dose and duration of this IIT protocol has been recommended by the JSDT guidelines [5]. All patients simultaneously received a CERA (epoetin β pegol) during the study period. The response to OIT or IIT was defined by the change in Hb levels before and after iron supplementation (ΔHb) of $\geq$200 g/L above baseline or maintenance of target Hb (tHb; 120~130 g/L). Since ΔHb of $\geq$10 g/L was used as an index of the response to iron therapy [4], the number of the patients with ΔHb of <20 g/L, but $\geq$10 g/L were also presented.

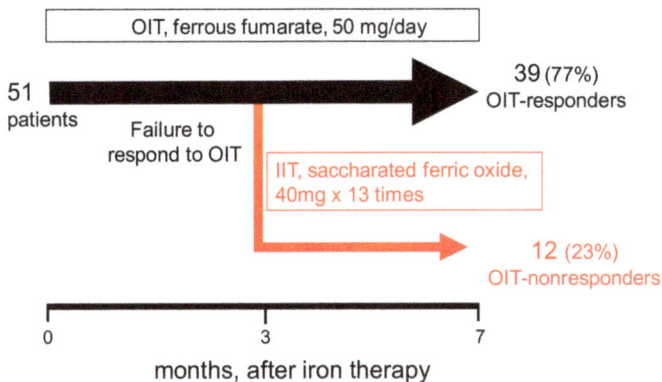

Figure 1. Protocol of iron therapy. Fifty-one consecutive hemodialysis (HD) patients with iron deficiency anemia (IDA) and minor inflammation were first treated with oral ferrous fumarate (50 mg/day). At 3 months after oral iron therapy (OIT), the patients were classified into two groups; OIT-responders and OIT-nonresponders. OIT was continued in 39 OIT-responders for another 4 months. OIT was switched to intravenous iron therapy (IIT; saccharated ferric oxide: 40 mg × 13 times for another 4 months) in the remaining 12 OIT-nonresponders. All patients simultaneously received a continuous erythropoietin receptor activator (CERA) during the study period.

The levels of Hb and serum levels of ferritin, as measured by standard laboratory methods, were analyzed every month after the initiation of iron supplementation. Serum levels of hepcidin-25, a key regulatory hormone of iron metabolism, were measured by liquid chromatography tandem-mass spectrometry (LC-MS/MS) at 0, 6, and 7 months after iron supplementation as described in our previous study [25]. To determine optimal levels of serum ferritin in OIT-responders, correlation between the levels of Hb and serum ferritin was determined, and then optimal serum levels of ferritin were calculated by the correlation efficient using tHb of 120–130 g/L. The dose of CERA was measured at 0, 3, and 6 months after iron supplementation, and compared between groups. Written informed consent was obtained from all participants prior to entering the study. Our institutional research and ethics review board approved the study (approval code: 28-1).

Statistical Analysis

Data are expressed as median (interquartile) in table, mean ± standard deviation (SD) in text and mean ± standard error of the mean (SEM) in figures. Comparison of two nonparametric data groups was performed using the Mann–Whitney U test. Comparison of nonparametric data in 3 groups was determined by Tukey–Kramer test, and that of two proportions was performed using the Fisher's exact test. The linear correlation between Hb and serum ferritin levels was determined using Pearson's correlation coefficient test. A p value < 0.05 was considered significant.

3. Results

Of the 51 HD patients, 39 patients (77%) responded to OIT (OIT-responders), and the remaining 12 patients (OIT-nonresponders) failed to respond to a 3-month-course of OIT (Figure 1 and Table 1). Demographic and baseline laboratory data before starting OIT in both the OIT-responders and the OIT-nonresponders are summarized in Table 1. There was no difference between the two groups in the variables except low Hb levels ($p < 0.05$) and high levels of serum triglycerides ($p < 0.05$) in the OIT-nonresponders. In the absence of apparent inflammation, serum hepcidin-25 is positively correlated with Hb till iron-repletion state is achieved. Thus, as Hb, the baseline hepcidin-25 levels tended to be lower in the OIT-nonresponders than in the OIT-responders. When ΔHb $\geq$ 10 g/L was used as criteria for the response to iron therapy, prevalence of OIT response was 44 of 51 patients (86.3%). At the end of the study, only one IIT-nonresponder achieved ΔHb <20 g/L but $\geq$10 g/L.

Table 1. Demographic and laboratory data in OIT-responders and OIT-nonresponders.

	OIT-Responders (*n* = 39)	OIT-Nonresponders (*n* = 12)	*p* Value
Age (years)	66.0 (18.0)	62.5 (13.8)	0.46
Female (%)	52	33	0.32
Body mass index (kg/m^2)	21.3 (4.0)	21.9 (3.6)	0.84
HD vintage (years)	4.5 (10.5)	4.0 (7.8)	0.50
spKt/V	1.49 (0.4)	1.35 (0.59)	0.65
Hb (g/L)	10.3 (1.4)	9.2 (1.3) *	0.04
MCV (fL)	84.8 (8.1)	85.9 (8.6)	0.49
Serum ferritin (pmol/L)	39.8 (51.2)	29.2 (53.4)	0.47
Serum iron (μmol/l)	12.5 (10.7)	8.3 (8.2)	0.13
TSAT (%)	18.2 (14.5)	15.5 (13.8)	0.71
Serum hepcidin (nmol/L)	5.1 (10.1)	2.8 (6.7)	0.25
Serum creatinine (μmol/L)	1034 (309)	919 (265)	0.50
Serum albumin (g/L)	35 (5)	36 (2)	0.34
Serum triglycerides (mmol/L)	0.95 (0.44)	1.42 (0.96) *	0.02
Serum calcium (mmol/L)	2.4 (0.1)	2.4 (0.4)	0.35
Serum phosphorus (mmol/L)	1.7 (0.6)	1.8 (0.5)	0.66
i-PTH (ng/L)	62.0 (82.0)	50.5 (84.5)	0.62
CRP (mg/L)	0.4 (0.9)	0.6 (0.8)	0.69
CERA dose (μg/week)	150 (50)	150 (62.5)	0.73
Comorbidities (%)			
Diabetes mellitus	32	33	
Hypertension	85	67	
Coronary artery disease	26	25	
Congestive heart failure	0	0	
Vascular disease	8	8	

Data are expressed as median (interquartile). OIT, oral iron therapy; CRP, C-reactive protein; HD, hemodialysis; CERA, continuous erythropoietin receptor activator; i-PTH, intact parathyroid hormone; MCV, mean corpuscular volume; TSAT, transferrin saturation. Comparison of two nonparametric data groups were determined by the Mann-Whitney U test. * p < 0.05, vs. OIT responders.

In the OIT-responders, mean levels of Hb rose from a baseline of 99 ± 11 g/L to 120 ± 6 g/L ($p < 0.05$) at 3 months and 126 ± 12 g/L ($p < 0.05$) at 6 months after OIT (Figure 2). The ΔHb at 3 and 6 months after OIT were 17 ± 6 g/L ($p < 0.01$) and 27 ± 19 g/L ($p < 0.01$), respectively, and the ΔHb at 6 months was higher ($p < 0.01$) than that at 3 months after OIT. The ΔHb were 30 ± 11 g/L at 3 months and 40 ± 13 g/L at 6 months after OIT in the 21 OIT-responders with ΔHb ≥ 20 g/L, and 10 ± 6 g/L at 3 months and 12 ± 11 g/L at 6 months after OIT in the remaining 18 OIT-responders who achieved the tHb but ΔHb < 20 g/L. In the 12 OIT-nonresponders, the baseline Hb was 92 ± 11 g/L, the Hb was 98 ± 8 g/L at 3 months after OIT, and the ΔHb remained unchanged (6 ± 12 g/L). In the OIT-nonresponders ($n = 12$), after switching to IIT, the ΔHb significantly rose at 6 months after OIT (16 ± 20 g/L, $p < 0.01$) compared to that at 3 months after OIT (6 ± 12 g/L).

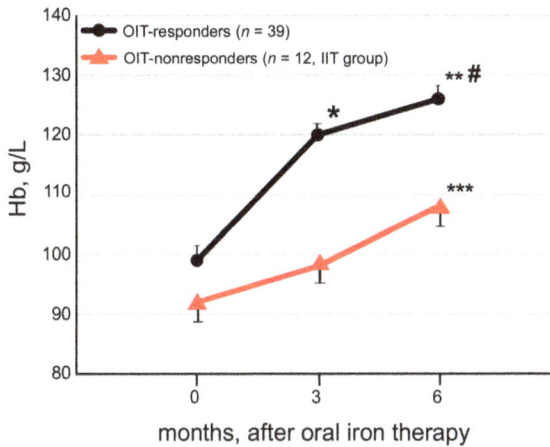

Figure 2. Change of Hb levels in OIT-responders and OIT-nonresponders. The Hb levels were increased at 3 and 6 months after OIT in OIT-responders. In OIT-nonresponders, the Hb levels remained unchanged at 3 months after OIT but increased with IIT at the end of the study as a whole IIT-group. Data are expressed as mean $\pm$ standard error of the mean (SEM). Comparison of two nonparametric data groups was analyzed by the Mann-Whitney U test. * $p < 0.01$, vs. data at 0 month, ** $p < 0.01$, vs. data at 3 months, *** $p < 0.05$, vs. data at 3 months, # $p < 0.05$, vs. OIT-nonresponders.

In the OIT-responders, the CERA dose significantly decreased from baseline of 135 ± 45 µg/4 weeks to 111 ± 49 µg/4 weeks ($p < 0.05$) at the end of the study, while it remained unchanged in the OIT-nonresponders (152 ± 57 µg/4 weeks at baseline vs. 160 ± 56 µg/4 weeks at 6 months).

Of the 12 OIT-nonresponders receiving IIT, seven patients (58%, IIT-responders) responded to IIT, and the remaining 5 failed to respond (IIT-nonresponders, Figure 3). In the IIT-responders, the ΔHb significantly rose from the value for 11 ± 13 g/L at 3 months to 17 ± 5 g/L ($p < 0.05$) at 6 months, respectively, whereas ΔHb at 3 and 6 months after iron therapy was 1 ± 9 g/L and -1 ± 10 g/L in the IIT-nonresponders.

To determine optimal serum levels of ferritin during OIT for the management of IDA in HD patients, we first analyzed sequential changes in the levels of Hb, serum ferritin and hepcidin-25 during OIT in the OIT-responders (Figure 4). The levels of Hb rose linearly with a peak at 5 months, and then slightly decreased till the end of the study. Serum levels of ferritin were decreased from the baseline at 1 month, and then rose continuously from 2 to 7 months after OIT. Serum levels of hepcidin-25 at 6 months (8.0 ± 7.2 nmol/L) were similar to the baseline data (8.1 ± 9.1 nmol/L) but significantly increased (21.6 ± 16.2 nmol/L, $p < 0.001$) at the end of the study. Serum levels of hepcidin-25 were positively correlated with those of ferritin in the OIT-responders ($r = 0.852$, $p < 0.0001$) at the start of OIT.

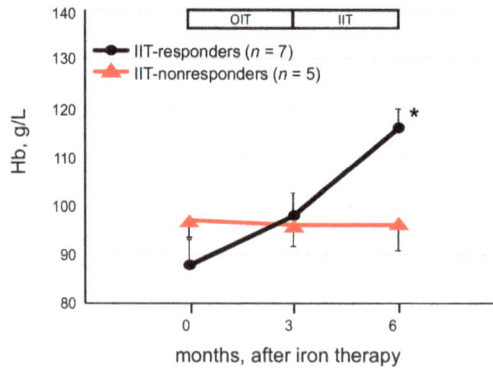

Figure 3. Change of Hb levels in IIT group before and after IIT. Of the 12 OIT-nonresponders, the levels of Hb were significantly increased in seven (58.3%) of the 12 patients at the end of the study, whereas the Hb levels remained unchanged in the five IIT-nonresponders. Data are expressed as mean ± SEM. Comparison of two nonparametric data groups was analyzed by the Mann–Whitney U test. * $p < 0.01$, vs. IIT-nonresponders.

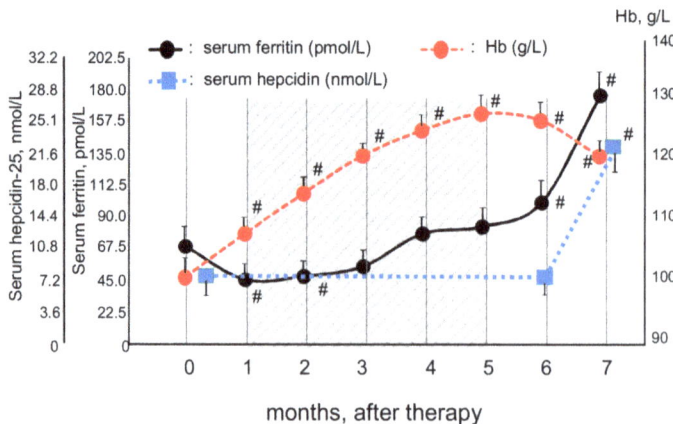

Figure 4. Sequential change in the levels of Hb, serum ferritin and hepcidin-25 in OIT-responders during OIT. The levels of Hb rose linearly with a peak at 5 months after OIT and then slightly decreased at the end of the study. Serum levels of ferritin were decreased from baseline at 1 month, and then rose continuously from 2 to 7 months after OIT. Serum levels of hepcidin-25 were similar to baseline at 6 months but significantly increased at the end of the study. Serum levels of hepcidin-25 were positively correlated with those of ferritin in the OIT-responders ($r = 0.869$, $p = 0.0002$). Data are expressed as mean ± SEM. Comparison of 2 means was determined by the Man–Whitney U test. # $p < 0.01$, vs. data at 0 month.

We next examined correlation between the levels of Hb and serum ferritin in the OIT-responders using mean values of Hb and serum ferritin in the OIT responders at every month during the study period. Despite no correlation was found between these parameters during 4–7 months after OIT, the levels of Hb were positively correlated with those of serum ferritin during 1 to 5 months after OIT

($r = 0.913$, $p = 0.03$, Figure 5). The correlation equation calculated by Peason's correlation coefficient test was y = 0.0945x + 9.23, where y = Hb and x = serum ferritin. Based on this equation, optimal levels of serum ferritin for the management of IDA were estimated to be 67.4–89.9 pmol/L when the tHb was 120–130 g/L.

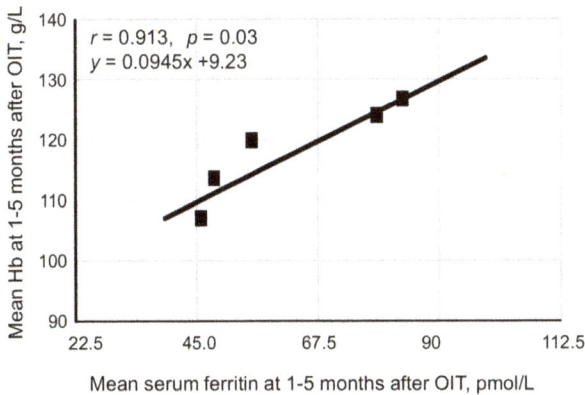

Figure 5. Correlation of Hb and serum ferritin between 1 and 5 months after OIT in OIT-responders. Ccorrelation between the levels of Hb and serum ferritin was analyzed in 39 OIT-responders using mean values for Hb and serum ferritin at every month obtained from OIT-responders as a whole. The levels of Hb were positively correlated with serum levels of ferritin till 5 months after OIT in 39 OIT-responders. The correlation equation calculated by Pearson's correlation coefficient test was y = 0.0945x + 9.23, where y = Hb: x = serum ferritin.

To determine whether high serum levels of ferritin are predictive of hyporesponsiveness to iron supplementation, serum levels of ferritin at 0 and 6 months after the initiation of iron supplementation were compared among the OIT-responders, IIT-responders, and IIT-nonresponders. Serum levels of ferritin at 6 months were significantly higher in the IIT-nonresponders (299.5 ± 247.8 pmol/L) than in the IIT-responders 142.0 ± 69.9 pmol/L, $p < 0.05$) and the OIT-responders (99.8 ± 54.8 pmol/L, $p < 0.01$, Figure 6). At the end of the study, serum iron levels were adequate and not statistically significant in the three groups; 13.3 ± 5.8 µmol/L in the OIT-responders, 9.8 ± 5.4 µmol/L in the IIT-responders, and 11.2 ± 3.3 µmol/L in the IIT-nonresponders. Despite no statistical difference in serum levels of hepcidin-25 between the groups at the start of the study, serum hepcidin-25 levels tended to be higher in the IIT-nonresponders (8.1 ± 10.5 nmol/L) than in the IIT-responders (4.1 ± 5.0 nmol/L). Similarly, at 6 months after iron therapy, serum levels of hepcidin-25 tended to be higher in the IIT-nonresponders (8.5 ± 9.0 nmol/L) than in the IIT-responders (2.0 ± 2.0 nmol/L). In addition, TSAT improved in the OIT-responders ($30.3 \pm 13.6\%$) and $20.1 \pm 12.5\%$ in the IT-responders, whereas it remained low ($15.2 \pm 0.9\%$) in the IIT-nonresponders at the end of the study.

We next examined whether the values for hepcidin-25 are predictive of the response to iron supplementation. In the 51 patients, serum levels of hepcidin-25 at the start of OIT were negatively correlated with ΔHb at 3 months ($r = -0.282$, $p < 0.05$, Figure 7A) and ΔHb at 6 months ($r = -0.392$, $p < 0.01$, Figure 7B), respectively. When correlation between the two parameters were determined only in the OIT-responders, a more significant correlation was noted between hepcidin-25 and ΔHb at 3 months ($r = -0.525$, $p < 0.01$) and 6 months ($r = -0.578$, $p < 0.01$).

Serum levels of hepcidin-25 were significantly lower in the 21 OIT-responders with ΔHb ≥ 20 g/L (5.1 ± 7.6 nmol/L, $p < 0.05$, Figure 8) than in the remaining 18 OIT-responders with ΔHb < 20 g/L (8.9 ± 2.2 nmol/L). Serum levels of hepcidin-25 at the start of OIT tended to be lower in the IIT-responders ($n = 7$, 4.1 ± 5.0 nmol/L) than in the IIT-nonresponders ($n = 5$, 8.1 ± 10.5 nmol/L). There was a similar trend for decreased serum levels of hepcidin-25 in the OIT-responders plus IIT-responders (*n* = 46, 4.6 ± 6.9 nmol/L) compared to those in the IIT-nonresponders (*n* = 5, 8.1 ± 10.5 nmol/L).

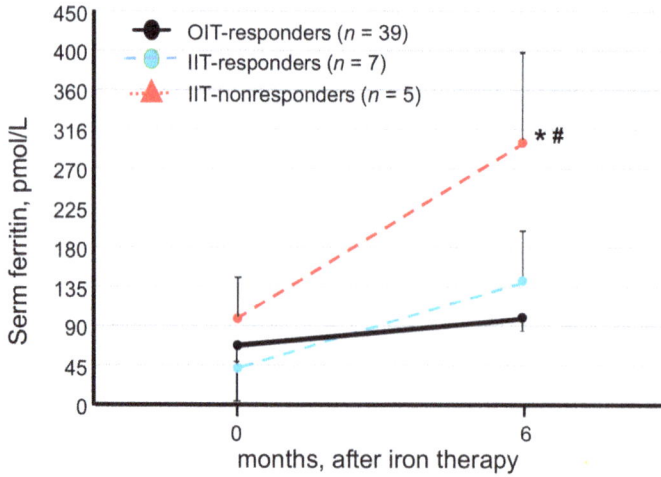

Figure 6. Change in serum levels of ferritin at 0 and 6 months after initiation of the study in OIT-responders, IIT-responders and IIT-nonresponders. Serum levels of ferritin were significantly higher in the IIT-nonresponders than in the OIT-responders and the IIT-responders, whereas there was no difference in serum ferritin levels between the OIT-responders and the IIT-responders. Comparison of three nonparametric data groups was analyzed by the Tukey–Kramer test. * $p < 0.05$, vs. IIT-responders, # $p < 0.01$, vs. OIT-responders.

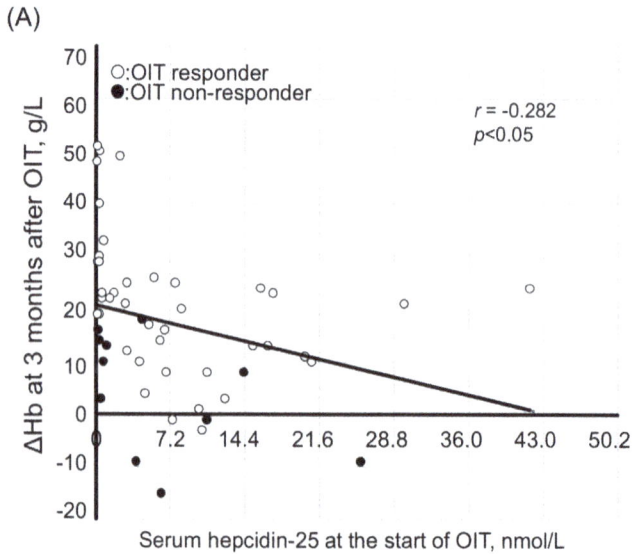

Figure 7. *Cont.*

(B)

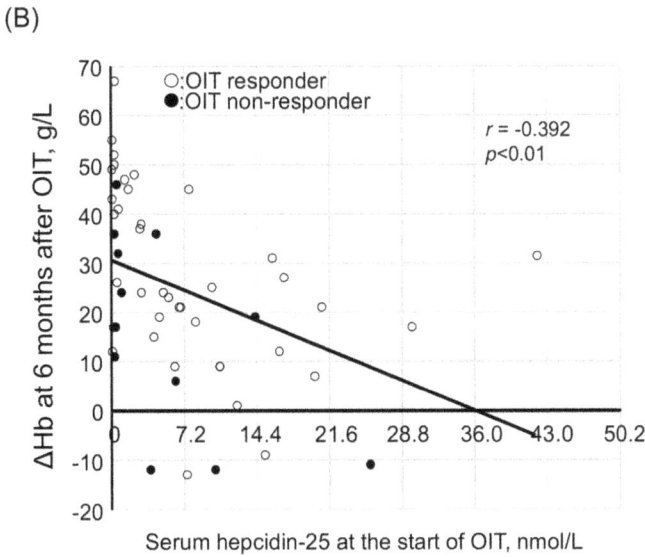

Figure 7. Correlation between serum levels of hepcidin-25 at the start of OIT and ΔHb at 3 and 6 months after OIT. Serum levels of hepcidin-25 at the start of OIT were negatively correlated with ΔHb at 3 months ($r = -0.282$, $p < 0.05$) (**A**) and at 6 months ($r = -0.392$, $p < 0.01$) (**B**) in 51 HD patients. The correlation equation was calculated by Pearson's correlation coefficient test. White circle: OIT-responders, black circle: OIT-nonreponders.

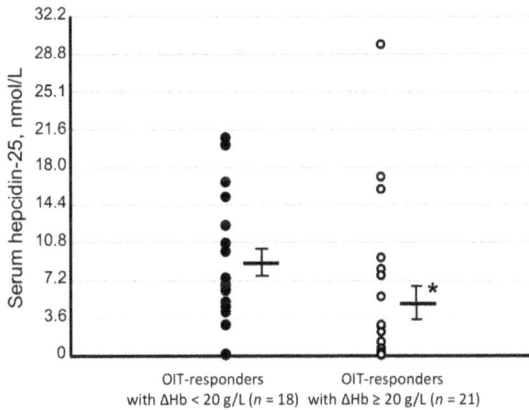

Figure 8. Serum levels of hepcidin-25 at the start of OIT between 21 OIT-responders with ΔHb ≥ 20 g/L and 18 OIT-responders achieving target Hb but ΔHb < 20 g/L at 3 months after OIT. Serum levels of hepcidin-25 at the start of OIT were significantly lower in the 21 OIT-responders with ΔHb ≥ 20 g/L than those in the 18 OIT responders who achieved target Hb (120–130 g/L) but ΔHb < 20 g/L. Comparison of two nonparametric data groups was analyzed by the Mann–Whitney U test. White circle: OIT-responders with ΔHb ≥ 20 g/L, black circle: the 18 OIT-responders with ΔHb < 20 g/L. * $p < 0.05$ vs. OIT-responders with ΔHb < 20 g/L.

Finally, we examined whether serum triglycerides can indicate the response to OIT due to higher serum triglycerides associated with the OIT-nonresponders (see Table 1). Despite a very weak negative correlation between serum triglycerides and hepcidin-25 ($r = -0.319$, $p = 0.02$), there was no significant correlation between serum triglycerides and ferritin ($r = 0.224$, $p = 0.08$) and ΔHb at 3 months ($r = -0.08$, $p = 0.59$).

There were no serious adverse effects associated with OIT or IIT and iron supplementation was well tolerated.

4. Discussion

There is a concern about a link between serum levels of ferritin and a risk of mortality in HD patients with IDA. Some investigators in the U.S. proposed that serum ferritin levels of 1123.5–2696.4 pmol/L were not associated with increased risk of mortality in HD patients receiving IIT and ESA if malnutrition and inflammation were controlled [27], while the same research group reported a trend for higher mortality in non-dialysis CKD patients with serum ferritin >561.8 pmol/L [28]. International guidelines for the management of IDA recommend that IV iron should be discontinued when serum ferritin is >1123.5–2696.4 pmol/L [3,29]. However, high levels of CRP [6,30] and serum ferritin of >179.8–1797.6 pmol/L were associated with worse outcome in HD patients [14,31–34]. In addition, serum ferritin levels of >1123.5–1797.6 pmol/L were associated with high mortality in HD patients in Europe, the U.S. [34,35] and Taiwan [31]. In these studies [31,34,35], the levels of CRP were high in the majority of the HD patients. In contrast, relatively lower serum ferritin levels (>179.8–1114.5 pmol/L) were associated with a significant risk of mortality in Japanese HD patients with minor inflammation receiving IIT and ESAs [14,32,33,36], suggesting that cutoff of serum ferritin to predict a risk of iron overload and mortality in HD patients may be lower in HD patients in the absence of inflammation. Aggressive IIT has been used in HD patients of Western countries probably due to high prevalence of inflammation, which increases serum ferritin and hepcidin-25, thereby inhibiting iron efflux and absorption for erythropoiesis and requiring higher dose of IV iron. In support of this finding, it was shown that if the CRP increased by 1 mg/L, possibilities to achieve tHb were reduced by 7.5% in HD patients with IDA [37]. High dose of IIT may increase a risk of infection-related mortality [38], cardiovascular events and high mortality in HD patients [12], although it was challenged [11]. On the other hand, low ferritin levels (<47.2–67.4 pmol/L) were also associated with a higher risk of mortality in HD patients receiving IIT and ESA [14,33], suggesting that both low and high serum ferritin are at a risk of mortality in HD patients.

The present study showed optimal serum ferritin levels of 67.4–89.9 pmol/L for the management of IDA with OIT in HD patients with minor inflammation. The serum ferritin levels in our patients are likely to represent more accurately iron status because of no overt inflammation. Further increment of serum ferritin was accompanied by increased levels of hepcidin-25 (see Figure 4), which can inhibit iron absorption and efflux, resulting in reduced iron availability for erythropoiesis and subsequent decrease in Hb levels [39]. This may explain a linear correlation between Hb and serum ferritin during 1–5 months in the OIT-responders, while no correlation was found when serum ferritin rose more than the threshold levels thereafter. In support of this finding, elevated iron indices failed to increase Hb in non-dialysis CKD patients with iron repletion (Hb > 110 g/L) [40]. The HD patients with serum ferritin of 67.4–179.8 pmol/L receiving IIT and ESA had better outcome than those with serum ferritin <67.4 pmol/L or >179.8 pmol/L [14]. The MRI study reported that optimal levels of serum ferritin were 359.5 pmol/L for liver iron content (LIC) >50 µmol/g (mild iron overload) and 651.6 pmol/L for LIC >200 µmol/g (severe iron overload) [10]. Thus, our optimal levels of serum ferritin in HD patients with minor inflammation receiving OIT and CERA are far less than these serum ferritin levels that might cause iron overload [10]. Our data support that therapeutic strategy for IDA in HD patients should include minimization of a risk of inflammation including infection that increases the required iron dose for IDA in HD patients [41].

Our study suggested that OIT was as effective as IIT in HD patients [23–25], that the response to OIT could reduce the dose of CERA in HD patients [8,24], and that in the absence of inflammation, low serum levels of ferritin and hepcidin-25 could be predictive of the response to OIT or IIT as reported in non-dialysis CKD [42] and our previous HD patients [25]. Iron absorption was not impaired in HD patients [43] but reduced when high inflammation was present [44]. This supports the efficacy of OIT for the management of IDA in our HD patients with minor inflammation. Of note is that the dose of OIT in our study is very low as compared to that in other studies showing similar benefit of OIT in HD patients [23,24]. Thus, in the absence of inflammation, low dose OIT may be adequate for the management of IDA in the majority of HD patients.

It remains elusive why some HD patients respond to OIT and others not. Inflammation is associated with obesity, diabetes mellitus and malnutrition, which are frequently seen in CKD patients. It is possible that these conditions could affect the response to iron therapy by increasing ferritin and hepcidin-25. In fact, increased levels of ferritin and hepcidin-25 were associated with obesity [45] and malnutrition [46]. In our study, however, no difference was found in prevalence of these conditions between the OIT-responders and the OIT-nonresponders. Our study confirmed our previous finding that ferritin and hepcidin-25 could be predictive factors for the response to OIT in HD patients in the absence of inflammation [25]. Serum levels of hepcidin-25 were positively correlated with triglycerides and interleukin (IL-6) and CRP in HD patients [47,48]. In addition, high serum levels of triglycerides were associated with hyporesponsiveness to IIT in HD patients [19]. Despite high levels of serum triglycerides in the OIT-responders compared to the OIT-nonresponders, no correlation was found between serum triglycerides and ferritin and ΔHb in our patients. Thus, it remains to be determined whether serum triglycerides is a predicting factor of the response to iron therapy in HD patients. Our study also showed that the IIT-nonresponders were associated with increased serum ferritin and adequate serum iron, whereas TSAT remained low at the end of the study, suggesting that the IIT-nonresponders may have non-inflammatory FIDA [49]. If this is the case, a more dose of IV iron may be required for the management of FIDA in these patients.

As other causes that may affect the response to iron therapy, reactive oxygen species (ROS) generation, reduced anti-oxidants, and increased IL-6 were associated with the HD patients who had even normal CRP [50,51]. These factors can increase ferritin and hepcidin-25, leading to reduced iron availability for erythropoiesis [39]. In fact, serum levels of IL-6 were correlated with those of ferritin and hepcidin-25 in CKD patients [17,46,48]. Regardless of ferritin and inflammation markers (CRP and IL-6), the levels of anti-oxidant glutathione peroxidase in erythrocytes were lower in the IIT-nonresponders than in the IIT-responders [52]. In HD patients, serum and erythrocyte folate concentrations were inversely correlated with serum ferritin in the IIT-responders [53]. CKD is associated with hypoxia which can increase hypoxia-inducible factor (HIF). HIF prolyl hydroxylase (HIF-PHD) inhibitors, which stabilize HIF, can increase Hb by inhibiting hepcidin-25 regardless of iron status in HD patients [54]. In fact, urine HIF-α mRNA was increased in CKD patients than controls [55]. Further studies are needed to determine the predictive values of these factors for the response to iron therapy in HD patients.

Little is known about early change of serum ferritin following iron supplementation in CKD patients. Our study demonstrated that serum ferritin first fell and started to rise at 2–3 months following OIT in HD patients. Kapoian et al. showed that despite an early increase in Hb levels, a decrease in ferritin levels was noted in HD patients at 1 month following IIT [56]. In CKD patients treated with oral ferric citrate or liposomal iron, decreased or unchanged serum ferritin was noted at 1 month after iron therapy [57]. In support of our finding, serum ferritin started to rise at 3 months after oral ferric citrate in HD patients and a decrease in the rate of rise of ferritin was noted among subjects on ferric citrate, probably due to stability of intestinal absorption of iron [58].

Although serum ferritin quickly rose after IIT in CKD patients due to direct infusion of iron into vessels [57], intestinal iron absorption after OIT was impaired in HD patients as compared to healthy controls [44]. Intestinal iron absorption became stable at 4 months after OIT in HD patients [59]. Bone marrow response to iron is limited to 20 mg/day of elemental iron, and an increase in Hb of 1 g/dL occurs every two to three weeks on iron therapy [60]. However, it may take up to 4 months for the iron stores to return to normal after the Hb has corrected [60]. In addition, intestinal absorption of oral iron fumarate used in our study is lower than oral ferrous sulphate [61]. In support of these findings, in healthy individuals receiving OIT after blood donation, serum ferritin recovered after 107 days [62]. These observations may explain a transient decrease in serum ferritin at early phase after starting OIT despite an increment of Hb in HD patients.

Finally, our study suggested that low dose of IIT could be a second line of iron supplementation for IDA in HD patients with minor inflammation who were resistant to OIT. IIT with ferrous saccharated (300–800 mg bolus once a month followed by 50 mg weekly for 3 months) were beneficial for IDA in 13 (76.4%) of the 17 HD patients who failed to maintain the tHb (10–11 g/dL) after the treatment with OIT and ESA [63]. However, higher dose of IV iron could increase a risk of systemic inflammation, cardiovascular events, infection and mortality in HD patients through iron overload-induced immune dysfunction, generation of reactive oxygen species and mitochondrial dysfunction [1,11,22]. Total doses of IIT in our protocol is lower than the low-dose maintenance IIT (31.25 mg/week over 1 year) that failed to prevent a risk of iron overload in HD patients with moderate anemia [64]. Our protocol (OIT and IIT) were well tolerated probably due to the low dose of iron used. However, the IIT-nonresponders who are likely to have non-inflammatory FIDA [49] may require higher dose of IV iron for the management of anemia.

5. Conclusions

OIT is beneficial for the management of IDA in Japanese HD patients with minor inflammation. Optimal levels of serum ferritin appear to be 67.4–89.9 pmol/L when tHb is 120–130 g/L, and further increment of serum ferritin is accompanied by increased levels of hepcidin-25, which inhibits iron availability for erythropoiesis, resulting in subsequent decrease in Hb. IIT can be a second choice of treatment for IDA in HD patients who are resistant to OIT. Limitations of our study include a small sample size and exclusion of HD patients with high inflammation and those with FIDA. Therapeutic strategy for IDA should be different among HD patients with high inflammation and those without, and include minimization of a risk of inflammation that increases ferritin and hepcidin-25, leading to hyporesponsiveness to iron therapy. Further studies using a large number of HD patients would be necessary to determine the benefit of OIT, optimal levels of serum ferritin to avoid a risk of iron overload, the benefit of IIT in patients who are resistant to OIT, and whether the response to iron therapy is different in HD patients with and without inflammation as well as whether predictive values of ferritin and hepcidin-25 for the response to iron therapy are dependent on inflammation.

Acknowledgments: The authors would like to thank Miyuki Tani for her assistance in collecting the data. This study has been supported by The Kidney Foundation, Japan (JKFB09-55).

Author Contributions: K.T. conceived and designed the analysis plan, analyzed the data, and contributed to the process of writing the first draft of the manuscript. C.T. and T.W. collected and analyzed the data. N.U. contributed to the study design, analysis and interpretation of results and wrote the first draft of the manuscript. All authors were involved in critically revising the manuscript. All authors have also read and approved the final manuscript.

Conflicts of Interest: The authors declare no conflict of interest.

References

1. Vaziri, N.D. Safety issues in iron treatment in CKD. *Semin. Nephrol.* **2016**, *36*, 112–118. [CrossRef] [PubMed]
2. Lopez, A.; Cacoub, P.; Macdougall, I.C.; Peyrin-Biroulet, L. Iron deficiency anaemia. *Lancet* **2016**, *387*, 907–916. [CrossRef]
3. The Kidney Disease: Improving Global Outcomes (KDIGO) Anemia Work Group. KDIGO clinical practice guideline for anemia in chronic kidney disease. *Kidney Int. Suppl.* **2012**, *2*, 279–335.
4. Macdougall, I.C.; Bock, A.H.; Carrera, F.; Eckardt, K.U.; Gaillard, C.; Van Wyck, D.; Roubert, B.; Nolen, J.G.; Roger, S.D.; FIND-CKD Study Investigators. FIND-CKD: A randomized trial of intravenous ferric carboxymaltose versus oral iron in patients with chronic kidney disease and iron deficiency anaemia. *Nephrol. Dial. Transplant.* **2014**, *29*, 2075–2084. [CrossRef] [PubMed]

5.   Tsubakihara, Y.; Nishi, S.; Akiba, T.; Hirakata, H.; Iseki, K.; Kubota, M.; Kuriyama, S.; Komatsu, Y.; Suzuki, M.; Nakai, S.; et al. 2008 Japanese Society for Dialysis Therapy: Guidelines for renal anemia in chronic kidney disease. *Ther. Apher. Dial.* **2010**, *14*, 240–275. [CrossRef] [PubMed]

6.   Bazeley, J.; Bieber, B.; Li, Y.; Morgenstern, H.; de Sequera, P.; Combe, C.; Yamamoto, H.; Gallagher, M.; Port, F.K.; Robinson, B.M. C-reactive protein and prediction of 1-year mortality in prevalent hemodialysis patients. *Clin. J. Am. Soc. Nephrol.* **2011**, *6*, 2452–2461. [CrossRef] [PubMed]

7.   Kawaguchi, T.; Tong, L.; Robinson, B.M.; Sen, A.; Fukuhara, S.; Kurokawa, K.; Canaud, B.; Lameire, N.; Port, F.K.; Pisoni, R.L. C-reactive protein and mortality in hemodialysis patients: The Dialysis Outcomes and Practice Patterns Study (DOPPS). *Nephron Clin. Pract.* **2011**, *117*, c167–c178. [CrossRef] [PubMed]

8.   Albaramki, J.; Hodson, E.M.; Craig, J.C.; Webster, A.C. Parenteral versus oral iron therapy for adults and children with chronic kidney disease. *Cochrane Database Syst. Rev.* **2012**, *18*, CD007857. [CrossRef] [PubMed]

9.   Rostoker, G.; Griuncelli, M.; Loridon, C.; Magna, T.; Janklewicz, P.; Drahi, G.; Dahan, H.; Cohen, Y. Maximal standard dose of parenteral iron for hemodialysis patients: An MRI-based decision tree learning analysis. *PLoS ONE* **2014**, *9*, e115096. [CrossRef] [PubMed]

10. Rostoker, G.; Griuncelli, M.; Loridon, C.; Magna, T.; Machado, G.; Drahi, G.; Dahan, H.; Janklewicz, P.; Cohen, Y. Reassessment of iron biomarkers for prediction of dialysis iron overload: An MRI study. *PLoS ONE* **2015**, *10*, e0132006. [CrossRef] [PubMed]

11. Bailie, G.R.; Larkina, M.; Goodkin, D.A.; Li, Y.; Pisoni, R.L.; Bieber, B.; Mason, N.; Tong, L.; Locatelli, F.; Marshall, M.R.; et al. Data from the Dialysis Outcomes and Practice Patterns Study validate an association between high intravenous iron doses and mortality. *Kidney Int.* **2015**, *87*, 162–168. [CrossRef] [PubMed]

12. Kuo, K.L.; Hung, S.C.; Lin, Y.P.; Tang, C.F.; Lee, T.S.; Lin, C.P.; Tarng, D.C. Intravenous ferric chloride hexahydrate supplementation induced endothelial dysfunction and increased cardiovascular risk among hemodialysis patients. *PLoS ONE* **2012**, *7*, e50295. [CrossRef] [PubMed]

13. Luo, J.; Jensen, D.E.; Maroni, B.J.; Brunelli, S.M. Spectrum and burden of erythropoiesis-stimulating agent hyporesponsiveness among contemporary hemodialysis patients. *Am. J. Kidney Dis.* **2016**, *68*, 763–771. [CrossRef] [PubMed]

14. Ogawa, C.; Tsuchiya, K.; Kanda, F.; Maeda, T. Low levels of serum ferritin lead to adequate hemoglobin levels and good survival in hemodialysis patients. *Am. J. Nephrol.* **2014**, *40*, 561–570. [CrossRef] [PubMed]

15. Del Vecchio, L.; Longhi, S.; Locatelli, F. Safety concerns about intravenous iron therapy in patients with chronic kidney disease. *Clin. Kidney J.* **2016**, *9*, 260–267. [CrossRef] [PubMed]

16. Nakanishi, T.; Kuragano, T.; Nanami, M.; Otaki, Y.; Nonoguchi, H.; Hasuike, Y. Importance of ferritin for optimizing anemia therapy in chronic kidney disease. *Am. J. Nephrol.* **2010**, *32*, 439–446. [CrossRef] [PubMed]

17. Łukaszyk, E.; Łukaszyk, M.; Koc-Żórawska, E.; Tobolczyk, J.; Bodzenta-Łukaszyk, A.; Małyszko, J. Iron status and inflammation in early stages of chronic kidney disease. *Kidney Blood Press. Res.* **2015**, *40*, 366–373. [CrossRef] [PubMed]

18. Kopelman, R.C.; Smith, L.; Peoples, L.; Biesecker, R.; Rizkala, A.R. Functional iron deficiency in hemodialysis patients with high ferritin. *Hemodial. Int.* **2007**, *11*, 238–246. [CrossRef] [PubMed]

19. Jenq, C.C.; Tian, Y.C.; Wu, H.H.; Hsu, P.Y.; Huang, J.Y.; Chen, Y.C.; Fang, J.T.; Yang, C.W. Effectiveness of oral and intravenous iron therapy in haemodialysis patients. *Int. J. Clin. Pract.* **2008**, *62*, 416–422. [CrossRef] [PubMed]

20. Kalra, P.A.; Bhandari, S.; Saxena, S.; Agarwal, D.; Wirtz, G.; Kletzmayr, J.; Thomsen, L.L.; Coyne, D.W. A randomized trial of iron isomaltoside 1000 versus oral iron in non-dialysis-dependent chronic kidney disease patients with anaemia. *Nephrol. Dial. Transplant.* **2016**, *31*, 646–655. [CrossRef] [PubMed]

21. Agarwal, R.; Kusek, J.W.; Pappas, M.K. A randomized trial of intravenous and oral iron in chronic kidney disease. *Kidney Int.* **2015**, *88*, 905–914. [CrossRef] [PubMed]

22. Fishbane, S.; Mathew, A.; Vaziri, N.D. Iron toxicity: Relevance for dialysis patients. *Nephrol. Dial. Transplant.* **2014**, *29*, 255–259. [CrossRef] [PubMed]

23. Lenga, I.; Lok, C.; Marticorena, R.; Hunter, J.; Dacouris, N.; Goldstein, M. Role of oral iron in the management of long-term hemodialysis patients. *Clin. J. Am. Soc. Nephrol.* **2007**, *2*, 688–693. [CrossRef] [PubMed]

24. Tsuchida, A.; Paudyal, B.; Paudyal, P.; Ishii, Y.; Hiromura, K.; Nojima, Y.; Komai, M. Effectiveness of oral iron to manage anemia in long-term hemodialysis patients with the use of ultrapure dialysate. *Exp. Ther. Med.* **2010**, *1*, 777–781. [CrossRef] [PubMed]

25. Takasawa, K.; Takaeda, C.; Maeda, T.; Ueda, N. Hepcidin-25, mean corpuscular volume, and ferritin as predictors of response to oral iron supplementation in hemodialysis patients. *Nutrients* **2015**, *7*, 103–118. [CrossRef] [PubMed]

26. Sanai, T.; Ono, T.; Fukumitsu, T. Beneficial effects of oral iron in Japanese patients on hemodialysis. *Intern. Med.* **2017**, *56*, 2395–2399. [CrossRef] [PubMed]

27. Kalantar-Zadeh, K.; Regidor, D.L.; McAllister, C.J.; Michael, B.; Warnock, D.G. Time-dependent associations between iron and mortality in hemodialysis patients. *J. Am. Soc. Nephrol.* **2005**, *16*, 3070–3080. [CrossRef] [PubMed]

28. Kovesdy, C.P.; Estrada, W.; Ahmadzadeh, S.; Kalantar-Zadeh, K. Association of markers of iron stores with outcomes in patients with nondialysis-dependent chronic kidney disease. *Clin. J. Am. Soc. Nephrol.* **2009**, *4*, 435–441. [CrossRef] [PubMed]

29. Ramanathan, G.; Olynyk, J.K.; Ferrari, P. Diagnosing and preventing iron overload. *Hemodial. Int.* **2017**, *21* (Suppl. 1), S58–S67. [CrossRef] [PubMed]

30. Chauveau, P.; Level, C.; Lasseur, C.; Bonarek, H.; Peuchant, E.; Montaudon, D.; Vendrely, B.; Combe, C. C-reactive protein and procalcitonin as markers of mortality in hemodialysis patients: A 2-year prospective study. *J. Ren. Nutr.* **2003**, *13*, 137–143. [CrossRef] [PubMed]

31. Jenq, C.C.; Hsu, C.W.; Huang, W.H.; Chen, K.H.; Lin, J.L.; Lin-Tan, D.T. Serum ferritin levels predict all-cause and infection-cause 1-year mortality in diabetic patients on maintenance hemodialysis. *Am. J. Med. Sci.* **2009**, *337*, 188–194. [CrossRef] [PubMed]

32. Hasuike, Y.; Nonoguchi, H.; Tokuyama, M.; Ohue, M.; Nagai, T.; Yahiro, M.; Nanami, M.; Otaki, Y.; Nakanishi, T. Serum ferritin predicts prognosis in hemodialysis patients: The Nishinomiya study. *Clin. Exp. Nephrol.* **2010**, *14*, 349–355. [CrossRef] [PubMed]

33. Maruyama, Y.; Yokoyama, K.; Yokoo, T.; Shigematsu, T.; Iseki, K.; Tsubakihara, Y. The different association between serum ferritin and mortality in hemodialysis and peritoneal dialysis patients using Japanese nationwide dialysis registry. *PLoS ONE* **2015**, *10*, e0143430. [CrossRef] [PubMed]

34. Kim, T.; Streja, E.; Soohoo, M.; Rhee, C.M.; Eriguchi, R.; Kim, T.W.; Chang, T.I.; Obi, Y.; Kovesdy, C.P.; Kalantar-Zadeh, K. Serum ferritin variations and mortality in incident hemodialysis patients. *Am. J. Nephrol.* **2017**, *46*, 120–130. [CrossRef] [PubMed]

35. Floege, J.; Gillespie, I.A.; Kronenberg, F.; Anker, S.D.; Gioni, I.; Richards, S.; Pisoni, R.L.; Robinson, B.M.; Marcelli, D.; Froissart, M.; et al. Development and validation of a predictive mortality risk score from a European hemodialysis cohort. *Kidney Int.* **2015**, *87*, 996–1008. [CrossRef] [PubMed]

36. Shoji, T.; Niihata, K.; Fukuma, S.; Fukuhara, S.; Akizawa, T.; Inaba, M. Both low and high serum ferritin levels predict mortality risk in hemodialysis patients without inflammation. *Clin. Exp. Nephrol.* **2017**, *21*, 685–693. [CrossRef] [PubMed]

37. Musanovic, A.; Trnacevic, S.; Mekic, M.; Musanovic, A. The influence of inflammatory markers and CRP predictive value in relation to the target hemoglobin level in patients on chronic hemodialysis. *Med. Arch.* **2013**, *67*, 361–364. [CrossRef] [PubMed]

38. Miskulin, D.C.; Tangri, N.; Bandeen-Roche, K.; Zhou, J.; McDermott, A.; Meyer, K.B.; Ephraim, P.L.; Michels, W.M.; Jaar, B.G.; Crews, D.C.; et al. Intravenous iron exposure and mortality in patients on hemodialysis. *Clin. J. Am. Soc. Nephrol.* **2014**, *9*, 1930–1939. [CrossRef] [PubMed]

39. Ueda, N.; Takasawa, K. Role of hepcidin-25 in chronic kidney disease: Anemia and beyond. *Curr. Med. Chem.* **2017**, *24*, 1417–1452. [CrossRef] [PubMed]

40. McMahon, L.P.; Kent, A.B.; Kerr, P.G.; Healy, H.; Irish, A.B.; Cooper, B.; Kark, A.; Roger, S.D. Maintenance of elevated versus physiological iron indices in non-anaemic patients with chronic kidney disease: A randomized controlled trial. *Nephrol. Dial. Transplant.* **2010**, *25*, 920–926. [CrossRef] [PubMed]

41. El-Khatib, M.; Duncan, H.J.; Kant, K.S. Role of C-reactive protein, reticulocyte haemoglobin content and inflammatory markers in iron and erythropoietin administration in dialysis patients. *Nephrology* **2006**, *11*, 400–404. [CrossRef] [PubMed]

42. Chand, S.; Ward, D.G.; Ng, Z.Y.; Hodson, J.; Kirby, H.; Steele, P.; Rooplal, I.; Bantugon, F.; Iqbal, T.; Tselepis, C.; et al. Serum hepcidin-25 and response to intravenous iron in patients with non-dialysis chronic kidney disease. *J. Nephrol.* **2015**, *28*, 81–88. [CrossRef] [PubMed]

43. Tovbin, D.; Schnaider, A.; Vorobiov, M.; Rogachev, B.; Basok, A.; Shull, P.; Novack, V.; Friger, M.; Avramov, D.; Zlotnik, M. Minor impairment of oral iron absorption in non-diabetic new dialysis patients. *J. Nephrol.* **2005**, *18*, 174–180. [PubMed]

44. Kooistra, M.P.; Niemantsverdriet, E.C.; van Es, A.; Mol-Beermann, N.M.; Struyvenberg, A.; Marx, J.J. Iron absorption in erythropoietin-treated haemodialysis patients: Effects of iron availability, inflammation and aluminium. *Nephrol. Dial. Transplant.* **1998**, *13*, 82–88. [CrossRef] [PubMed]

45. Sarafidis, P.A.; Rumjon, A.; MacLaughlin, H.L.; Macdougall, I.C. Obesity and iron deficiency in chronic kidney disease: The putative role of hepcidin. *Nephrol. Dial. Transplant.* **2012**, *27*, 50–57. [CrossRef] [PubMed]

46. Aydin, Z.; Gursu, M.; Karadag, S.; Uzun, S.; Sumnu, A.; Doventas, Y.; Ozturk, S.; Kazancioglu, R. The relationship of prohepcidin levels with anemia and inflammatory markers in non-diabetic uremic patients: A controlled study. *Ren. Fail.* **2014**, *36*, 1253–1257. [CrossRef] [PubMed]

47. Malyszko, J.; Malyszko, J.S.; Pawlak, K.; Mysliwiec, M. Hepcidin, iron status, and renal function in chronic renal failure, kidney transplantation, and hemodialysis. *Am. J. Hematol.* **2006**, *81*, 832–837. [CrossRef] [PubMed]

48. Samouilidou, E.; Pantelias, K.; Petras, D.; Tsirpanlis, G.; Bakirtzi, J.; Chatzivasileiou, G.; Tzanatos, H.; Grapsa, E. Serum hepcidin levels are associated with serum triglycerides and interleukin-6 concentrations in patients with end-stage renal disease. *Ther Apher Dial.* **2014**, *18*, 279–283. [CrossRef] [PubMed]

49. Mercadal, L.; Metzger, M.; Haymann, J.P.; Thervet, E.; Boffa, J.J.; Flamant, M.; Vrtovsnik, F.; Gauci, C.; Froissart, M.; Stengel, B.; et al. A 3-marker index improves the identification of iron disorders in CKD anaemia. *PLoS ONE* **2014**, *9*, e84144. [CrossRef] [PubMed]

50. Tutal, E.; Sezer, S.; Bilgic, A.; Aldemir, D.; Turkoglu, S.; Demirel, O.; Ozdemir, N.; Haberal, M. Influence of oxidative stress and inflammation on rHuEPO requirements of hemodialysis patients with CRP values "in normal range". *Transplant. Proc.* **2007**, *39*, 3035–3040. [CrossRef] [PubMed]

51. Shinzato, T.; Abe, K.; Furusu, A.; Harada, T.; Shinzato, K.; Miyazaki, M.; Kohno, S. Serum pro-hepcidin level and iron homeostasis in Japanese dialysis patients with erythropoietin (EPO)-resistant anemia. *Med. Sci. Monit.* **2008**, *14*, CR431–CR437. [PubMed]

52. Prats, M.; Font, R.; García, C.; Muñoz-Cortés, M.; Cabré, C.; Jariod, M.; Romeu, M.; Giralt, M.; Martinez-Vea, A. Oxidative stress markers in predicting response to treatment with ferric carboxymaltose in nondialysis chronic kidney disease patients. *Clin. Nephrol.* **2014**, *81*, 419–426. [CrossRef] [PubMed]

53. Sakellariou, G. Do serum and red blood cell folate levels indicate iron response in hemodialysis patients? *ASAIO J.* **2006**, *52*, 163–168.

54. Besarab, A.; Chernyavskaya, E.; Motylev, I.; Shutov, E.; Kumbar, L.M.; Gurevich, K.; Chan, D.T.; Leong, R.; Poole, L.; Zhong, M.; et al. Roxadustat (FG-4592): Correction of anemia in incident dialysis patients. *J. Am. Soc. Nephrol.* **2016**, *27*, 1225–1233. [CrossRef] [PubMed]

55. Movafagh, S.; Raj, D.; Sanaei-Ardekani, M.; Bhatia, D.; Vo, K.; Mahmoudieh, M.; Rahman, R.; Kim, E.H.; Harralson, A.F. Hypoxia inducible factor 1: A urinary biomarker of kidney disease. *Clin. Transl. Sci.* **2017**, *10*, 201–207. [CrossRef] [PubMed]

56. Kapoian, T.; O'Mara, N.B.; Carreon, M.; Gajary, A.; Rizkala, A.; Lefavour, G.; Sherman, R.A.; Walker, J. Iron indices and intravenous ferumoxytol: Time to steady-state. *Ann. Pharmacother.* **2012**, *46*, 1308–1314. [CrossRef] [PubMed]

57. Pisani, A.; Riccio, E.; Sabbatini, M.; Andreucci, M.; Del Rio, A.; Visciano, B. Effect of oral liposomal iron versus intravenous iron for treatment of iron deficiency anaemia in CKD patients: A randomized trial. *Nephrol. Dial. Transplant.* **2015**, *30*, 645–652. [CrossRef] [PubMed]

58. Lewis, J.B.; Sika, M.; Koury, M.J.; Chuang, P.; Schulman, G.; Smith, M.T.; Whittier, F.C.; Linfert, D.R.; Galphin, C.M.; Athreya, B.P.; et al. Ferric citrate controls phosphorus and delivers iron in patients on dialysis. *J. Am. Soc. Nephrol.* **2015**, *26*, 493–503. [CrossRef] [PubMed]

59. Deira, J.; Martín, M.; Sánchez, S.; Garrido, J.; Núñez, J.; Tabernero, J.M. Evaluation of intestinal iron absorption by indirect methods in patients on hemodialysis receiving oral iron and recombinant human. *Am. J. Kidney Dis.* **2002**, *39*, 594–599. [CrossRef]

60. Killip, S.; Bennett, J.M.; Chambers, M.D. Iron deficiency anemia. *Am. Fam. Physician* **2007**, *75*, 671–678. [PubMed]

61. Zariwala, M.G.; Somavarapu, S.; Farnaud, S.; Renshaw, D. Comparison study of oral iron preparations using a human intestinal model. *Sci. Pharm.* **2013**, *81*, 1123–1139. [CrossRef] [PubMed]

62. Kiss, J.E.; Brambilla, D.; Glynn, S.A.; Mast, A.E.; Spencer, B.R.; Stone, M.; Kleinman, S.H.; Cable, R.G.; National Heart, Lung, and Blood Institute (NHLBI) Recipient Epidemiology and Donor Evaluation Study-III (REDS-III). Oral iron supplementation after blood donation: A randomized clinical trial. *JAMA* **2015**, *313*, 575–583. [CrossRef] [PubMed]

63. Al-Hawas, F.; Abdalla, A.H.; Popovich, W.; Mousa, D.H.; Al-Sulaiman, M.H.; Al-Khader, A.A. Use of i.v. iron saccharate in haemodialysis patients not responding to oral iron and erythropoietin. *Nephrol. Dial. Transplant.* **1997**, *12*, 2801–2802. [CrossRef] [PubMed]

64. Canavese, C.; Bergamo, D.; Ciccone, G.; Burdese, M.; Maddalena, E.; Barbieri, S.; Thea, A.; Fop, F. Low-dose continuous iron therapy leads to a positive iron balance and decreased serum transferrin levels in chronic haemodialysis patients. *Nephrol. Dial. Transplant.* **2004**, *19*, 1564–1570. [CrossRef] [PubMed]

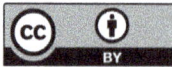

nutrients

MDPI

Article

Serum Hepcidin Concentration in Individuals with Sickle Cell Anemia: Basis for the Dietary Recommendation of Iron

Juliana Omena [1], Cláudia dos Santos Cople-Rodrigues [1], Jessyca Dias do Amaral Cardoso [1], Andrea Ribeiro Soares [2], Marcos Kneip Fleury [3], Flávia dos Santos Barbosa Brito [1], Josely Correa Koury [1] and Marta Citelli [1,*]

[1] Instituto de Nutrição, Universidade do Estado do Rio de Janeiro, Rio de Janeiro 20550-900, Brazil; omenaju@gmail.com (J.O.); claudiacople@gmail.com (C.d.S.C.-R.); jessycadiaxs@hotmail.com (J.D.d.A.C.); barbosaflavia@bol.com.br (F.d.S.B.B.); jckoury@gmail.com (J.C.K.)

[2] Faculdade de Ciências Médicas, Universidade do Estado do Rio de Janeiro, Rio de Janeiro 20550-900, Brazil; andrearsoares@hotmail.com

[3] Faculdade de Farmácia, Universidade Federal do Rio de Janeiro, Rio de Janeiro 21941-590, Brazil; marcos.fleury@yahoo.com.br

* Correspondence: martacitelli@gmail.com; Tel.: +55-21-2234-0679

Received: 6 March 2018; Accepted: 10 April 2018; Published: 17 April 2018

Abstract: Dietary iron requirements in patients with sickle cell disease (SCD) remain unclear. SCD is a neglected hemoglobinopathy characterized by intense erythropoietic activity and anemia. Hepcidin is the hormone mainly responsible for iron homeostasis and intestinal absorption. Intense erythropoietic activity and anemia may reduce hepcidin transcription. By contrast, iron overload and inflammation may induce it. Studies on SCD have not evaluated the role of hepcidin in the presence and absence of iron overload. We aimed to compare serum hepcidin concentrations among individuals with sickle cell anemia, with or without iron overload, and those without the disease. Markers of iron metabolism and erythropoietic activity such as hepcidin, ferritin, and growth differentiation factor 15 were evaluated. Three groups participated in the study: the control group, comprised of individuals without SCD (C); those with the disease but without iron overload (SCDw); and those with the disease and iron overload (SCDio). Results showed that hepcidin concentration was higher in the SCDio > C > SCDw group. These data suggest that the dietary iron intake of the SCDio group should not be reduced as higher hepcidin concentrations may reduce the intestinal absorption of iron.

Keywords: sickle cell anemia; hepcidin; iron overload

---

1. Introduction

Sickle cell disease (SCD) is an inherited hemoglobinopathy caused by the substitution of glutamic acid by valine at the 6th position of the beta globin chain. This modification induces the formation of hemoglobin S (Hb S), causing red blood cells to acquire the sickle shape and, consequently, leading to chronic hemolysis and the occurrence of vessel occlusion phenomena, pain episodes, and injury of organs and tissues [1].

Blood transfusions are administered in order to treat manifestations of the disease, improve the capacity of oxygen transport and minimize hemolysis, as in splenic sequestration crises [2], or to prevent complications and disease progression, as in the prevention of stroke in children [3,4]. Despite the benefits, regular transfusions can lead to iron overload, since each unit of transfused blood contains about 200–250 mg of this mineral [5,6]. In healthy people, the body's iron content is around 4 g [7], while chronically transfused individuals can store 5 g to 10 g per year [8]. With the progression of iron overload, iron becomes potentially toxic, due to its tendency to catalyze the formation of reactive oxygen species, consequently leading to oxidative stress and culminating in cellular damage [9].

Hepcidin—a polypeptide hormone formed by a sequence of 25 amino acids, from the transcription of the HAMP (hepcidin antimicrobial peptide) gene—plays a significant role in iron homeostasis through its binding to ferroportin, a protein responsible for the export of iron from various cell types, especially enterocytes and macrophages of the reticuloendothelial system [10]. The hepcidin–ferroportin complex is internalized by these cells, and ferroportin undergoes degradation, blocking iron output and consequently leading to a reduction in the absorption of intestinal iron and its bioavailability [11,12].

The intense but ineffective erythropoiesis and anemia inherent to the SCD are factors that potentially lead to reduced hepcidin concentration [13], leading to increased intestinal absorption of this micronutrient. In contrast, the characteristic inflammatory feature as well as the increased serum iron concentration can induce the transcription of this hormone [14], reducing iron absorption.

As the factors that activate and inhibit hepcidin synthesis may be simultaneously present in patients with SCD, the common nutritional approach used by health professionals to treat individuals with iron overload is the restriction of the most abundant food sources of this mineral, such as meats, mainly viscera, and legumes. However, these actions may also reduce the bioavailability of other minerals, such as zinc, present in foods that are also sources of iron. Patients with the disease usually have reduced plasma zinc concentrations [15].

Hepcidin has not yet been sufficiently studied in SCD. A few existing studies present inconclusive data regarding hepcidin concentration, as most studies do not differentiate patients with SCD in relation to the presence or absence of iron overload, nor do they compare these concentrations with healthy control groups [16–23]. Thus, it is difficult to define the appropriate iron-related nutritional care for this group as data regarding the behavior of hepcidin are limited. Hence, this study aimed to compare the serum hepcidin concentration in people with sickle cell anemia, with or without iron overload, and to a control group without the disease. Markers of iron metabolism and erythropoietic activity were also evaluated.

2. Materials and Methods

2.1. Study Participants

Adult patients aged 18–59 years old, of both genders, with sickle cell anemia (Hb SS genotype) were recruited from the hematology and hemolytic anemia outpatient clinics, respectively, at the Pedro Ernesto University Hospital and Arthur Siqueira de Cavalcanti State Institute of Hematology (Hemorio) (Rio de Janeiro, Brazil). The control group was composed of healthy volunteers without sickle cell anemia (Hb AA genotype).

Participants with sickle cell trait, those with other hemoglobinopathies and hematological diseases, pregnant women, patients with SCD who had been hospitalized, and/or those who received blood transfusions 15 days prior to blood collection were excluded from this study.

In patients without SCD (control group), those with serum ferritin <10 ng/mL (for women) and <20 ng/mL (for men) were excluded from the study. Participants who used medications for treatment of diabetes and hypo/hyperthyroidism were also excluded.

Participants were divided into three groups: sickle cell disease with iron overload (SCDio) group, consisting of patients with SCD and serum ferritin ≥1000 ng/mL; sickle cell disease without iron overload (SCDw) group, those with SCD and ferritin <1000 ng/mL; and the control (C) group, composed of individuals without SCD. To compare the results without differentiating the presence of iron overload, the SCDio and SCDw groups were merged and named sickle cell disease group (SCD). Serum ferritin ≥1000 ng/mL was adopted based on the cut-off point referenced by the study by Porter and Garbowski [24].

All study participants received and signed the informed consent form before taking part in the study. The study was approved by the Research Ethics Committees of Pedro Ernesto University Hospital (number: 758.174) and Arthur de Siqueira Cavalcanti State Institute of Hematology (number: 391/15).

2.2. Anthropometry and Nutritional Assessment

Body mass and height were determined using a 0.1 kg portable precision scale (Filizola, São Paulo, Brazil). The participants' body mass index (BMI) was calculated (body mass/height^2). Participants with BMI between 18.5 kg/m^2 and 24.9 kg/m^2 were considered eutrophic [25].

2.3. Blood Sampling and Analysis

Participants' blood was collected by venipuncture in the morning for routine hematological and biochemical analyses. For hematological analysis, the blood was collected in tubes with anticoagulant ethylenediamine tetraacetic acid (EDTA). For serological and biochemical analyses, collection tubes with clot activator gel were used to extract the serum.

Except for the samples collected in EDTA tubes, the others were centrifuged at $700 \times g$ for 10 min, aliquoted into microtubes, and stored in a freezer at a temperature of $-80\,^{\circ}$C until analysis.

2.4. Hematological Measurements and Biochemical Analysis

Hemoglobin, hematocrit, and leukocytes were analyzed using the automated counter Horiba$^{\circledR}$ Pentra 60 C$^+$ (Horiba ABX Diagnostics, Pentra 60 C$^+$, Montpellier, France), which combines the principles of electrical impedance, flow cytometry, cytochemistry, and spectrophotometry.

To confirm the genotypes of the study participants, the determination and quantification of normal hemoglobin and variants were performed through ion-exchange high-performance liquid chromatography using the Variant^{TM} equipment (Bio-Rad Laboratories, Hercules, CA, USA).

Serum ferritin levels were analyzed using a commercially available enzyme-linked immunosorbent assay (ELISA) kit (Symbiosys, ALKA Tecnologia$^{\circledR}$, São Paulo, Brazil).

The serum concentration of bioactive hepcidin-25 (DRG Instruments GmbH, Marburg, Germany), growth differentiation factor 15 (GDF-15) (Sigma Aldrich Inc., Saint Louis, MO, USA) and Interleukin 6 (IL-6) (Merck Millipore, Darmstadt, Germany) were also analyzed using ELISA.

Serum iron and total iron-binding capacity (TIBC) were analyzed by a colorimetric method using Ferrozine$^{\circledR}$(Labtest, Belo Horizonte, Brazil). Transferrin saturation (TS) index is calculated as follows: serum iron/TIBC$\times$ 100.

The lactate dehydrogenase (LDH) analysis was performed by continuous ultraviolet kinetics method (pyruvate-lactate method) using the Labmax Plenno automatic analyzer (Labtest, Belo Horizonte, Brazil).

Analyses were performed according to the manufacturers' instructions.

2.5. Statistical Analysis

The distribution of variables was analyzed for normality using the Shapiro–Wilk test. As most of the variables did not present a Gaussian distribution, we chose to use non-parametric tests.

Measures of central tendency and dispersion were expressed as median and interquartile ranges (1st–3rd quartile). In the descriptive analysis, data were expressed as frequencies (*n*) and percentages (%).

The Mann–Whitney U test was used to assess the differences of continuous variables between the two groups and the Kruskal–Wallis test for the three study groups ($p < 0.05$). Subsequently, the Mann–Whitney U test with Bonferroni correction ($p < 0.017$) was used to compare the pairs of groups.

The statistical analysis was performed using the Statistical Package for Social Science software (IBM SPSS$^{\circledR}$ Inc., version 22.0, Chicago, IL, USA).

3. Results

A total of 158 individuals participated in the study; 115 met the inclusion criteria, 72 had SCD (54.2%, male), and 43 were included as a control group (41.9%, male).

The median age of patients with SCD was 29.5 years (Interquartile Range, IQR: 18–59 years), while the control group was 26.0 years (IQR: 19–54 years), denoting homogeneity among individuals. However, the median age of the SCDio group was higher than the other groups (38.5; IQR: 22–59 years).

Most of the participants with SCD (62.5%) were classified as eutrophic, whereas those in the control group had similar percentages of eutrophy and overweight (48.8%) (Table 1).

Table 1. Frequency of the general characteristics of patients with sickle cell disease (*n* = 72) and the control group (*n* = 43).

General Characteristics	Patients with SCD *n* (%)	Control *n* (%)
Gender, male	39 (54.2%)	18 (41.9%)
Underweight	14 (19.4%)	1 (2.4%)
Eutrophic	45 (62.5%)	21 (48.8%)
Overweight	10 (13.9%)	16 (37.2%)
Obese type I	3 (4.2%)	4 (9.3%)
Obese type II	0 (0%)	0 (0%)
Obese type III	0 (0%)	1 (2.3%)

Biochemical data obtained from a single group of individuals with SCD, without separation of the groups into SCDw and SCDio, are presented in Table 2. As expected, individuals with SCD presented lower hematocrit and hemoglobin concentrations when compared with the control group. However, the SCD group had significantly lower serum hepcidin concentrations. Regarding other markers of iron metabolism, ferritin, serum iron, and TS levels were higher in the SCD group than in the control group, while the TIBC values were higher in the control group than in the SCD group. Regarding parameters related to hemolysis and erythropoietic activity, the SCD group had higher median values for both LDH and GDF-15 than the control group. This result was expected, since SCD is a disease that presents with intense hemolysis and erythropoiesis.

Table 2. Comparison of laboratorial parameters between the control and SCD groups (SCDw + SCDio).

Laboratorial Parameters	Control Group *n* = 43		SCD Groups *n* = 72		*p* Value
	Median	IQR (P25–P75)	Median	IQR (P25–P75)	
Hemoglobin (g/dL)	13.5	12.8–14.7	8.0	7.1–9.3	<0.001
Hematocrit (%)	40.1	38.7–44.1	23.6	21.4–28.1	<0.001
Leukocytes ($\times 10^3$/mm^3)	5.8	4.9–6.6	10.7	7.6–13.9	<0.001
Lymphocytes (%)	37.1	33.0–42.1	38.4	30.8–46.0	0.676
Hepcidin (ng/mL)	7.2	5.6–11.6	5.3	2.5–10.9	0.014
Ferritin (ng/mL)	29.8	17.1–68.5	228.7	69.4–703.5	<0.001
Ferritin/Leukocytes ratio	6.3	3.1–13.2	27.5	7.2–77.0	<0.001
Serum iron (µg/dL)	105.0	69.0–129.0	119.0	92.0–158.8	0.012
TIBC (µg/dL)	333.0	301.0–383.0	293.0	233.3–347.0	0.001
TS (%)	31.4	20.5–41.8	43.1	30.1–62.5	<0.001
LDH (U/L)	349.0	293.0–391.0	818.0	619.8–1198.0	<0.001
GDF-15 (pg/mL)	504.8	396.0–652.4	1299.2	618.4–1553.1	<0.001
IL-6 (pg/mL)	0.0	0.0–2.5	3.8	2.4–8.9	<0.001

Results are expressed as median and interquartile ranges (IQR); P25–P75: 25th–75th percentile. Differences were tested using Mann–Whitney U test, *p* < 0.05. SCD: sickle cell disease groups, SCDw: sickle cell disease without iron overload, SCDio: sickle cell disease with iron overload, TIBC: total iron-binding capacity, TS: transferrin saturation, LDH: lactate dehydrogenase, GDF-15: growth differentiation factor 15, IL-6: interleukin-6.

Regarding serum ferritin levels, participants with SCD were then divided into SCDio group (individuals with SCD and ferritin $\geq$1000 ng/mL; $n = 14$) and SCDw group (individuals with SCD and ferritin <1000 ng/mL; $n = 58$) (Table 3). The concentrations of hemoglobin and hematocrit markers in the SCDw and SCDio groups were lower than in the control group ($p < 0.001$), in agreement with what had already been observed in the SCD group. These parameters did not differ between the SCDw and SCDio groups. The same was observed for leukocytes, which presented higher medians in both SCDw and SCDio groups ($10.7 \times 10^3/mm^3$ vs. $10.9 \times 10^3/mm$, respectively) than the control group ($5.8 \times 10^3/mm^3$) but did not present statistical difference when compared among them.

Table 3. Comparison of laboratorial parameters between the control, SCDw, and SCDio groups.

Laboratorial Parameters	Control $n = 43$		SCDw $n = 58$		SCDio $n = 14$		*p* Value
	Median	IQR (P25–P75)	Median	IQR (P25–P75)	Median	IQR (P25–P75)	
Hemoglobin (g/dL)	13.5 [a]	12.8–14.7	8.2 [b]	7.2–9.4	7.3 [b]	6.0–8.3	<0.001
Hematocrit (%)	40.1 [a]	38.7–44.1	24.4 [b]	21.7–28.3	22.2 [b]	18.5–26.1	<0.001
Leukocytes ($\times 10^3/mm^3$)	5.8 [a]	4.9–6.6	10.7 [b]	7.2–13.7	10.9 [b]	9.5–14.6	<0.001
Lymphocytes (%)	37.1 [a]	33.0–42.1	39.5 [a]	31.0–47.7	35.0 [a]	26.7–41.5	0.167
Hepcidin (ng/mL)	7.2 [a]	5.6–11.6	4.2 [b]	2.2–7.8	11.6 [c]	9.8–23.0	<0.001
Ferritin (ng/mL)	29.8 [a]	17.1–68.5	167.8 [b]	60.3–436.3	1986.4 [c]	1379.7–2261.6	<0.001
Ferritin/Leukocytes ratio	6.3 [a]	3.1–13.2	14.1 [b]	6.4–33.8	172.7 [c]	127.0–249.3	<0.001
Serum iron (µg/dL)	105.0 [a]	69.0–129.0	111.5 [a,b]	92.0–146.8	158.5 [b]	97.3–204.0	0.006
TIBC (µg/dL)	333.0 [a]	301.0–383.0	293.0 [b]	244.8–349.0	270.5 [b]	202.8–321.0	0.001
TS (%)	31.4 [a]	20.5–41.8	38.4 [b]	29.3–58.0	55.6 [b]	38.7–81.4	<0.001
LDH (U/L)	349.0 [a]	293.0–391.0	894.0 [b]	596.5–1328.5	730.5 [b]	684.3–997.5	<0.001
GDF-15 (pg/mL)	504.8 [a]	396.0–652.4	1227.3 [b]	593.7–1496.7	1643.7 [c]	1299.8–1702.3	<0.001
IL-6 (pg/mL)	0.0 [a]	0.0–2.5	3.7 [b]	2.4–8.3	4.3 [b]	2.9–15.2	<0.001

Results are expressed as median and interquartile ranges (IQR); P25–P75: 25th–75th percentile. Differences between three groups were tested using Kruskal–Wallis test ($p < 0.05$). Post hoc analysis was performed using the Mann–Whitney U test for two groups with Bonferroni correction ($p < 0.017$), different letters indicate statistical difference between groups; SCDw: sickle cell disease without iron overload, SCDio: sickle cell disease with iron overload, TIBC: total iron binding capacity, TS: transferrin saturation, LDH: lactate dehydrogenase, GDF-15: growth differentiation factor 15.

Furthermore, the three groups had significantly different serum hepcidin concentrations. The SCDio group presented the highest levels of this hormone (11.6 ng/mL) in comparison to the other groups, while the SCDw group had the lowest median values (4.2 ng/mL), both in relation to SCDio and in the control group (7.2 ng/mL). This result could only be evidenced by the separation of the groups into SCDio and SCDw (Table 3).

The concentration of serum iron in the SCDio group was higher than that in the control group, due to the excessive iron load to which they were exposed due to blood transfusions. However, no difference was observed between the SCDw and SCDio groups and neither between the SCDw group and control group.

The values of TIBC and TS variables (Table 3) in the control group were lower than those presented by the SCDio and SCDw groups, the same as observed in Table 2.

LDH levels were higher in the SCDw and SCDio groups than in the control group (Table 3). However, the GDF-15 marker presented a statistically significant difference between the three groups analyzed, with higher concentrations in the SCDio group (1643.7 pg/mL) than in the SCDw (1227.3 pg/mL) and control groups (504.8 pg/mL).

SCD is characterized by the presence of low-grade chronic inflammation, which may be evidenced by interleukin-6 (IL-6) and leukocyte concentrations (Table 2). For this reason, we evaluated whether the differences in ferritin concentrations between the control group and the SCD groups would be maintained when corrected for the leukocyte (ferritin/leukocyte ratio) value. The comparative analysis showed that the ferritin/leukocyte ratio is higher in the SCD groups (Tables 2 and 3).

4. Discussion

Transfusional iron overload has frequently been reported in studies of sickle cell anemia. Although the data on its prevalence are still limited, it is known that the increase in the life expectancy of individuals with sickle cell anemia may lead to a greater number of blood transfusions and, consequently, an increase in cases of iron overload.

This study showed that patients with SCD and iron overload had serum hepcidin concentrations higher than those in patients with SCD without iron overload and individuals of the control group. However, when all patients with SCD were merged in a single group, serum hepcidin concentration in the SCD appeared to be lower than that in the control group.

Previous studies reported various hepcidin concentrations in patients with sickle cell disease, which can be explained by the heterogeneity of the studied groups. Most of the studies analyzed the sickle cell group without considering the signs of iron overload observed among the participants; additionally, other studies compared the hepcidin concentrations of people with sickle cell disease with that of other hematological diseases [16,17]. To our knowledge, this is the first study to evaluate hepcidin concentration in the two groups of adults with SCD, with the main difference being the presence or absence of iron overload, identified by serum ferritin values.

The findings of this study corroborate those found by Nemeth [14], who showed increased urinary hepcidin excretion in two patients with SCD and signs of iron overload when compared with healthy individuals.

In some previous studies that considered the SCD group as a whole, hepcidin concentrations in these patients were lower [18], equal [19–22], or even higher [23] than in the control group. Such variations are probably due to the fact that several of the studies do not distinguish the participants regarding their transfusion behavior, that is, they include individuals who never received blood transfusion and the polytransfused ones, and/or do not distinguish iron overload by ferritin concentration (>1000 ng/mL).

In this study, the history and frequency of blood transfusions of the participants varied; all patients had already been transfused, and about 36.1% of them reported having had an average of 10 or more transfusions (simple or blood exchange) (data not shown).

As observed in our study, the analysis of all individuals with SCD who present characteristics so different from each other can interfere in the results found, since the group comprised of patients with SCD presented a serum hepcidin concentration smaller than the one observed in the control group. Thus, the serum hepcidin concentration of the SCDio group was masked and could only be revealed when the separation between groups with and without iron overload was performed.

These results show that the behavior of hepcidin in SCD may be influenced by various changes in this hemoglobinopathy, whether linked to iron metabolism or factors inherent to the disease itself. Regarding inflammation, as revealed by IL-6 and leukocyte concentrations, it was increased in patients with SCD, with and without iron overload, when compared to individuals in the control group. It is known that inflammation is one of the factors capable of increasing hepcidin concentration. In inflammation, the interaction of IL-6 with its receptor (IL-6R) activates JAK tyrosine kinases, triggering the formation of STAT3 (Signal transducer and transcription activator 3) complexes that bind to the hepcidin promoter in the nucleus [26]. Additionally, obesity seems to be another factor capable of exerting influence on serum hepcidin concentrations [27]. However, in the present study, the percentage of individuals with excess of adiposity was lower in the SCD group.

Karafin et al. [28] also investigated the relationship between possible factors that could contribute to changes in the hepcidin concentration in SCD and observed that erythropoiesis markers were the strongest factors capable of influencing its serum concentration, followed by serum ferritin. These results were in line with the findings of this study, since the concentration of GDF-15 in the SCD group was 2.5-fold higher than that in the control group, which could explain the reduced hepcidin concentration in the group with SCD. Increase in the concentration of this marker was already expected.

In the iron overload group, high levels of iron, identified by the high concentration of serum ferritin, overlapped the elevation of GDF-15 levels, possibly leading to higher hepcidin concentration.

This study revealed the heterogeneity of the characteristics of the SCDw and SCDio groups. The behavior of hepcidin in SCD needs to be interpreted considering the presence or absence of iron overload, since iron regulates the synthesis of several molecules involved in its own homeostasis.

In many countries, including Brazil, some public policies have been developed to prevent iron deficiency, such as mandatory fortification of wheat and corn flours [29]. Although these actions can help prevent iron-deficiency anemia and are aimed at the entire Brazilian population, the safety of these actions is still unknown for individuals with diseases caused by iron overload such as hereditary hemochromatosis, thalassemia, and SCD. To date, data on intestinal iron absorption in sickle cell disease are limited, making it impossible to guarantee that these actions do not cause harm to this group.

However, some authors have observed iron deficiency in people with SCD. Kassim et al. [30] observed that 13.3% of the SCD participants presented iron deficiency—most of them had never undergone transfusion previously. In this case, the diagnosis of iron deficiency was established if all the following four criteria were present: low serum iron <45 µg/ dL, low transferrin saturation (TS) <16%, high TIBC ≥450 µg/dL, and low MCV for age.

5. Conclusions

Differences in hepcidin concentrations between groups may suggest an increase (in the case of the SCD and SCDw groups) or decrease (SCDio) in the intestinal absorption of iron. These data suggest that individuals with iron overload may not need to reduce intake of foods rich in iron. However, these results are not sufficient to the establishment of a nutritional approach to be adopted. Future studies evaluating the intestinal absorption of iron in patients with sickle cell anemia must be conducted to address this question. Regarding the participants in the group without overload, suppression of hepcidin appears to occur possibly due to the increase of erythropoiesis in response to anemia, which is characteristic of the disease and, consequently, could lead to increased intestinal absorption of iron.

Acknowledgments: The authors thank Viviane Fernandes de Meneses for excellent technical assistance. This study was funded by Fundação Carlos Chagas Filho de Amparo à Pesquisa do Estado do Rio de Janeiro, Conselho Nacional de Desenvolvimento Científico e Tecnológico, Ministério da Saúde do Brasil and Coordenação de Aperfeiçoamento de Pessoal de Nível Superior.

Author Contributions: M.C. and C.d.S.C.-R. conceived and designed the experiments; J.O., J.D.d.A.C., A.R.S. and M.K.F. performed the experiments; M.C., J.O., J.C.K. and F.d.S.B.B. analyzed the data; M.C., M.K.F., J.C.K. and C.d.S.C.-R. contributed reagents/materials/analysis tools; M.C. and J.O. wrote the paper.

Conflicts of Interest: The authors declare no conflict of interest.

References

1. Ballas, S.K. Sickle cell anaemia: Progress in pathogenesis and treatment. *Drugs* **2002**, *62*, 1143–1172. [CrossRef] [PubMed]
2. Josephson, C.D.; Su, L.L.; Hillyer, K.L.; Hillyer, C.D. Transfusion in the patient with sickle cell disease: A critical review of the literature and transfusion guidelines. *Transfus. Med. Rev.* **2007**, *21*, 118–133. [CrossRef] [PubMed]
3. Adams, R.J.; McKie, V.C.; Hsu, L.; Files, B.; Vichinsky, E.; Pegelow, C.; Abboud, M.; Gallagher, D.; Kutlar, A.; Nichols, F.T.; et al. Prevention of a first stroke by transfusions in children with sickle cell anemia and abnormal results on transcranial Doppler ultrasonography. *N. Engl. J. Med.* **1998**, *339*, 5–11. [CrossRef] [PubMed]
4. Adams, R.J.; Brambilla, D. Optimizing Primary Stroke Prevention in Sickle Cell Anemia (STOP 2) Trial Investigators. Discontinuing prophylactic transfusions used to prevent stroke in sickle cell disease. *N. Engl. J. Med.* **2005**, *353*, 2769–2778. [CrossRef] [PubMed]

5. Inati, A.; Khoriaty, E.; Musallam, K.M. Iron in sickle-cell disease: What have we learned over the years? *Pediatr. Blood Cancer* **2011**, *56*, 182–190. [CrossRef] [PubMed]
6. Remacha, A.; Sanz, C.; Contreras, E.; De Heredia, C.D.; Grifols, J.R.; Lozano, M.; Nuñez, G.M.; Salinas, R.; Corral, M.; Villegas, A. Guidelines on haemovigilance of post-transfusional iron overload. *Blood Transfus.* **2013**, *11*, 128–139. [CrossRef] [PubMed]
7. Ganz, T. Molecular control of iron transport. *J. Am. Soc. Nephrol.* **2007**, *18*, 394–400. [CrossRef] [PubMed]
8. Hoffbrand, A.V.; Taher, A.; Capellini, M.D. How I treat transfusional iron overload. *Blood* **2012**, *120*, 3657–3669. [CrossRef] [PubMed]
9. Ward, R. An update on disordered iron metabolism and iron overload. *Hematology* **2010**, *15*, 311–317. [CrossRef] [PubMed]
10. Ganz, T.; Nemeth, E. Hepcidin and iron homeostasis. *Biochim. Biophys. Acta* **2012**, *1823*, 1434–1443. [CrossRef] [PubMed]
11. Mena, N.P.; Esparza, A.; Tapia, V.; Valdés, P.; Núñez, M.T. Hepcidin inhibits apical iron uptake in intestinal cells. *Am. J. Physiol. Gastrointest. Liver Physiol.* **2008**, *294*, G192–G198. [CrossRef] [PubMed]
12. Bergamaschi, G.; Di Sabatino, A.; Pasini, A.; Ubezio, C.; Costanzo, F.; Grataroli, D.; Masotti, M.; Alvisi, C.; Corazza, G.R. Intestinal expression of genes implicated in iron absorption and their regulation by hepcidin. *Clin. Nutr.* **2017**, *36*, 1427–1433. [CrossRef] [PubMed]
13. Nemeth, E. Iron regulation and erythropoiesis. *Curr. Opin. Hematol.* **2008**, *15*, 169–175. [CrossRef] [PubMed]
14. Nemeth, E.; Valore, E.V.; Territo, M.; Schiller, G.; Lichtenstein, A.; Ganz, T. Hepcidin, a putative mediator of anemia of inflammation, is a type II acute-phase protein. *Blood* **2003**, *101*, 2461–2463. [CrossRef] [PubMed]
15. Zemel, B.S.; Kawchak, D.A.; Fung, E.B.; Ohene-Frempong, K.; Stallings, V.A. Effect of zinc supplementation on growth and body composition in children with sickle cell disease. *Am. J. Clin. Nutr.* **2002**, *75*, 300–307. [CrossRef] [PubMed]
16. Sayani, F.; Bansal, S.; Evans, P.; Weljie, A.; Hilder, R.C.; Porter, J.B. Disease specific modulation of serum hepcidin: Impact of GDF-15 and iron metabolism markers in thalassemia major, thalassemia intermedia and sickle cell disease: A univariate and multivariate analysis. *Blood* **2008**, *112*, 3850.
17. El Beshlawy, A.; Alaraby, I.; Abdel Kader, M.S.; Ahmed, D.H.; Abdelrahman, H.E. Study of serum hepcidin in hereditary hemolytic anemias. *Hemoglobin* **2012**, *36*, 555–570. [CrossRef] [PubMed]
18. Fertrin, K.Y.; Lanaro, C.; Franco-Penteado, C.F.; Albuquerque, D.M.; Mello, M.R.B.; Pallis, F.R.; Bezerra, M.A.; Hatzhofer, B.L.; Olbina, G.; Saad, S.T.; et al. Erythropoiesis-driven regulation of hepcidin in human red cell disorders is better reflected through concentrations of soluble transferrin receptor rather than growth differentiation factor 15. *Am. J. Hematol.* **2014**, *89*, 385–390. [CrossRef] [PubMed]
19. Ezeh, C.; Ugochukwu, C.C.; Weinstein, J.; Okpala, I. Hepcidin, haemoglobin and ferritin levels in sickle cell anaemia. *Euro. J. Haematol.* **2005**, *74*, 86–88. [CrossRef] [PubMed]
20. Kearney, S.L.; Nemeth, E.; Neufeld, E.J.; Thapa, D.; Ganz, T.; Weinstein, D.A.; Cunningham, M.J. Urinary hepcidin in congenital chronic anemias. *Pediatr. Blood Cancer* **2007**, *48*, 57–63. [CrossRef] [PubMed]
21. Kroot, J.J.; Laarakkers, C.M.; Kemna, E.H.; Biemond, B.J.; Swinkels, D.W. Regulation of serum hepcidin levels in sickle cell disease. *Haematologica* **2009**, *94*, 885–887. [CrossRef] [PubMed]
22. Shen, J.; Wongtong, N.; Nouboussie, D.; Elsherif, L.; Zhou, Q.; Cai, J.; Ataga, K.I. Lack of difference in hepcidin levels in sickle cell anemia and sickle cell beta thalassemia. *Blood* **2015**, *126*, 4591.
23. Nnodim, J.; Uche, U.B.; Ifeoma, U.H.; Chidozie, N.J.; Ifeanyi, O.E.; Oluchi, A.A. Hepcidin and erythropoietin level in sickle cell disease. *Br. J. Med. Med. Res.* **2015**, *8*, 261–265. [CrossRef]
24. Porter, J.; Garbowski, M. Consequences and management of iron overload in sickle cell disease. *Hematology* **2013**, *2013*, 447–456. [CrossRef] [PubMed]
25. World Health Organization. *Physical Status: The Use and Interpretation of Anthropometry*; Report of a WHO Expert Committee; Technical Report Series No. 854; World Health Organization: Geneva, Switzerland, 1995.
26. Muckenthaler, M.U.; Rivella, S.; Hentze, M.W.; Galy, B. A red carpet for iron metabolism. *Cell* **2017**, *168*, 344–361. [CrossRef] [PubMed]
27. Citelli, M.; Fonte-Faria, T.; Nascimento-Silva, V.; Renovato-Martins, M.; Silva, R.; Luna, A.S.; Silva, S.V.; Barja-Fidalgo, C. Obesity promotes alterations in iron recycling. *Nutrients* **2015**, *7*, 335–348. [CrossRef] [PubMed]

28. Karafin, M.S.; Koch, K.L.; Rankin, A.B.; Nischik, D.; Rahhal, G.; Simpson, P.; Field, J.J. Erythropoietic drive is the strongest predictor of hepcidin level in adults with sickle cell disease. *Blood Cells Mol. Dis.* **2015**, *55*, 304–307. [CrossRef] [PubMed]

29. Brasil. Ministério da Saúde. Agência Nacional de Vigilância Sanitária (ANVISA). Aprova o Regulamento Técnico Para a Fortificação de Farinhas de Trigo e Das Farinhas de Milho com Ferro e Ácido Fólico. Resolução n. 344, de 13 de Dezembro de 2002b. Publicada no DOU n. 244 em 18 de Dezembro de 2002. Available online: http://portal.anvisa.gov.br/documents/10181/2718376/RDC_344_2002_COMP.pdf/b4d87885-dcb9-4fe3-870d-db57921cf73f (accessed on 10 January 2018).

30. Kassim, A.; Thabet, S.; Al-Kabban, M.; Al-Nihari, K. Iron deficiency in Yemeni patients with sickle-cell disease. *East. Mediterr. Health J.* **2012**, *18*, 241–245. [CrossRef] [PubMed]

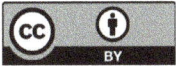

nutrients

Review

Impact of Inflammation on Ferritin, Hepcidin and the Management of Iron Deficiency Anemia in Chronic Kidney Disease

Norishi Ueda [1,*] and Kazuya Takasawa [2,3]

[1] Department of Pediatrics, Public Central Hospital of Matto Ishikawa, 3-8 Kuramitsu, Hakusan, Ishikawa 924-8588, Japan
[2] Department of Internal Medicine, Public Central Hospital of Matto Ishikawa, 3-8 Kuramitsu, Hakusan, Ishikawa 924-8588, Japan; kazuya@takasawa.org
[3] Department of Internal Medicine, Public Tsurugi Hospital, Ishikawa 920-2134, Japan
* Correspondence: nueda@mattohp.com; Tel.: +81-76-275-2222; Fax: +81-76-274-5974

Received: 26 June 2018; Accepted: 17 August 2018; Published: 27 August 2018

Abstract: Iron deficiency anemia (IDA) is a major problem in chronic kidney disease (CKD), causing increased mortality. Ferritin stores iron, representing iron status. Hepcidin binds to ferroportin, thereby inhibiting iron absorption/efflux. Inflammation in CKD increases ferritin and hepcidin independent of iron status, which reduce iron availability. While intravenous iron therapy (IIT) is superior to oral iron therapy (OIT) in CKD patients with inflammation, OIT is as effective as IIT in those without. Inflammation reduces predictive values of ferritin and hepcidin for iron status and responsiveness to iron therapy. Upper limit of ferritin to predict iron overload is higher in CKD patients with inflammation than in those without. However, magnetic resonance imaging studies show lower cutoff levels of serum ferritin to predict iron overload in dialysis patients with apparent inflammation than upper limit of ferritin proposed by international guidelines. Compared to CKD patients with inflammation, optimal ferritin levels for IDA are lower in those without, requiring reduced iron dose and leading to decreased mortality. The management of IDA should differ between CKD patients with and without inflammation and include minimization of inflammation. Further studies are needed to determine the impact of inflammation on ferritin, hepcidin and therapeutic strategy for IDA in CKD.

Keywords: chronic kidney disease; ferritin; C-reactive protein; hepcidin; inflammation; iron deficiency anemia

1. Introduction

Iron deficiency (ID) occurs in two major forms; absolute ID as defined by a decrease in the body iron stores and functional ID (FID), a disorder in which the total body iron stores are normal or increased but the iron supply to the bone marrow is inadequate [1]. ID anemia (IDA) is frequently associated with chronic inflammatory conditions, in which inflammation is pathogenically involved, including inflammatory bowel disease (IBD, e.g., ulcerative colitis, Crohn's disease), chronic heart failure, chronic liver disease, obesity, rheumatoid arthritis (RA) and chronic kidney disease (CKD) [1]. IDA is a global public health problem affecting 7.2–13.96 per 1000 person-years and accounting for 800,000 deaths per year worldwide [2]. IDA also has an impact on mortality in children and adults with CKD [3,4]. Thus, appropriate management of IDA is crucial for improving quality of life (QOL) and mortality in CKD patients.

Iron is a component of heme proteins (hemoglobin; Hb and myoglobin), which carry or store oxygen and essential for the functioning of all organs. Iron is also present in heme enzymes, non-heme iron enzymes and iron-sulfur proteins that regulate various cell functions including electron transport in mitochondrial respiration, redox reactions and DNA synthesis [5]. However, excessive iron leaves a fraction of free iron (known as "labile" iron) and makes redox active, forming reactive oxygen species that cause oxidant stress. Because of no excretion system for iron from the body, iron homeostasis is tightly regulated via a network of proteins involved in the import, storage, export and transport of iron within the body.

There are two major molecules that regulate iron metabolism and iron availability for erythropoiesis. Ferritin binds iron as a ferric complex within a protein shell, in which iron fluxes in and out and functions as iron storage site and ferroxidase [5,6]. Thus, alteration of serum ferritin may be a determinant of mortality in adults on maintenance hemodialysis (HD) [7–9]. While iron supplementation reduced mortality in HD adults [9], excess iron therapy increased ferritin levels, leading to high mortality [7]. To date, optimal levels of serum ferritin during iron therapy for IDA remain to be determined in CKD patients. On the other hand, hepcidin-25 (referred to as hepcidin), a 25 amino acid peptide, is a major iron-regulatory hormone that binds to ferroportin (FPN) and inhibits iron export from enterocytes, hepatocytes and macrophages through the internalization and degradation of FPN, thereby regulating iron metabolism in various diseases, including CKD [10–12].

Inflammation as defined by the innate immune response to stimuli such as pathogens, cellular injury and metabolic stress [13] is part of the complex biologic response to tissue injury, infection, ischemia and autoimmune diseases. It is characterized by the acute-phase response including elevated inflammation markers such as C-reactive protein (CRP, >0.3 mg/dL) [14] and pro-inflammatory cytokines which promote CRP synthesis [15]. Inflammation is characteristic feature of CKD and caused by multiple factors of the toxic uremic milieu and the dialysis procedure itself. The interpretation of iron biomarkers is hindered by inflammation, which can directly affect the concentrations of most iron biomarkers [14], including ferritin and hepcidin [16–18]. Inflammation-mediated increase in hepcidin leads to iron trapping within the macrophages and hepatocytes, resulting in FID [19]. This leads to high association of inflammation with FID anemia (FIDA) in CKD patients [16–18], requiring higher dose of IV iron to maintain Hb targets [20]. Inflammation also induces hyporesponsiveness to iron therapy [20–22] and erythropoiesis-stimulating agents (ESA) in HD patients [21,23] by increasing ferritin and hepcidin. Conversely, aggressive intravenous iron therapy (IIT) may enhance inflammation in patients with end-stage renal disease (ESRD) [16], leading to further disturbance of iron metabolism. Thus, inflammation has an impact on the expression of ferritin and hepcidin as well as therapeutic strategy for the management of IDA in CKD patients.

The aim of this review is to provide an overview of clinical and experimental studies regarding a role of ferritin, hepcidin and inflammation in the regulation of IDA, efficacy of oral iron therapy (OIT) and IIT, predictive values of ferritin and hepcidin for the response to iron therapy, upper limit of ferritin levels to predict iron overload, optimal ferritin levels during iron therapy, complications and outcome in CKD patients. This review especially focuses on the impact of inflammation on these issues in CKD patients.

2. Ferritin Regulation by Iron Status and Inflammation

Ferritin has two isoforms; the heavy chain (FtH) and the light chain of ferritin (FtL). In contrast to FtH, FtL lacks detectable ferroxidase activity but can store more iron [6]. Ferritin sequesters iron in a nontoxic form, whereas the levels of free iron regulate cellular ferritin levels [6]. Cytoplasmic ferritin synthesis is stimulated by an increase of iron, while it is decreased by iron depletion. This process is mediated by the interaction between the two RNA-binding proteins (iron regulatory proteins 1 and 2; IRP1/2) and a region in the 5_untranslated region of FtH and FtL mRNA, termed the iron responsive element (IRE) that has a "stem-loop" structure. Binding of IRP1/2 to the IRE inhibits mRNA ferritin translation. IRP1 and IRP2 are differentially regulated, depending on iron status. When iron is abundant, IRP1 exists as a cytosolic aconitase, whereas under iron depletion, it assumes an open configuration associated with the loss of iron atoms in the iron-sulfur cluster and can bind to the IRE stem loop, thereby suppressing ferritin translation. IRP2 protein is abundant in iron depletion status but is rapidly degraded in iron excess. IRP1 and IRP2 have distinct tissue-specific roles [6].

Synthesis of FtH and FtL is activated by pro-inflammatory cytokines such as interleukin (IL)-1β and tumor necrosis factor (TNF)-α [6,24] via nuclear factor (NF)-κB pathway [25]. Interferon (INF)-γ and lipopolysaccharide (LPS) induce degradation of IRP2 in nitric oxide (NO)-dependent manner, leading to ferritin synthesis in macrophages [26]. IL-6 also enhances synthesis of FtH and FtL in hepatocytes [24]. FtH transcription is predominantly active in inflammatory conditions, whereas transcription of FtL can be induced only after exposure to very high concentration of iron [27]. Pro-inflammatory cytokines modulate the relative ratio of ferritin to body iron storage by increasing ferritin synthesis [27].

3. Hepcidin and Iron Metabolism

3.1. Hepcidin-Ferroporin Axis Regulates Iron Homeostasis

Dietary iron containing heme and non-heme iron is absorbed by the divalent metal transporter (DMT1) located at the apical membrane of duodenal enterocytes [10–12] (Figure 1), which transports only Fe^{2+} but most dietary iron is Fe^{3+}. Thus, Fe^{3+} should be reduced to Fe^{2+} before iron transport by DMT1. This reduction step is mediated by the ferrireductase duodenal cytochrome b (DCYTB) at the apical membrane of duodenal enterocytes. Hepcidin binds to FPN and triggers its internalization, ubiquitination and subsequent lysosomal degradation, leading to inhibition of iron export by FPN from enterocytes, hepatocytes and macrophages into the circulation. Heme absorbed by the enterocytes is degraded by heme oxygenase-1 (HO-1) and the liberated iron is processed in a similar manner as the absorbed inorganic iron. The export of enterocytic iron by FPN requires hephaestin, a multicopper oxidase homologous to ceruloplasmin (CP), which oxidizes Fe^{2+} to Fe^{3+} for loading onto transferrin (Tf) [10]. Once exported by FPN into the circulation, Fe^{2+} is oxidized into Fe^{3+} by a ferrioxidase CP in hepatocytes and macrophages. Iron-loaded (diferric) transferrin (Tf-Fe$_2$, holo-Tf) is transported to other cells or tissues for iron metabolism or storage [10–12].

Hepatocytes sense iron stores and regulate hepcidin promotor activity, thereby releasing hepcidin accordingly. In ID (Figure 1A), hepcidin is low and thus iron is released by FPN into the circulation from enterocytes, hepatocytes and macrophages, facilitating iron availability for erythropoiesis [10–12]. Under iron overload (Figure 1B), increased hepcidin in hepatocytes is released [10–12]. Increased hepcidin binds to FPN and inhibits FPN-mediated iron export into the circulation to reduce Tf saturation (TSAT), leading to subsequent inhibition of duodenal iron absorption.

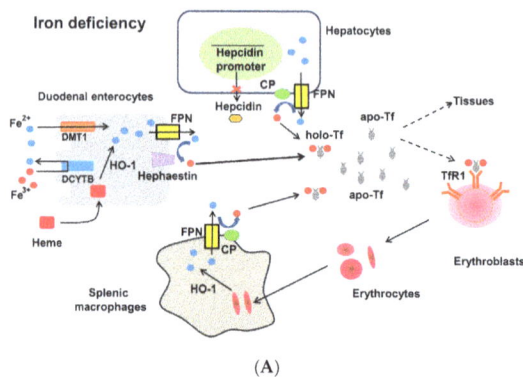

(A)

Figure 1. *Cont.*

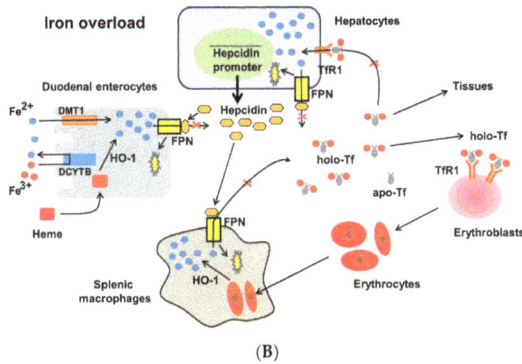

(B)

Figure 1. Regulation of systemic iron homeostasis. Divalent metal transporter 1 (DMT1) at the apical membrane of enterocytes takes up Fe^{2+} from the lumen after duodenal cytochrome b (DCYTB) reduces dietary Fe^{3+} to Fe^{2+}. Ferroportin (FPN) at the basolateral membrane exports Fe^{2+} into the circulation. FPN cooperates with hephaestin that oxidizes Fe^{2+} to Fe^{3+}. In hepatocytes and macrophages, Fe^{2+} is oxidized by a ferroxidase, ceruloplasmin (CP). Diferric ($Fe^{3+}{}_2$) transferrin (holo-Tf) supplies iron to all cells and tissues through binding to Tf receptor 1 (TfR1) and endocytosis. Erythrocytes are phagocytized by macrophages. Hemoglobin-derived heme in enterocytes and macrophages is catabolized by heme oxygenase-1 (HO-1). After sensing iron, hepatocytes produce and release hepcidin. In iron deficiency (**A**), low hepcidin facilitates iron export by FPN into the circulation. In iron overload (**B**), high hepcidin binds to FPN and inhibits iron export from enterocytes, hepatocytes and macrophages by triggering internalization and degradation of FPN, leading to reduction of iron storage. Dashed line indicates less iron supply. x: inhibition. Figures adapted from [12].

3.2. Hepcidin Regulation by Iron Status

After sensing iron, bone morphogenetic protein (BMP)-6 is produced in the liver [28] and increases hepcidin via BMP/small mothers against decapentaplegic (SMAD) proteins-mediated signaling pathway [28] (Figure 2). Holo-Tf displaces the interaction of hereditary hemochromatosis protein (HFE)-TfR1 and stabilizes the association of HFE-TfR2 with membrane-anchored hemojuvelin (mHJV), forming a complex of HFE/TfR2/HJV which is dispensable for hepcidin transcription [10,11,28]. mHJV exclusively expressed in hepatocytes acts as a co-receptor for BMP-6, leading to activation of BMP/SMAD-mediated hepcidin transcription [28]. Neogenin acts as a scaffold to facilitate assembly of HJV/BMP/BMP receptor (BMPR) complex [29] and maintains proper mHJV function [28]. Matriptase (MT)-2 (also known as TMPRSS6) functions as a negative regulator of hepcidin-related BMP/SMAD signaling by cleaving mHJV into soluble HJV (sHJV) [11].

ID reduces BMP-6, leading to inhibition of BMP/SMAD-dependent hepcidin transcription. Decreased holo-Tf in ID destabilizes the TfR2-HFE interaction, thereby inhibiting hepcidin transcription [28]. Decreased holo-Tf and non-Tf-bound iron increase sHJV, leading to inhibition of hepcidin, while increased holo-Tf and non-Tf-bound iron have the opposite effect [28]. ID stabilizes MT-2, thereby suppressing hepcidin [28,30]. Furin, which cleaves mHJV into sHJV, is upregulated by ID and inhibits hepcidin [31]. In iron overload, increased holo-Tf stabilizes the TfR2-HFE interaction [10,11,28] and decreases furin [32], thereby increasing hepcidin translation.

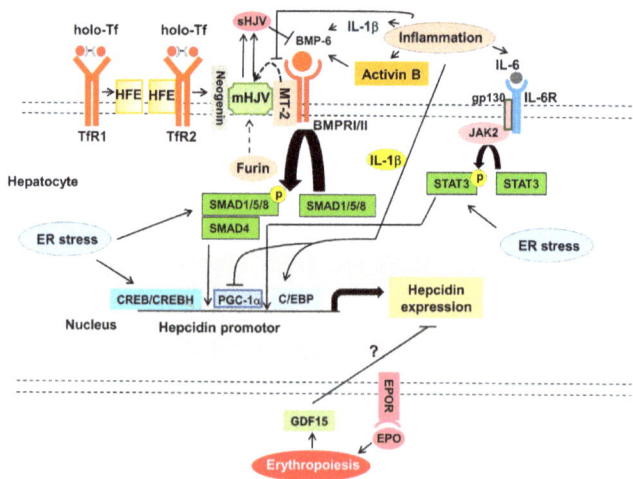

Figure 2. Regulation of hepcidin by iron status and inflammation. Under high iron conditions, increased holo-Tf induces bone morphogenetic protein (BMP)-6 in non-parenchymal cells in the liver, disrupts hereditary hemochromatosis protein (HFE)-transferrin receptor (TfR)1 interaction to promote HFE-TfR2 interaction and its association with membrane-anchored hemojuvelin (mHJV), forming a complex of HFE/TfR2/BMP-6/BMPR/HJV/neogenin, which is dispensable for hepcidin transcription via BMP/small mothers against decapentaplegic (SMAD) signaling. In iron overload, furin, which cleaves mHJV, is downregulated, thereby increasing hepcidin. Low iron conditions increase matriptase (MT)-2 and furin, which cleaves mHJV, reduces BMP-6 production and facilitates the HFE-TfR1 interaction, leading to inhibition of BMP/SMAD-dependent hepcidin transcription. Pro-inflammatory cytokines such as interleukin (IL)-1β and IL-6 stimulate hepcidin expression via the Janus kinase (JAK)/signal transducers and activators of transcription (STAT)3 signaling. Inflammation induces other cytokine, activin B, which stimulates BMP/SMAD signaling, synergically with IL-6 and STAT3 signaling, leading to hepcidin expression. Endoplasmic reticulum (ER) stress associated with inflammation increases hepcidin via SMAD1/5/8 and cyclic-AMP-responsive-element-binding protein (CREB)H that binds and activates hepcidin promoter activity. Inflammation increases hepcidin by inhibiting MT-2 via decreased STAT5 and peroxisome proliferator-activated receptor γ coactivator (PGC)-1α which antagonizes lipopolysaccharide-induced hepcidin transcription via the interaction with hepatocyte nuclear factor 4α. Inflammation-induced IL-1β enhances hepcidin transcription by inducing CCAT enhancer-binding protein (C/EBP)δ. Hepcidin translation is mediated indirectly through erythropoietin (EPO)/EPOR-induced erythropoiesis and possibly growth differentiation factor (GDF)15. gp130: glycoprotein 130. Dashed line: cleavage, →: activation, ⊢: inhibition.

3.3. Inflammation Increases Hepcidin Expression

Pro-inflammatory cytokines are increased in CKD [17,18]. Pro-inflammatory cytokines such as IL-1β and IL-6 stimulate hepcidin expression via the Janus kinase (JAK)/signal transducer and activator of transcription 3 (STAT3) pathways [10–12,28] (Figure 2). Inflammation induces other cytokine activin B which stimulates BMP-6/SMAD pathway synergically with IL-6 and STAT3, leading to hepcidin expression [11]. Endoplasmic reticulum (ER) stress associated with inflammation increases hepcidin by activating SMAD1/5/8 [33], IL-6-dependent phosphorylated STAT3 [34] and ER stress-activated transcription factor, cyclic AMP response element–binding protein H (CREBH), which bind and activate hepcidin promoter activity [35]. Inflammation inhibits MT-2 by suppressing STAT5 [36] and peroxisome proliferator-activated receptor γ coactivator-1α (PGC-1α) which antagonizes LPS-induced hepcidin transcription via the interaction with hepatocyte nuclear factor 4α [37], leading to activation of hepcidin translation. Inflammation-induced IL-1β also activates hepcidin expression by inducing CCAAT enhancer-binding protein (C/EBP)δ in hepatocytes [38].

4. Biomarkers of Iron Status and Inflammation in CKD

A number of biomarkers of iron status have been used in a clinical setting. However, traditional biochemical iron parameters such as serum iron, Tf and serum ferritin are influenced by inflammation [14], making them less suitable indicators. Due to confounding effects of the acute-phase response on the interpretation of most iron indicators, the assessment of iron status is challenging when concomitant inflammation is present. In fact, serum levels of ferritin were positively correlated with CRP, a measure of inflammation, in children and adults on HD [16,39,40]. Under minor inflammation, serum ferritin appears to be a most reliable biomarker of total body iron stores and ID is diagnosed below the cutoff serum ferritin levels of <15 ng/mL in individuals older than 5 years [1]. However, serum ferritin levels of 50 ng/mL or higher could still be ID when apparent inflammation is present [1]. Thus, the interpretation of serum ferritin, an acute phase reactant, is complicated by concomitant inflammation [1,14,41].

As negative acute phase reactants, concentrations of serum iron and Tf, an iron transport protein, are decreased in response to inflammation [14,41–43]. Low TSAT (<20%) with low serum ferritin is diagnostic of IDA [1,44]. Low TSAT combined with normal or elevated serum ferritin is diagnostic of FIDA [44]. As discussed later, many international guidelines for the management of IDA in CKD use the combination of low serum ferritin and TSAT for diagnosis of IDA. TSAT represents the percentage of binding sites on all Tf molecules occupied with iron molecules and is calculated as the ratio of serum iron to Tf or serum iron to total iron-binding capacity (TIBC) which indicates the maximum amount of iron necessary to saturate all available transferrin iron-binding sites [1,44]. TIBC is a negative acute-phase reactant and reduction in TIBC induced by inflammation leads to higher TSAT levels independent of iron status [41]. Thus, reliability of TSAT as a measure of iron status is reduced by inflammation associated with CKD. Soluble TfR (sTfR), which is produced by proteolysis of the membrane TfR, is increased in HD patients with ID and inversely correlated with the amount of iron available for erythropoiesis [44]. As a marker of iron status, sTfR is not an acute-phase reactant and less influenced by inflammation than serum ferritin is, while it is increased in individuals with general inflammation [14]. In addition, sTfR appears to represent erythropoietic activity more than iron-restricted erythropoiesis in CKD patients receiving ESA [44]. Thus, the interpretation of sTfR is also confounded by the use of ESA [1,41]. Thus, it is an inferior marker to cellular measures such as the content of Hb in reticulocytes (CHr) or the percentage of hypochromic red blood cells (%Hypo) [41,44]. Other limitations of sTfR measurement include cost for the measurement and lack of standard cutoff and widespread availability [1,41]. The interpretation of total body iron (TBI), the log ratio of sTfR to serum ferritin, is also complicated by the same confounding factors as for serum ferritin and sTfR concentrations [14].

Other laboratory markers of iron status include CHr and %Hypo. Both iron biomarkers are influenced by inflammation [45,46]. CHr is inversely related to log CRP [45] and there is a positive correlation between %Hypo and CRP [46]. CHr is a very early index of iron available for erythropoiesis within 3–4 days [1,41,44]. The CHr of <27.2 pg is diagnostic of ID, while false normal values are frequently encountered [1]. The measurement of %Hypo as a proportion of hypochromic cells defined as erythrocytes with mean cellular Hb concentration less than 28 g/dL in total red blood cells is the most sensitive marker of ID in CKD (cutoff, <6%) [1] and FID [41]. However, it is not suitable for the assessment of short-term changes in iron status [1,41,44]. Furthermore, a fresh blood sample is needed and automated analyzers are not widely available in clinical setting. Currently, none of the measurements are adequate and accurate indicators of iron status, especially when concomitant inflammation is present.

It is controversial about whether hepcidin is a reliable biomarker of iron status in CKD patients. Serum hepcidin has been shown to be positively correlated with serum ferritin, percent iron saturation,

CRP and sTfR and negatively with glomerular filtration rate (GFR) in CKD patients [47]. As GFR decreased, serum hepcidin levels were increased in non-dialysis (ND)-CKD patients [48]. Dialysis can remove hepcidin [49] and inflammation increases hepcidin like ferritin [18,48,50]. A significant intra-individual variability of hepcidin was dependent on short-term fluctuations in the inflammatory condition [50]. Thus, short-term measurement of serum hepcidin should not be used as a biomarker of iron status in HD patients [50]. Interpretation of the data for serum hepcidin should be with caution due to the confounding factors as described. However, hepcidin could be a good biomarker of iron status in CKD patients in the absence of apparent inflammation.

5. IDA in CKD

5.1. Impact of Inflammation on Diagnosis of IDA

The cutoff levels of Hb for diagnosis of anemia depend on age, sex and pregnancy [1] (Table 1). In general, low serum ferritin (<15 ng/mL) and TSAT (<16%) are used for diagnosis of IDA in individuals without inflammatory conditions [1]. However, IDA could be diagnosed based on higher cutoff levels of serum ferritin and TSAT in the presence of chronic inflammatory condition such as CKD [1]. Table 2 summarizes diagnostic criteria for IDA in ND-CKD and HD patients used by international guidelines for the management of IDA in CKD patients [51–60]. Some guidelines in Canada, the US [51,52,54] and Taiwan [57] recommend higher cutoff levels of serum ferritin ≤200–500 ng/mL and TSAT ≤30% [54,57] for diagnosis of IDA and initiation of iron supplementation in ND-CKD and HD patients than those (serum ferritin <100 ng/mL and TSAT <20%) recommended by the Japanese Society for Dialysis Therapy (JSDT) guidelines [53] and other guidelines from Europe and Australia [55,56,58–60]. The Japanese nationwide study showed low cutoff levels of serum ferritin (<50–100 ng/mL) and TSAT (<20%) to diagnose IDA in HD patients with low CRP (median, 1.0 mg/mL) [61]. The reason for the difference in the criteria for diagnosis of IDA and the initiation of iron therapy in CKD patients between Japan and some Western countries is unclear. However, it may be in part due to lower prevalence of inflammation associated with HD patients in Japan than those in Western countries [15,61,62]. While the specific biologic basis underlying differences by race and ethnicity is unclear [62], one of the reasons may be higher prevalence of arteriovenous (AV) fistula and lower prevalence of. catheter use and AV graft in Japan [15,63,64] that are associated with higher levels of CRP [65] as compared to Western countries. Nonetheless, the impact of inflammation could increase the cutoff levels of serum ferritin and TSAT for diagnosis of IDA to initiate iron therapy in CKD patients.

Table 1. Cutoff of hemoglobin (Hb) for diagnosis of anemia.

Age/Gender Groups	Hb Below (g/dL)
Children	
6 months to 4 years	<11.0
5 to 11 years	<11.5
12 to 14 years	<12.0
Adults	
Non-pregnant women ≥15 years	<12.0
Pregnant women ≥15 years	<11.0
Men ≥15 years	<13.0

Table 2. International clinical guidelines for diagnosis of IDA and upper limit of serum ferritin and TSAT in CKD patients.

Organization (Year)	Origin	ID/IDA	Recommended ID Cutoff Serum Ferritin (ng/mL)		TSAT (%)		Upper Limit of Serum Ferritin (ng/mL)	TSAT (%)	Reference
			ND	HD	ND	HD			
KDOQI (2007)	USA	ID/IDA	≤100	≤200	≤20	≤20	≤500	NA	[51]
CSN (2008)	Canada	ID/IDA	≤100	≤200	≤20	≤20	≤800	NA	[52]
JSDT (2008)	Japan	ID/IDA	≤100	≤100	≤20	≤20	≤800	≤50	[53]
		Children	≤100	≤100	≤20	≤20	NA	NA	
KDIGO (2012)	International	ID/IDA	≤500	≤500	≤30	≤30	≤500–800	NA	[54]
		Children	≤100	≤100	≤20	≤20	≤500–800	NA	
ERBP (2016)	Europe	ID/IDA	<100	<100	<20	<20	≤500	≤30	[55]
KHA-CARI (2013)	Australia	ID	<100	<100	<20	<20	≤500	NA	[56]
TPG (1996)	Taiwan	ID/IDA	≤300	≤300	≤30	≤30	≤800	≤50	[57]
NICE (2015)	UK	ID/IDA	≤100	≤100	≤20	≤20	<800	NA	[58,59]
UKRA (2017)	UK	ID/IDA	≤100	≤100	≤20	≤20	≤500–800	NA	[60]
		Children	≤100	≤100	≤20	≤20	≤500–800	NA	

CKD: chronic kidney disease; CSN: Canadian Society of Nephrology; ERBP: European Renal Best Practice; HD: hemodialysis; ID: iron deficiency; IDA: ID anemia; JSDT: The Japanese Society for Dialysis Therapy; KDIGO: The Kidney Disease, Improving Global Outcomes; KDOQI: The Kidney Disease Outcomes Quality Initiative; KHA-CARI: Kidney Health Australia-Caring for Australians with Renal Impairment; ND: non-dialysis; NICE: The National Institute for Health and Care Excellence; TPG: Taiwan Practice Guidelines; TSAT: transferrin saturation; UKRA: United Kingdom Renal Association. ID is defined as a decrease in the body iron stores. NA: not available.

5.2. IDA, Inflammation and Clinical Outcome in CKD

IDA and FIDA are frequently associated with chronic inflammation, including CKD. IDA occurs in 42.0% in children with CKD [66] and 1.2–13.9% in those without [67,68] as well as in 24.0–85.0% of adults with CKD [69,70] and 1.0–4.5% of those without [67,71], suggesting that IDA is more frequently associated with CKD patients than general population. IDA is more prevalent in both girls and women than boys and men and in patients with advanced CKD than in those with low grade CKD [66,69]. FIDA occurs in 12.0–21.4% of ND-CKD adults [18,48] and 23.0–42.9% of HD adults [17,72] although prevalence of FIDA remains unknown in CKD children and general population. Thus, both IDA and FIDA more frequently occur as CKD advances.

IDA increases a risk of hospitalization [73] and mortality, including all-cause and cardiovascular-related mortality in ND-CKD [4,73,74] and HD adults [75,76]. Several short-term studies showed that Hb < 10 g/dL was a risk factor of mortality in ND-CKD [77] and HD adults [78,79]. The long-term studies showed that Hb levels of <10–12 g/dL [80–82] were a risk factor of mortality in HD adults. On the other hand, in HD children, Hb <12 g/dL was associated with increased risk of hospitalization and mortality [83]. These data suggest that the levels of Hb of < 12 g/dL are a risk factor of mortality in both children and adults with ND-CKD and HD. Additionally, longer time required to reach the tHb level was associated with higher risk of hospitalization and mortality in HD adults [84]. Thus, early intervention with iron therapy for IDA can improve QOL and mortality in CKD patients.

Little is known whether inflammation affects the cutoff levels of ferritin deficiency as a risk factor of mortality in CKD patients. The study from Europe reported that in HD adults, mortality rate was 13.8/100 patient-years and that serum ferritin levels of <100 ng/mL were a risk factor of cardiovascular-related mortality in HD patients with positive CRP [76]. However, the Japanese study showed that low serum ferritin levels of either <30 ng/mL or <50 ng/mL were associated with a significant risk of mortality in Japanese HD patients with normal CRP receiving IIT and ESA [8,85]. These data suggest that low levels of serum ferritin are a risk factor of mortality in CKD patients, whereas the cutoff levels of ferritin deficiency to predict mortality is lower in HD patients without than those with apparent inflammation.

In addition to low ferritin, low serum iron (<45.3 µg/dL) [86], TSAT (≤20%) [74,87,88] and TIBC [75] have been shown to be risk factors of hospitalization and mortality in ND-CKD and HD adults. IDA induces resistance to ESA [88] which aggravates renal anemia, leading to worse outcome in HD patients [89]. These data suggest that IDA is a significant risk factor of mortality in CKD patients. As discussed earlier, inflammation affects these indicators of iron status, especially the cutoff levels of serum ferritin deficiency to predict mortality in CKD patients.

5.3. Inflammation, Increased Serum Ferritin and Mortality in CKD

The management of IDA with iron supplementation is crucial for better outcome in CKD patients. However, aggressive iron therapy causes iatrogenic iron overload, leading to inflammation and increasing a risk of mortality. In support of this hypothesis, inflammation and hyperferritinemia (>500 ng/mL) were associated with cardiovascular and all-cause mortality in HD adults [90]. In addition, in dialysis children and adolescents with iron overload, ferritin levels showed a positive correlation with inflammation markers (CRP and IL-6) and left ventricular mass (LVM) [39].

It is controversial whether iron overload is associated with a risk of infection or infection-related mortality [91]. High serum ferritin has been shown to be an independent risk factor of infection-related mortality in HD patients [7,92–95]. Bolus dosing of ferric gluconate could increase a risk of infection-related mortality and hospitalization in HD patients with catheter [96]. However, no relation has been reported between ferritin and a risk of infection-related mortality in HD patients [97].

To reduce a risk of iron overload-mediated toxicity, international guidelines for the management of IDA in CKD recommend that upper limit of serum ferritin and TSAT should be maintained at <500–800 ng/mL [51–60] and <30–50% [53,55,57], respectively (Table 2). Other study groups in Europe and the US recommend that serum ferritin should be maintained at 400–600 ng/mL [98] and

200–1200 ng/mL [99] in HD patients. The percentage of US facilities with an upper ferritin target of 1200 ng/mL increased from 20% to 40% from 2010 to 2011 and more than 90% facilities had an upper ferritin target of 800 ng/mL in 2014 [100]. Upper ferritin targets of 500 ng/mL remained common in Europe and no European facility had upper ferritin targets of 1200 ng/mL in 2014. In Japan, upper ferritin targets were lower, with most facilities targeting upper limits of 300 ng/mL [100]. In this study, the data for CRP were negative in Japanese facilities although data for CRP in US facilities are not available. These guidelines and the studies described here except for those from Japan are likely to be based on the data obtained from inflamed CKD patients as suggested by other studies [15,61,62]. Thus, inflammation significantly affects upper serum ferritin targets to avoid iron overload for the management of IDA in CKD patients. In support of this hypothesis, in the setting of concomitant inflammation, serum ferritin levels of ≥500–800 ng/mL are found to be predictive of high mortality in HD patients of Europe [9,101] and Taiwan [92] and USA [95]. High CRP levels alone may predict high mortality in HD patients [62,102]. Taken together, these data suggest that iron overload as reflected by high serum ferritin and concomitant inflammation independently or synergically can increase a risk of mortality in CKD patients.

By contrast, in the absence of inflammation, even slight increase in serum ferritin (≥200 ng/mL) is associated with a risk of mortality in Japanese HD patients [85]. Thus, the cutoff levels of serum ferritin to predict iron overload and a risk of mortality are significantly lower in HD patients without than in those with apparent inflammation. Since inflammation increases ferritin independent of iron status, upper serum ferritin targets to predict iron overload and mortality may be lower than >500–800 ng/mL in HD patients with apparent inflammation. Further studies would be necessary to determine what are true levels of upper serum ferritin targets to predict iron overload in CKD patients when concomitant inflammation is present.

6. Impact of Inflammation on Therapeutic Strategy with Iron Supplementation in CKD

Iron supplementation has been used in 57.3–78.0% of dialysis children [103–105] and its use is less prevalent in those not receiving than in those receiving ESA [104,105]. Thus, iron therapy is likely to be more frequently used in severe anemic CKD children receiving ESA. There is a similar trend in CKD adults; iron therapy has been used in 48.1–56.3% of ND-CKD [4,106], 68.0% of peritoneal dialysis (PD) and 76.0–84.4% of HD adults [104,107]. The use of IIT has recently been increased to >70% of HD adults [108] and serum ferritin targets and IV iron doses have been increased in HD adults [108,109]. Maintenance IIT can improve the response to ESA with a reduction of ESA dose and early survival in ND-CKD [73] and HD adults [110]. However, Hb levels of >13 g/dL following IIT is associated with worse outcome in CKD patients [111]. Thus, the target Hb (tHb) of 10–13 g/dL is recommended for the management of IDA in CKD patients [112–114]. We herein discuss the impact of inflammation on some therapeutic issues to maintain tHb for the management of IDA in CKD patients.

6.1. Inflammation and the Response to Iron Supplementation in CKD

IIT is generally superior to OIT to improve IDA in children and adults with CKD [115,116], while some patients fail to respond to iron therapy. In support of this, Qunibi et al. showed that the tHb levels were more maintained in ND-CKD patients (60.4%) after IV ferric carboxymaltose than in those (34.7%) receiving OIT [117]. One of the reasons accounting for superiority of ITT over OIT to maintain tHb in CKD patients may be difference in the efficacy of IIT and OIT in CKD patients in the presence of concomitant inflammation that increases ferritin and hepcidin. Table 3 summarizes data regarding the impact of inflammation on the effect of OIT versus IIT for IDA in CKD patients, in whom the data for CRP are available. The efficacy of IIT is generally better than OIT for the management of IDA in inflamed ND-CKD patients with positive CRP [98,118–122]. Stoves et al. showed no significant difference in the Hb levels at the end of OIT and IIT in ND-CKD adults with positive CRP, while the levels of Hb achieved tended to be higher in the IIT group than those in the OIT group [123]. In contrast, in HD patients with normal CRP, OIT and low dose of IIT is as effective as the standard IIT [124–126]. HD adults responding to OIT showed lower CRP levels (mean, 0.8 mg/dL) compared to those in the OIT-non-responders (mean, 5.6 mg/dL) [122]. These data suggest that superiority of IIT over OIT for the management of IDA in CKD patients [115–117] is true in the presence of apparent inflammation but not under minor inflammation and that inflammation may induce hyporesponsiveness to iron therapy, especially to OIT. The HD patients with high CRP levels had lower intestinal iron absorption [127] probably due to inflammation-induced increase in ferritin and hepcidin that block iron absorption [128]. Thus, inflammation makes OIT less effective to maintain tHb in CKD patients. Due to an alteration of ferritin and hepcidin by inflammation, higher dose of IV iron may be required to maintain tHb for IDA in CKD patients with concomitant inflammation.

In support of this hypothesis, an inflammation marker CRP was inversely correlated with Hb in HD patients [129–131]. In HD patients receiving IIT and ESA, below tHb was associated with high CRP [132]. In addition, high CRP with low CHr and TSAT led to a lack of response to further increment of IV iron dose in HD patients [21]. Serum hepcidin and inflammation markers (CRP, IL-6 and TNF-α) were more increased as CKD advanced [18,133–135], in which more severe IDA occurs. Furthermore, serum hepcidin was positively correlated with inflammation markers (CRP, IL-6 and TNF-α) and ferritin but inversely correlated with TIBC, Hb, Ht and GFR [50,134,135]. In contrast, relatively low CRP (≤6.5 mg/dL) was associated with more achievement of tHb and if CRP increased by 1 mg/dL, possibility to maintain tHb was reduced by 7.5% in HD patients [136]. These data suggest that inflammation is a confounding factor for maintenance of tHb probably due to increased ferritin and hepcidin which inhibit iron absorption and efflux, leading to reduced iron bioavailability for erythropoiesis.

Other supportive findings for an impact of inflammation on the response to iron therapy come from the case of FIDA in CKD patients accompanied by inflammation [18]. Serum inflammation markers (CRP and IL-6), ferritin and hepcidin were increased in HD patients with FIDA [17,18]. Iron absorption was reduced in HD patients with FIDA, in particular in those with high CRP [127]. FIDA in HD adults could be managed by IIT [20,137] but not OIT [137]. However, the overall response rate to IIT was only 46.3% in HD adults with FIDA, while IIT produced a significant but only small increase in Hb (mean, 0.54 g/dL) [20]. In addition, in CKD patients, IIT increased serum hepcidin levels, which in turn exacerbated FIDA, requiring higher doses of IV iron to maintain tHb [128]. Taken together, these clinical observations indicate that as CKD advances, inflammation worsens and increases ferritin and hepcidin, leading to inhibition of iron absorption and efflux and subsequent hyporesponsiveness to iron therapy. As a result, higher dose of IV iron may be required for the management of IDA in CKD patients with apparent inflammation.

6.2. Does Autoimmune Disease and Inflammatory Disorders That Lead to CKD/ESRD Affect the Response to Iron Therapy?

If inflammation could induce hyporesponsiveness to iron therapy by increasing ferritin and hepcidin, question arises as to whether inflammation associated with autoimmune and inflammatory disorders coexisting or underlying CKD has similar effects. The following clinical observations may answer this question. First, IDA and FIDA frequently occur in autoimmune and inflammatory disorders such as systemic lupus erythematosus (SLE) [138], RA [139,140] and IBD [141,142]. These disorders are frequently associated with CKD, leading to ESRD [143,144]. In addition, serum levels of ferritin and inflammation markers (CRP and IL-6) were higher in patients with active than in those with inactive SLE and controls [145–147] and IL-6 inversely correlated with Hb between active and inactive SLE [147,148]. Serum ferritin was positively correlated with SLE disease activity index, anti-dsDNA, IFN-γ, IL-6, proteinuria and renal dysfunction and negatively correlated with C3, C4 and Hb [140,145–147]. Thus, inflammation increases ferritin and worsens anemia in SLE [148]. Furthermore, urine levels of hepcidin were higher in adults with lupus nephritis (LN) than in lupus patients without LN and controls [149] and in LN patients with severe renal histology compared to those with mild lesions [149,150]. The kidney biopsy specimens from LN patients revealed infiltration of interstitial leukocytes expressing hepcidin [150]. Thus, hepcidin levels increase as LN advances, leading to further inhibition of iron absorption and efflux which may worsen anemia.

As other autoimmune disease, in active RA patients, serum levels of ferritin and hepcidin were significantly higher than those in inactive patients [140] and positively correlated with CRP and negatively with Ht or Hb [140,151]. In addition, serum levels of hepcidin were increased in IBD patients with iron malabsorption and positively correlated with serum levels of ferritin and CRP [152]. Furthermore, patients with IBD having higher levels of CRP achieved a lower Hb response with OIT than those with lower levels of CRP [153]. Thus, IIT has been more efficacious than OIT in patients with RA, SLE [154,155] and IBD [142]. Taken together, these data suggest that inflammation in autoimmune disorders and IBD leading to CKD/ESRD may have an impact on the expression of ferritin and hepcidin, the response to iron therapy and mode of iron therapy as well. Future studies would be necessary to address whether inflammation in autoimmune disease and IBD coexisting or underlying CKD has similar impact on the response to iron therapy as in CKD patients.

6.3. Inflammation May Reduce Predictive Values of Ferritin and Hepcidin for the Response to Iron Therapy

It is controversial whether baseline serum ferritin is predictive of the response to iron therapy in CKD patients with concomitant inflammation. Inflammation was associated with high serum ferritin ($\geq$500 ng/mL) and conversely, this ferritin level and low TSAT (<25%) had higher odds ratio for serum CRP levels of $\geq$10 mg/dL in HD adults [156]. In addition, the levels of CRP were positively correlated with those of serum ferritin in HD patients [157] and higher levels of CRP and ferritin were associated with lower Hb levels in ESRD patients [129]. These data suggest that under concomitant inflammation, ferritin is not a predictor of the response to iron therapy. In support of this, Musanovic et al. reported that the predictive values of CRP to achieve tHb following IIT was $\leq$6.5 mg/dL and that serum ferritin levels failed to predict the response to IIT in highly inflamed HD patients with higher CRP levels [136]. In addition, in HD patients with high levels of serum ferritin (500–1200 ng/mL) and CRP (>20 mg/dL) and low TSAT (<25%), none of the iron indices (ferritin, CHr, TSAT or sTfR) was predictive of the response to IIT, while lower CRP levels of $\leq$14.0 mg/dL were predictive of the response to IIT [22]. Furthermore, in HD patients with moderately increased levels of serum ferritin (mean, 146 ng/mL) and CRP (mean, 4.1 mg/dL), %Hypo and CHr but neither ferritin nor TSAT were predictors of the response to IIT in HD patients [158]. These data suggest that the values of CRP but not ferritin may be predictive of the response to iron therapy in inflamed CKD patients.

In contrast, Macdougall et al. showed that in ND-CKD adults with relatively low CRP levels (mean, 4.5 mg/dL), the response rate to OIT was very limited (21.6%), whereas both low baseline ferritin and CRP may be predictive of the response to OIT [121]. In addition, serum ferritin levels were higher in HD patients with minor inflammation not responding to IIT than in those responding to IIT and OIT as described in our previous study [124]. Thus, basal ferritin may be predictive of the response to IIT in CKD patients with minor inflammation.

Regarding an impact of inflammation on predictive value of hepcidin for the response to iron therapy, serum hepcidin and prohepcidin were positively correlated with ferritin and CRP in HD patients [47,50,134,158]. Prohepcidin was negatively correlated with Hb and Ht in ND-CKD and dialysis patients with positive CRP and hyperferritinmia [134]. No correlation was found between hepcidin and TSAT and Hb in inflamed ND-CKD [159] and HD patients with FIDA [18]. In addition, serum levels of hepcidin failed to predict the response to IIT in adults on HD receiving ESA, in whom the levels of CRP and serum ferritin were relatively high [158] or in ND-CKD adults not receiving ESA with relatively high levels of CRP (mean, 6.7 mg/dL) [159]. The latter study also showed a correlation between hepcidin and ferritin levels at baseline and at the study endpoint, whereas an association between hepcidin and ferritin was plateaued at higher ferritin levels [159]. These data suggest that hepcidin is not a good predictor of the response to iron therapy in inflamed CKD patients.

Table 3. Impact of inflammation on the effect of intravenous and oral iron therapy for IDA in CKD patients.

Reference	Mode of Iron Therapy	Patients	Baseline Mean CRP (mg/dL)		Baseline Mean Ferritin (ng/mL)		ESA Use		Definition of Response to Iron Therapy	Response Rate or Maintained Hb Levels after Iron Therapy	
			OIT	IIT	OIT	IIT	OIT	IIT		OIT	IIT
Macdougall et al. [99,121]	OIT/IIT	ND-CKD	5.2	6.2; HFG, 6.7; LFG	57.3	56.4; HFG, 57.7; LFG	–	–	ΔHb ≥ 1 g/dL	32.1%	34.2% (LFG), 56.9% (HFG) *
Pisani et al. [118]	OIT/IIT	ND-CKD	1.2	1.3	71.4	67.7	+	+	ΔHb ≥ 0.6 g/dL	ΔHb 0.6 g/dL, 8.7%	ΔHb 1.0 g/dL, 33.7% **
Agarwal et al. [119]	OIT/IIT	ND-CKD	6.9	8.2	66.4	72.5	–	–	NA	ΔHb 0.2 g/dL	ΔHb 0.4 g/dL ***
Kalra et al. [120]	OIT/IIT	ND-CKD	8.6	9	98.8	95	–	–	NA	ΔHb 0.49 g/dL	ΔHb 0.94 g/dL *
Jenq et al. [122]	OIT/IIT	HD	4.8	12.4	181	348	+	+	ΔHt ≥ 3% from BL	12.5%	50% *
Stoves et al. [123]	OIT/IIT	ND-CKD	6	6	74	100	+	+	tHb 12 g/dL	Hb 12.2 (10.6–12.8) g/dL	Hb12.5 (11.6–13.3) g/dL
Takasawa et al. [124]	OIT	HD	0.11		29.5		+		ΔHb ≥ 2 g/dL	76.5%	
Ogawa et al. [125]	IIT	HD	0.06		50.6			+	tHb 10–11 g/dL	79.3%	
Sanai et al. [126]	OIT	HD	0.32		38		+		ΔHb ≥ 1 g/dL	100%	

BL: baseline, CKD: chronic kidney disease, CRP: C-reactive protein, ESA: erythropoiesis-stimulating agents, Hb: hemoglobin, HD: hemodialysis, Ht: hematocrit, IIT: intravenous iron therapy, ND: non-dialysis, OIT: oral iron therapy, tHb: target Hb. NA: not available. ΔHb and Ht are defined as the change in Hb and Ht before and after iron supplementation. HFG = high target ferritin group (400–600 ng/mL) receiving high dose of IIT (500–100 mg iron), LFG = low target ferritin group (100–200 ng/mL) receiving low dose of IIT (200 mg iron). * statistically significant vs. OIT. ** IIT produced a more rapid Hb increase than OIT. *** ΔHb did not differ between OIT and IIT groups but was only significant in IIT group.

Under minor inflammation, correlation between iron indicators (ferritin and TSAT) is more robust in HD patients [160]. In this condition, there was a negative association between hepcidin and Hb in ND-CKD adults with sufficient iron stores (serum ferritin ≥ 91 ng/mL) and in contrast, a positive association in those with ID (serum ferritin < 91 ng/mL) [161]. This finding suggests that under minor inflammation, the values of hepcidin to predict the response to iron therapy in CKD patients may be dependent on the levels of ferritin. In support of this hypothesis, hepcidin was positively correlated with ferritin (mean, 50.6 ng/mL) and TSAT in HD adults with minor inflammation [125]. In addition, low levels of serum hepcidin and ferritin with normal or slightly positive CRP levels were able to predict a greater response to OIT or IIT in ND-CKD [162] and HD patients [113,124]. Furthermore, lower levels of hepcidin and higher sTfR and sTfR/hepcidin ratio were predictive of the response to IIT in ND-CKD patients with relatively low CRP (mean, 3.8 mg/dL) [163]. Taken together, under minor inflammation in which correlation between hepcidin, ferritin and Hb is more robust, hepcidin may be predictive of the response to iron therapy in CKD patients, depending on ferritin levels. When concomitant inflammation is present, ferritin and hepcidin are unlikely to predict the response to iron therapy since an increase in these parameters independent of iron status may induce hyporesponsiveness to iron supplementation [128]. Thus, measurement of CRP should be part of the routine hematological assessment of HD patients to allow the correct interpretation of data and therapeutic approach for IDA in CKD patients.

7. What Are Optimal Levels of Serum Ferritin for the Management of IDA in CKD Patients with Minor Inflammation?

Optimal levels of serum ferritin during iron therapy remain to be determined in CKD patients with and without apparent inflammation. Due to a lack of data in CKD patients with apparent inflammation, we herein discuss data reported in the literature for optimal serum ferritin levels to maintain tHb during iron therapy in CKD patients with IDA and minor inflammation. Table 4 summarizes data from studies reporting optimal serum ferritin levels in ND-CKD and dialysis patients with either minor inflammation [124–126] or low serum ferritin levels (<100 ng/mL) [105,164–166]. The patients in these studies were treated with either OIT or low dose of IIT and the majority of patients simultaneously received ESA. Based on the data, OIT or very low dose of IIT is as effective as the standard IIT to improve IDA in HD patients with minor inflammation or low serum ferritin levels. Optimal ferritin levels are both low in HD patients receiving OIT (30–115 ng/mL) and in those receiving IIT (<300 ng/mL), while they were lower in the OIT group than in the IIT group. In dialysis children, serum ferritin levels of 25–50 ng/mL were associated with an achievement of highest Hb levels, although mode of iron therapy and data for CRP are not available [105]. Our previous study showed that optimal serum ferritin levels were estimated to be 30–40 ng/mL in HD patients with normal CRP and that further increment of serum ferritin was associated with increased levels of serum hepcidin and decreased Hb levels [124]. As shown in Table 4, optimal serum ferritin levels are significantly lower in HD patients with minor inflammation receiving IIT than achieved serum ferritin targets in those with apparent inflammation receiving IIT (mean serum ferritin, 340–810 ng/mL) [114,120,123,136,167] but similar to those (mean, 238.5 ng/mL) in ND-CKD patients with weakly positive CRP (mean, 1.3 mg/dL) receiving IIT [118]. Thus, concomitant inflammation increases serum ferritin targets to maintain tHb, making IIT more preferable than OIT to maintain tHb in CKD patients. Of note is that optimal levels of serum ferritin in HD patients with minor inflammation receiving OIT or low dose of IIT (Table 4) are less than the cutoff serum ferritin levels of 160 ng/mL and 290 ng/mL to predict mild and severe iron overload in HD adults with positive CRP evaluated on magnetic resonance imaging (MRI) [168]. Taken together, these data suggest that optimal levels of serum ferritin during iron therapy for the management of IDA are quite low in CKD patients with minor inflammation as compared to those with apparent inflammation. Due to a small sample size, further studies are necessary to determine optimal levels of serum ferritin for the management of IDA in CKD patients with minor inflammation.

Table 4. Optimal levels of serum ferritin during iron therapy in CKD patients with minor inflammation or lower serum ferritin levels.

Reference	Patients	Mode of Iron Therapy	Target Hb (g/dL)	ESA Dose Reduction after Iron Therapy	Mean Baseline CRP (mg/dL)	Mean Baseline Ferritin (ng/mL)	Optimal Serum Ferritin Levels after Iron Therapy (ng/mL)
Children							
van Stralen et al. [105]	PD/HD	57.3% received iron therapy †	10.5–12.5	NA	NA	122	25–50
Adults							
Takasawa et al. [124]	HD	OIT	12–13	+	0.11	29.5	30–40
Ogawa et al. [125]	HD	Low dose IIT *	10–11	NA	0.06	50.6	<90
Sanai et al. [126]	HD	OIT	10–11	+	0.32	38	67.5 ± 44.0 #
Lenga et al. [164]	HD	OIT	≥11	+	NA	72	≥100 (target)
Tsuchida et al. [165]	HD	OIT/IIT	10–11	+	NA	32.6; OIT 57.8; IIT	115.3 ± 28.1 #; OIT 183.5 ± 47.5 #; IIT
Nagaraju et al. [166]	ND–CKD	OIT **/IIT	10.5–13	+	NA	71; OIT 67; IIT	85.5 (44–104) #; OIT 244 (71.5–298) #; IIT

CKD: chronic kidney disease, CRP: C-reactive protein, ESA: erythropoiesis-stimulating agents, Hb: hemoglobin, HD: hemodialysis, IIT: intravenous iron therapy, ND: non-dialysis, OIT: oral iron therapy, PD: peritoneal dialysis. † Mode of iron therapy is unknown. * 40 mg of ferric saccharate/week for 2–6 weeks. ** Oral heme iron polypeptide. # Serum levels of ferritin achieved at the end of OIT or IIT and the data are expressed as mean ± SD. NA: not available.

8. Role of Ferritin, Hepcidin and Inflammation for the Development of Complications in CKD

Ferritin deficiency is a risk factor for increased LVM index in ND-CKD patients [169]. In HD patients, high serum levels of ferritin were associated with progressive arterial stiffness, leading to atherosclerosis, in particular when serum ferritin was >500 ng/mL [170]. Higher levels of serum ferritin induced by aggressive IIT may be a cause of increased incidence of atherosclerosis in HD patients [171]. In dialysis children and adolescents with iron overload, ferritin levels showed a positive correlation with CRP, IL-6 and LVM [39]. On the other hand, decreased levels of serum hepcidin were associated with a higher LVM index in ND-CKD patients [172]. However, serum hepcidin levels were increased and positively correlated with brachial-ankle pulse wave velocity as the measurement of arterial stiffness in HD adults [173]. Similarly, carotid artery intima media thickness was positively correlated with serum hepcidin and CRP in diabetic HD patients, in whom hepcidin positively correlated with ferritin and inflammation markers (CRP, TNF-α and IL-6) [174]. Despite no relation between hepcidin, CRP, IL-6 and LVM [175], increased levels of serum hepcidin were associated with fatal and non-fatal cardiovascular events and inflammation was a significant confounder in the relation between hepcidin and all-cause mortality in HD patients [176]. These data suggest that both low and high levels of ferritin and hepcidin may be risk factors for the development of complications associated with CKD.

9. Safety Issues of Iron Therapy

9.1. Which is First Either OIT or IIT?

The French National Agency for the Safety of Medicines and Health Product (ANSM, Saint-Denis, France), Canadian guidelines and other investigators recommend that it is appropriate to use OIT in first intention due to its lower toxicity, regardless of ND-CKD or HD patients [52,126,177,178]. Several international guidelines also recommend that OIT should be administered first in ND-CKD patients [52,58,59], while other guidelines recommend that IIT be firstly used in HD patients [51,54,55,58,59]. Our previous study demonstrated that low dose of IIT could be a second line of iron supplementation for the management of IDA in HD patients with minor inflammation who failed to respond to OIT [124]. In support of our finding, IIT with ferrous saccharated (300–800 mg bolus once a month followed by 50 mg weekly for 3 months) was beneficial in 13 (76.4%) of the 17 HD patients with IDA who failed to maintain the tHb (10–11 g/dL) following OIT and ESA [179]. Total doses of IIT in our protocol [124] are lower than the low maintenance dose of IIT (iron gluconate 31.25 mg/week over 1 year) which could not prevent a risk of iron overload in HD patients [180] and far less than <250 mg of iron/month to avoid iron overload evaluated on MRI [181]. In our view, OIT should be first administered in CKD patients, in particular in those with minor inflammation, and be switched to IIT when patients fail to respond to OIT or severe adverse effects of OIT are present.

9.2. Adverse Effects of OIT and IIT

While oral iron is safer than IV iron, it is associated with reduced treatment adherence, due to gastrointestinal side effects [182,183]. The short-term studies reported no significant difference in prevalence of acute adverse effects between IIT and OIT in CKD patients [115,116]. However, IIT is more frequently associated with serious adverse events than OIT in ND-CKD patients [184]. IV iron, especially with high weekly doses, significantly increased a risk of infection and hospitalization and promoted oxidant stress, cardiovascular events and all-cause mortality in CKD patients [7,182,184–186]. Infection-related mortality was high in HD adults receiving IV iron dose of >1050 mg in 3 months or >2100 mg in 6 months [187]. Thus, the Kidney Disease Improving Global Outcomes (KDIGO) guidelines recommend not administering IIT during active infection [54]. Similarly, atherosclerotic change was correlated with serum levels of ferritin and doses of IV iron in HD patients [188]. OIT improved anemia in ND-CKD patients without affecting renal function [189], while IV iron sucrose increased proteinuria in ND-CKD patients, indicating that high doses of IV iron may aggravate kidney injury [190]. Repeated administration of IV iron in HD patients increased oxidative DNA injury and serum ferritin, suggesting that excess body iron stores caused by aggressive IIT might promote oxidative stress [191].

9.3. Iron Overload in CKD

Serum levels of ferritin are generally higher in HD patients receiving IIT compared to those receiving OIT [120,192]. In recent years, there is a trend for decreasing the use of ESA and increasing the use of IIT for CKD patients in the US [109]. Like CRP [15,62], serum ferritin levels and the doses of IV iron used were generally higher in HD patients of Western countries than in those of Japan [193,194]. Serum ferritin levels were increased in HD patients of Canada, Europe and the US from 1997 to 2011, compared to those of Japan [195]. Karaboyas et al. recently reported that during 2009–2015, median ferritin levels in HD adults were 718 ng/mL in the US, 405 ng/mL in Europe and 83 ng/mL in Japan [100]. In addition, mean serum ferritin levels of HD patients in the US in 2013 exceeded 800 ng/mL, with 18% of the patients exceeding ferritin of 1200 ng/mL [109]. Kalantar-Zadeh et al. defined iron overload as serum ferritin levels of >2000 ng/mL since serum ferritin may be increased up to 2000 ng/mL due to non-iron-related factors, including malnutrition-inflammation complex syndrome [40]. However, no clear evidence for iron overload was presented in this study.

Recently, several approaches using imaging for the quantification of liver iron concentration have been used to detect iron overload in CKD patients. Using superconducting quantum interference device for direct noninvasive magnetic measurements of non-heme hepatic iron content, 32.5% and 37.5% of HD patients had mild (liver iron content; LIC 400 to 1000 µg/g liver tissue) and severe iron overload (LIC > 1000 µg/g liver tissue), while 70% of these patients had serum ferritin levels of <500 ng/mL [196]. In this study, the best specificity/sensitivity ratio for serum ferritin to identify iron overload was proposed as >340 ng/mL [196]. Ghoti et al. showed that iron overload in the liver was detected using MRI in HD patients with serum ferritin levels of >1000 ng/mL receiving IIT [197]. However, Rostoker et al. using MRI showed that in HD adults with positive CRP, cutoff levels of serum ferritin were 160 ng/mL for mild (LIC > 50 µmol/g liver tissue) and 290 ng/mL for severe iron overload (LIC > 200 µmol/g liver tissue) [168]. Despite the presence of inflammation, these cutoff levels of serum ferritin to detect iron overload using MRI are significantly lower than upper limit of serum ferritin to avoid iron overload proposed by international guidelines (Table 2) [51–60]. The same research group using MRI recommended that the maximum amount of IV iron should be lowered to 250 mg/month to avoid iron overload [181]. In support of this recommendation, Bailie et al. reported that mortality was significantly higher in HD adults receiving IV iron dose of >300 mg/month than those receiving iron dose of <299 mg/month [186]. Thus, it remains to be determined whether international guidelines for the use of IV iron are safe enough to avoid a risk of iron overload [198].

To answer this question, accurate, noninvasive, rapid and inexpensive methods for evaluation of iron overload would be mandatory. In our view, international guidelines for upper limit of serum ferritin to avoid a risk of iron overload in CKD patients may need a revision according to the presence or absence of inflammation. Vaziri stated in his review [182] that compared with Western countries, the JSDT guidelines [53] for iron therapy in dialysis patients are far more conservative, while outcomes of the Japanese dialysis patients are as good as or better than those in American counterparts and that an approach with more conservative iron therapy should be considered. Efforts should be directed towards lowering serum ferritin targets to avoid the long-term adverse effects of iron overload-mediated toxicity especially in CKD patients with apparent inflammation.

9.4. Safer Treatment with Iron and Non-Iron Agents for the Management of IDA in CKD

There are a number of oral iron salts including ferrous sulphate, ferrous fumarate and ferrous gluconate, of which ferrous sulphate has been most frequently used in ND-CKD patients [183]. Recently, several oral iron agents have been used to reduce adverse effects for the management of IDA in CKD patients. Oral liposomal iron, a preparation of ferric pyrophosphate conveyed within a phospholipid membrane associated with ascorbic acid, is well absorbed from the gut and demonstrates high bioavailability with low side effects [118]. It is a safe and efficacious alternative to IV iron gluconate for the management of IDA in ND-CKD patients [118]. Oral heme iron polypeptide, a compound that uses the heme porphyrin ring to supply iron, can increase iron store and has similar efficacy to IV iron sucrose in ND-CKD [166] and HD patients [199]. As a new agent, low dose of oral ferric citrate, a compound comprising trivalent iron with citrate that functions as a phosphate binder, has been shown to improve IDA without inducing iron overload in hyperphosphatemic HD patients [200].

To avoid potential serious adverse effects of IIT, safer regimens with low dose of IV iron have been used for the management of IDA in CKD patients. Maintenance IV iron regimen in smaller doses at frequent intervals has been more efficacious and safer than large intermittent doses [201]. Continuous low dose of IV iron sucrose was more effective in maintaining tHb compared to the regimen with bolus high dose of IV iron in HD patients [202]. Low dose of iron sucrose (20 mg) at the end of every HD session was effective to maintain functional iron levels and ESA dose, thereby reducing iron overload in HD patients without serious adverse effects [203]. Weekly low dose (50 mg) of IV iron sucrose for 6 months maintained tHb and reduced the ESA dose without induction of high serum ferritin levels in HD patients [204]. In addition, low dose of IV ferric carboxymaltose appeared to be safe for the management of IDA in ND-CKD patients [98]. The efficacy and safety of IV ferumoxytol was comparable to IV iron sucrose in patients with varying degrees of renal function [205]. Intravenous low-molecular-weight iron dextran for 12 months was effective even in iron-pretreated HD patients [206]. Furthermore, ferric pyrophosphate citrate, a water-soluble iron salt administered via dialysate at a dose of 2 μmol/L (110 mg/L of Fe^{3+}) to supply ∼5–7 mg of iron during the course of each dialysis session, was able to decrease the amount of IV iron needed for maintenance of tHb with a reduction of the ESA dose in HD patients [207].

As alternative treatment, non-iron agents that can inhibit hepcidin have recently been used for the management of IDA in CKD patients. Pentoxifylline, a methylxanthine derivative, inhibited phosphodiesterase, resulting in increased intracellular cyclic AMP, activation of protein kinase A and inhibition of IL and TNF synthesis as well as inflammation. Pentoxifylline reduced expression of IL-6 and ferritin and increased Hb and TSAT possibly through modulation of hepcidin in ND-CKD adults [208].

As other agents, an oral hypoxia-inducible factor (HIF)-prolyl hydroxylases (PHD) inhibitor—vadadustat (AKB-6548, Akebia Therapeutics Inc, Cambridge, MA, USA)—has been shown to increase Hb, mean absolute reticulocyte count and TIBC and reduced hepcidin and ferritin by stabilizing HIF in iron-replete ND-CKD patients receiving a minimum dose of OIT with or without ESA [209,210]. Roxadustat (FG-4592, FibroGen, San Francisco, CA, USA), other oral HIF-PHD inhibitor, decreased hepcidin, ferritin and TSAT and increased Hb and TIBC in iron-replete ND-CKD patients not receiving IIT and ESA [211]. Regardless of CRP and iron repletion, roxadustat increased Hb and decreased hepcidin in HD patients [212]. In this study, an increase in Hb was greater in HD patients receiving OIT or IIT than in those not receiving iron, while TSAT and CHr were decreased in the patients with no iron but unchanged in those receiving OIT or IIT. In addition, serum ferritin levels did not change in HD patients receiving OIT or IIT but decreased in those not receiving iron. Roxadustat can be used even in the presence of inflammation and leads to sufficiency of low-dose oral iron for anemia correction in CKD patients [212]. Other oral HIF-PHD inhibitor, daprodustat (GSK127886, GlaxoSmithKline, Philadelphia, PA, USA), decreased hepcidin, ferritin, serum iron and TSAT and increased Hb, total reticulocyte counts, TIBC and unsaturated iron-binding capacity in ND-CKD and dialysis patients [213]. In addition, HIF-PHD inhibitors can reduce iron dose to maintain tHb in HD patients and minimize iatrogenic iron overload from IV iron [212]. These non-iron agents can increase iron availability for effective erythropoiesis by decreasing ferritin and hepcidin and this effect is not affected by inflammation. Thus, they have a benefit for the management of IDA/FIDA even in CKD patients with apparent inflammation.

10. Minimizing a Risk of Inflammation as Therapeutic Strategy for IDA in CKD

Minimization of a risk of inflammation may reduce the required dose of iron therapy in HD patients [21]. Correctible causes of inflammation in CKD include tunneled dialysis catheters, AV grafts, catheter infection, periodontal disease, poor water quality and dialyzer incompatibility [62,214]. Ultrapure dialysate reduced serum levels of CRP and ferritin and improved iron utilization in HD patients [215]. Thus, OIT was as effective as IIT for the management of IDA in HD patients using ultrapure dialysate [165]. HD patients with catheters and AV grafts were associated with high inflammation markers and required a higher dose of ESA as compared to those with AV fistulae [21]. Obesity is frequently associated with IDA and inflammation in CKD patients [216,217]. Despite IDA, obesity increases the expression of hepcidin due to inflammation-induced hepcidin synthesis by adipose tissues [216]. Obese CKD patients frequently developed hyporesponsiveness to OIT due to increased hepcidin [217]. Therapeutic strategy for the management of IDA should include minimization of these risk factors of inflammation in CKD patients.

11. Conclusions

IDA induces resistance to ESA, poor QOL and increased mortality in CKD patients. Inflammation highly associated with CKD increases ferritin and hepcidin, which block iron absorption and efflux, leading to reduced iron availability for erythropoiesis and subsequent hyporesponsiveness to iron therapy and ESA. In the absence of inflammation, correlation between ferritin and hepcidin is robust to predict iron status and responsiveness to iron therapy. Diagnosis of IDA, criteria for initiation of iron therapy and upper limit of ferritin to predict iron overload are different among international guidelines for the management of IDA in CKD patients. Inflammation-mediated increase in ferritin and hepcidin independent of iron status affect these issues and reduces the predictive values of ferritin and hepcidin for the response to iron therapy. IIT has been considered to be superior to OIT for the management of IDA in CKD patients. While this may be true in the presence of apparent inflammation, OIT is as effective as IIT under minor inflammation. Many short-term studies show that aggressive IIT in CKD patients, especially in those with high inflammation, has been considered safe based on appearance of iron overload symptoms. Thus, iron overload can silently progress, leading to a risk of mortality in CKD patients. Currently, there is no evidence for how much iron is accumulated in the tissues and the long-term adverse effects of aggressive IIT including mortality in CKD patients. Upper limit of serum ferritin to predict iron overload using MRI is far less than that proposed by international guidelines for IDA in CKD patients. Accurate, non-invasive and rapid methods to detect iron overload other than MRI need to be established. Alteration of iron status such as IDA and iatrogenic iron overload and of expression of ferritin and hepcidin as well as inflammation may affect the development of complications and mortality in CKD patients. The management of IDA in CKD patients should differ, depending on the absence or presence of inflammation and include minimization of a risk of inflammation. Future well-powered studies using a large number of CKD patients with or without inflammation would be necessary to address the impact of inflammation on therapeutic strategies for the management of IDA in CKD patients.

Author Contributions: N.U. wrote the first draft of the manuscript. K.T. contributed to the process of writing the first draft of the manuscript. All authors were involved in critically revising the manuscript, read and approved the final manuscript.

Acknowledgments: The authors are grateful to Maiko Ueda for her critical reading of this manuscript. This study has been supported by The Kidney Foundation, Japan (JKFB09-55).

Conflicts of Interest: The authors declare no conflict of interest.

Abbreviations

AV	arteriovenous
BMP	bone morphogenetic protein
BMPR	BMP receptor
C/EBP	CCAAT enhancer-binding protein
CHr	content of hemoglobin in reticulocytes
CKD	chronic kidney disease
CP	ceruloplasmin
CREBH	cyclic-AMP-responsive-element-binding protein H
CRP	C-reactive protein
DCYTB	duodenal cytochrome b
DMT1	divalent metal transporter1
EPO	erythropoietin
ESA	erythropoiesis-stimulating agents
ESRD	end-stage renal disease
FIDA	functional IDA
FPN	ferroportin
FtH	heavy chain of ferritin
FtL	light chain of ferritin
GDF15	growth differentiation factor 15
GFR	glomerular filtration rate
Hb	hemoglobin
HD	hemodialysis
HIF	hypoxia-inducible factor
HO-1	heme oxygenase-1
HFE	hereditary hemochromatosis protein
HIF	hypoxia-inducible factor
Ht	hematocrit
IBD	inflammatory bowel disease
IDA	iron deficiency anemia
IIT	intravenous iron therapy
IL	interleukin
INF	interferon
IRE	iron responsive element
IRP	iron regulatory protein
JAK	Janus kinase
LN	lupus nephritis
LPS	lipopolysaccharide
LVM	left ventricular mass
mHJV	membrane-anchored hemojuvelin
MRI	magnetic resonance imaging
MT-2	matriptase-2
ND	non-dialysis
NF	nuclear factor
NO	nitric oxide
OIT	oral iron therapy
%Hypo	percentage of hypochromic red cells
PD	peritoneal dialysis
PHD	prolyl hydroxylase
PGC-1α	peroxisome proliferator-activated receptor γ coactivator-1α
QOL	quality of life
RA	rheumatoid arthritis
sHJV	soluble HJV

SLE	systemic lupus erythematosus
SMAD	small mothers against decapentaplegic proteins
STAT	signal transducers and activators of transcription
sTfR	soluble transferrin receptor
Tf	transferrin
tHb	target Hb
TIBC	total iron binding capacity
TNF	tumor necrosis factor
TSAT	Tf saturation

References

1. Lopez, A.; Cacoub, P.; Macdougall, I.C.; Peyrin-Biroulet, L. Iron deficiency anaemia. *Lancet* **2016**, *387*, 907–916. [CrossRef]
2. Levi, M.; Rosselli, M.; Simonetti, M.; Brignoli, O.; Cancian, M.; Masotti, A.; Pegoraro, V.; Cataldo, N.; Heiman, F.; Chelo, M.; et al. Epidemiology of iron deficiency anaemia in four European countries: A population-based study in primary care. *Eur. J. Haematol.* **2016**, *97*, 583–593. [CrossRef] [PubMed]
3. Atkinson, M.A.; Furth, S.L. Anemia in children with chronic kidney disease. *Nat. Rev. Nephrol.* **2011**, *7*, 635–641. [CrossRef] [PubMed]
4. Iimori, S.; Naito, S.; Noda, Y.; Nishida, H.; Kihira, H.; Yui, N.; Okado, T.; Sasaki, S.; Uchida, S.; Rai, T. Anaemia management and mortality risk in newly visiting patients with chronic kidney disease in Japan: The CKD-ROUTE study. *Nephrology (Carlton)* **2015**, *20*, 601–608. [CrossRef] [PubMed]
5. Geissler, C.; Singh, M. Iron, meat and health. *Nutrients* **2011**, *3*, 283–316. [CrossRef] [PubMed]
6. Torti, F.M.; Torti, S.V. Regulation of ferritin genes and protein. *Blood* **2002**, *99*, 3505–3516. [CrossRef] [PubMed]
7. Kuragano, T.; Matsumura, O.; Matsuda, A.; Hara, T.; Kiyomoto, H.; Murata, T.; Kitamura, K.; Fujimoto, S.; Hase, H.; Joki, N.; et al. Association between hemoglobin variability, serum ferritin levels, and adverse events/mortality in maintenance hemodialysis patients. *Kidney Int.* **2014**, *86*, 845–854. [CrossRef] [PubMed]
8. Ogawa, C.; Tsuchiya, K.; Kanda, F.; Maeda, T. Low levels of serum ferritin lead to adequate hemoglobin levels and good survival in hemodialysis patients. *Am. J. Nephrol.* **2014**, *40*, 561–570. [CrossRef] [PubMed]
9. Zitt, E.; Sturm, G.; Kronenberg, F.; Neyer, U.; Knoll, F.; Lhotta, K.; Weiss, G. Iron supplementation and mortality in incident dialysis patients: An observational study. *PLoS ONE* **2014**, *9*, e114144. [CrossRef] [PubMed]
10. Hentze, M.W.; Muckenthaler, M.U.; Galy, B.; Camaschella, C. Two to tango: Regulation of mammalian iron metabolism. *Cell* **2010**, *142*, 24–38. [CrossRef] [PubMed]
11. Ganz, T. Systemic iron homeostasis. *Physiol. Rev.* **2013**, *93*, 1721–1741. [CrossRef] [PubMed]
12. Ueda, N.; Takasawa, K. Role of hepcidin-25 in chronic kidney disease: Anemia and beyond. *Curr. Med. Chem.* **2017**, *24*, 1417–1452. [CrossRef] [PubMed]
13. Antonelli, M.; Kushner, I. It's time to redefine inflammation. *FASEB J.* **2017**, *31*, 1787–1791. [CrossRef] [PubMed]
14. Suchdev, P.S.; Williams, A.M.; Mei, Z.; Flores-Ayala, R.; Pasricha, S.R.; Rogers, L.M.; Namaste, S.M. Assessment of iron status in settings of inflammation: Challenges and potential approaches. *Am. J. Clin. Nutr.* **2017**, *106* (Suppl. 6), 1626S–1633S. [CrossRef]
15. Kawaguchi, T.; Tong, L.; Robinson, B.M.; Sen, A.; Fukuhara, S.; Kurokawa, K.; Canaud, B.; Lameire, N.; Port, F.K.; Pisoni, R.L. C-reactive protein and mortality in hemodialysis patients: The Dialysis Outcomes and Practice Patterns Study (DOPPS). *Nephron Clin. Pract.* **2011**, *117*, c167–c178. [CrossRef] [PubMed]
16. Jairam, A.; Das, R.; Aggarwal, P.K.; Kohli, H.S.; Gupta, K.L.; Sakhuja, V.; Jha, V. Iron status, inflammation and hepcidin in ESRD patients: The confounding role of intravenous iron therapy. *Indian J. Nephrol.* **2010**, *20*, 125–131. [PubMed]
17. Małyszko, J.; Koc-Żórawska, E.; Levin-Iaina, N.; Małyszko, J.; Koźmiński, P.; Kobus, G.; Myśliwiec, M. New parameters in iron metabolism and functional iron deficiency in patients on maintenance hemodialysis. *Pol. Arch. Med. Wewn.* **2012**, *122*, 537–542. [CrossRef] [PubMed]

18. Łukaszyk, E.; Łukaszyk, M.; Koc-Żórawska, E.; Tobolczyk, J.; Bodzenta-Łukaszyk, A.; Małyszko, J. Iron status and inflammation in early stages of chronic kidney disease. *Kidney Blood Press. Res.* **2015**, *40*, 366–373. [CrossRef] [PubMed]

19. Gangat, N.; Wolanskyj, A.P. Anemia of chronic disease. *Semin. Hematol.* **2013**, *50*, 232–238. [CrossRef] [PubMed]

20. Susantitaphong, P.; Alqahtani, F.; Jaber, B.L. Efficacy and safety of intravenous iron therapy for functional iron deficiency anemia in hemodialysis patients: A meta-analysis. *Am. J. Nephrol.* **2014**, *39*, 130–141. [CrossRef] [PubMed]

21. El-Khatib, M.; Duncan, H.J.; Kant, K.S. Role of C-reactive protein, reticulocyte haemoglobin content and inflammatory markers in iron and erythropoietin administration in dialysis patients. *Nephrology (Carlton)* **2006**, *11*, 400–404. [CrossRef] [PubMed]

22. Singh, A.K.; Coyne, D.W.; Shapiro, W.; Rizkala, A.R.; DRIVE Study Group. Predictors of the response to treatment in anemic hemodialysis patients with high serum ferritin and low transferrin saturation. *Kidney Int.* **2007**, *71*, 1163–1171. [CrossRef] [PubMed]

23. Malyszko, J.; Malyszko, J.S.; Mysliwiec, M. Hyporesponsiveness to erythropoietin therapy in hemodialyzed patients: Potential role of prohepcidin, hepcidin, and inflammation. *Ren. Fail.* **2009**, *31*, 544–548. [CrossRef] [PubMed]

24. Naz, N.; Moriconi, F.; Ahmad, S.; Amanzada, A.; Khan, S.; Mihm, S.; Ramadori, G.; Malik, I.A. Ferritin L is the sole serum ferritin constituent and a positive hepatic acute-phase protein. *Shock* **2013**, *39*, 520–526. [CrossRef] [PubMed]

25. Pham, C.G.; Bubici, C.; Zazzeroni, F.; Papa, S.; Jones, J.; Alvarez, K.; Jayawardena, S.; De Smaele, E.; Cong, R.; Beaumont, C.; et al. Ferritin heavy chain upregulation by NF-kB inhibits TNFα-induced apoptosis by suppressing reactive oxygen species. *Cell* **2004**, *119*, 529–542. [CrossRef] [PubMed]

26. Recalcati, S.; Taramelli, D.; Conte, D.; Cairo, G. Nitric oxide-mediated induction of ferritin synthesis in J774 macrophages by inflammatory cytokines: Role of selective iron regulatory protein-2 downregulation. *Blood* **1998**, *91*, 1059–1066. [PubMed]

27. Nakanishi, T.; Kuragano, T.; Nanami, M.; Otaki, Y.; Nonoguchi, H.; Hasuike, Y. Importance of ferritin for optimizing anemia therapy in chronic kidney disease. *Am. J. Nephrol.* **2010**, *32*, 439–446. [CrossRef] [PubMed]

28. Zhao, N.; Zhang, A.S.; Enns, C.A. Iron regulation by hepcidin. *J. Clin. Investig.* **2013**, *123*, 2337–2343. [CrossRef] [PubMed]

29. Zhao, N.; Maxson, J.E.; Zhang, R.H.; Wahedi, M.; Enns, C.A.; Zhang, A.S. Neogenin facilitates the induction of hepcidin expression by hemojuvelin in the liver. *J. Biol. Chem.* **2016**, *291*, 12322–12335. [CrossRef] [PubMed]

30. Zhao, N.; Nizzi, C.P.; Anderson, S.A.; Wang, J.; Ueno, A.; Tsukamoto, H.; Eisenstein, R.S.; Enns, C.A.; Zhang, A.S. Low intracellular iron increases the stability of matriptase-2. *J. Biol. Chem.* **2015**, *290*, 4432–4446. [CrossRef] [PubMed]

31. Silvestri, L.; Pagani, A.; Camaschella, C. Furin-mediated release of soluble hemojuvelin: A new link between hypoxia and iron homeostasis. *Blood* **2008**, *111*, 924–931. [CrossRef] [PubMed]

32. Wichaiyo, S.; Yatmark, P.; Morales Vargas, R.E.; Sanvarinda, P.; Svasti, S.; Fucharoen, S.; Morales, N.P. Effect of iron overload on furin expression in wild-type and β-thalassemic mice. *Toxicol. Rep.* **2015**, *2*, 415–422. [CrossRef] [PubMed]

33. Canali, S.; Vecchi, C.; Garuti, C.; Montosi, G.; Babitt, J.L.; Pietrangelo, A. The SMAD pathway is required for hepcidin response during endoplasmic reticulum stress. *Endocrinology* **2016**, *157*, 3935–3945. [CrossRef] [PubMed]

34. Shin, D.Y.; Chung, J.; Joe, Y.; Pae, H.O.; Chang, K.C.; Cho, G.J.; Ryter, S.W.; Chung, H.T. Pretreatment with CO-releasing molecules suppresses hepcidin expression during inflammation and endoplasmic reticulum stress through inhibition of the STAT3 and CREBH pathways. *Blood* **2012**, *119*, 2523–2532. [CrossRef] [PubMed]

35. Vecchi, C.; Montosi, G.; Zhang, K.; Lamberti, I.; Duncan, S.A.; Kaufman, R.J.; Pietrangelo, A. ER stress controls iron metabolism through induction of hepcidin. *Science* **2009**, *325*, 877–880. [CrossRef] [PubMed]

36. Meynard, D.; Sun, C.C.; Wu, Q.; Chen, W.; Chen, S.; Nelson, C.N.; Waters, M.J.; Babitt, J.L.; Lin, H.Y. Inflammation regulates TMPRSS6 expression via STAT5. *PLoS ONE* **2013**, *8*, e82127. [CrossRef] [PubMed]

37. Qian, J.; Chen, S.; Huang, Y.; Shi, X.; Liu, C. PGC-1α regulates hepatic hepcidin expression and iron homeostasis in response to inflammation. *Mol. Endocrinol.* **2013**, *27*, 683–692. [CrossRef] [PubMed]

38. Kanamori, Y.; Murakami, M.; Sugiyama, M.; Hashimoto, O.; Matsui, T.; Funaba, M. Interleukin-1β (IL-1β) transcriptionally activates hepcidin by inducing CCAAT enhancer-binding protein δ (C/EBPδ) expression in hepatocytes. *J. Biol. Chem.* **2017**, *292*, 10275–10287. [CrossRef] [PubMed]

39. Ruiz-Jaramillo Mde, L.; Guízar-Mendoza, J.M.; Amador-Licona, N.; Gutiérrez-Navarro Mde, J.; Hernández-González, M.A.; Dubey-Ortega, L.A.; Solorio-Meza, S.E. Iron overload as cardiovascular risk factor in children and adolescents with renal disease. *Nephrol. Dial. Transplant.* **2011**, *26*, 3268–3273. [CrossRef] [PubMed]

40. Kalantar-Zadeh, K.; Rodriguez, R.A.; Humphreys, M.H. Association between serum ferritin and measures of inflammation, nutrition and iron in haemodialysis patients. *Nephrol. Dial. Transplant.* **2004**, *19*, 141–149. [CrossRef] [PubMed]

41. Hayes, W. Measurement of iron status in chronic kidney disease. *Pediatr. Nephrol.* **2018**. [CrossRef] [PubMed]

42. Kemna, E.; Pickkers, P.; Nemeth, E.; van der Hoeven, H.; Swinkels, D. Time-course analysis of hepcidin, serum iron, and plasma cytokine levels in humans injected with LPS. *Blood* **2005**, *106*, 1864–1866. [CrossRef] [PubMed]

43. Formanowicz, D.; Formanowicz, P. Transferrin changes in haemodialysed patients. *Int. Urol. Nephrol.* **2012**, *44*, 907–919. [CrossRef] [PubMed]

44. Gaweda, A.E. Markers of iron status in chronic kidney disease. *Hemodial. Int.* **2017**, *21* (Suppl. 1), S21–S27. [CrossRef]

45. Hackeng, C.M.; Beerenhout, C.M.; Hermans, M.; Van der Kuy, P.H.; Van der Dussen, H.; Van Dieijen-Visser, M.P.; Hamulyák, K.; Van der Sande, F.M.; Leunissen, K.M.; Kooman, J.P. The relationship between reticulocyte hemoglobin content with C-reactive protein and conventional iron parameters in dialysis patients. *J. Nephrol.* **2004**, *17*, 107–111. [PubMed]

46. Bovy, C.; Tsobo, C.; Crapanzano, L.; Rorive, G.; Beguin, Y.; Albert, A.; Paulus, J.M. Factors determining the percentage of hypochromic red blood cells in hemodialysis patients. *Kidney Int.* **1999**, *56*, 1113–1119. [CrossRef] [PubMed]

47. Zaritsky, J.; Young, B.; Wang, H.J.; Westerman, M.; Olbina, G.; Nemeth, E.; Ganz, T.; Rivera, S.; Nissenson, A.R.; Salusky, I.B. Hepcidin—A potential novel biomarker for iron status in chronic kidney disease. *Clin. J. Am. Soc. Nephrol.* **2009**, *4*, 1051–1056. [CrossRef] [PubMed]

48. Mercadal, L.; Metzger, M.; Haymann, J.P.; Thervet, E.; Boffa, J.J.; Flamant, M.; Vrtovsnik, F.; Houillier, P.; Froissart, M.; Stengel, B.; et al. The relation of hepcidin to iron disorders, inflammation and hemoglobin in chronic kidney disease. *PLoS ONE* **2014**, *9*, e99781. [CrossRef] [PubMed]

49. Zaritsky, J.; Young, B.; Gales, B.; Wang, H.J.; Rastogi, A.; Westerman, M.; Nemeth, E.; Ganz, T.; Salusky, I.B. Reduction of serum hepcidin by hemodialysis in pediatric and adult patients. *Clin. J. Am. Soc. Nephrol.* **2010**, *5*, 1010–1014. [CrossRef] [PubMed]

50. Ford, B.A.; Eby, C.S.; Scott, M.G.; Coyne, D.W. Intra-individual variability in serum hepcidin precludes its use as a marker of iron status in hemodialysis patients. *Kidney Int.* **2010**, *78*, 769–773. [CrossRef] [PubMed]

51. National Kidney Foundation. KDOQI Clinical practice guidelines and clinical practice recommendations for anemia in chronic kidney disease. *Am. J. Kidney Dis.* **2006**, *47* (5 Suppl. 3), S11–S145.

52. Madore, F.; White, C.T.; Foley, R.N.; Barrett, B.J.; Moist, L.M.; Klarenbach, S.W.; Culleton, B.F.; Tonelli, M.; Manns, B.J.; Canadian Society of Nephrology. Clinical practice guidelines for assessment and management of iron deficiency. *Kidney Int. Suppl.* **2008**, *110*, S7–S11. [CrossRef] [PubMed]

53. Tsubakihara, Y.; Nishi, S.; Akiba, T.; Hirakata, H.; Iseki, K.; Kubota, M.; Kuriyama, S.; Komatsu, Y.; Suzuki, M.; Nakai, S.; et al. 2008 Japanese Society for Dialysis Therapy: Guidelines for renal anemia in chronic kidney disease. *Ther. Apher. Dial.* **2010**, *14*, 240–275. [CrossRef] [PubMed]

54. The Kidney Disease: Improving Global Outcomes (KDIGO) Anemia Work Group. KDIGO clinical practice guideline for anemia in chronic kidney disease. *Kidney Int. Suppl.* **2012**, *2*, 279–335.

55. Locatelli, F.; Bárány, P.; Covic, A.; De Francisco, A.; Del Vecchio, L.; Goldsmith, D.; Hörl, W.; London, G.; Vanholder, R.; Van Biesen, W.; et al. Kidney disease: Improving global outcomes guidelines on anaemia management in chronic kidney disease: A European Renal Best Practice position statement. *Nephrol. Dial. Transplant.* **2013**, *28*, 1346–1359. [CrossRef] [PubMed]

56. Macginley, R.; Walker, R.; Irving, M. KHA-CARI Guideline: Use of iron in chronic kidney disease patients. *Nephrology (Carlton)* **2013**, *18*, 747–749. [CrossRef] [PubMed]

57. Hung, S.C.; Kuo, K.L.; Tarng, D.C.; Hsu, C.C.; Wu, M.S.; Huang, T.P. Anaemia management in patients with chronic kidney disease: Taiwan practice guidelines. *Nephrology (Carlton)* **2014**, *19*, 735–739. [CrossRef] [PubMed]

58. National Clinical Guideline Centre (UK). Anaemia Management in Chronic Kidney Disease: Partial Update 2015. In *National Institute for Health and Care Excellence (NICE): Clinical Guideline*; Loyal College of Physicians: London, UK, 2015.

59. Ratcliffe, L.E.; Thomas, W.; Glen, J.; Padhi, S.; Pordes, B.A.; Wonderling, D.; Connell, R.; Stephens, S.; Mikhail, A.I.; Fogarty, D.G.; et al. Diagnosis and management of iron deficiency in CKD: A summary of the NICE Guideline Recommendations and Their Rationale. *Am. J. Kidney Dis.* **2016**, *67*, 548–558. [CrossRef] [PubMed]

60. Mikhail, A.; Brown, C.; Williams, J.A.; Mathrani, V.; Shrivastava, R.; Evans, J.; Isaac, H.; Bhandari, S. Renal association clinical practice guideline on anaemia of chronic kidney disease. *BMC Nephrol.* **2017**, *18*, 345. [CrossRef] [PubMed]

61. Hamano, T.; Fujii, N.; Hayashi, T.; Yamamoto, H.; Iseki, K.; Tsubakihara, Y. Thresholds of iron markers for iron deficiency erythropoiesis-finding of the Japanese nationwide dialysis registry. *Kidney Int. Suppl.* **2015**, *5*, 23–32. [CrossRef] [PubMed]

62. Bazeley, J.; Bieber, B.; Li, Y.; Morgenstern, H.; de Sequera, P.; Combe, C.; Yamamoto, H.; Gallagher, M.; Port, F.K.; Robinson, B.M. C-reactive protein and prediction of 1-year mortality in prevalent hemodialysis patients. *Clin. J. Am. Soc. Nephrol.* **2011**, *6*, 2452–2461. [CrossRef] [PubMed]

63. Ethier, J.; Mendelssohn, D.C.; Elder, S.J.; Hasegawa, T.; Akizawa, T.; Akiba, T.; Canaud, B.J.; Pisoni, R.L. Vascular access use and outcomes: An international perspective from the Dialysis Outcomes and Practice Patterns Study. *Nephrol. Dial. Transplant.* **2008**, *23*, 3219–3226. [CrossRef] [PubMed]

64. Pisoni, R.L.; Arrington, C.J.; Albert, J.M.; Ethier, J.; Kimata, N.; Krishnan, M.; Rayner, H.C.; Saito, A.; Sands, J.J.; Saran, R.; et al. Facility hemodialysis vascular access use and mortality in countries participating in DOPPS: An instrumental variable analysis. *Am. J. Kidney Dis.* **2009**, *53*, 475–491. [CrossRef] [PubMed]

65. Banerjee, T.; Kim, S.J.; Astor, B.; Shafi, T.; Coresh, J.; Powe, N.R. Vascular access type, inflammatory markers, and mortality in incident hemodialysis patients: The Choices for Healthy Outcomes in Caring for End-Stage Renal Disease (CHOICE) Study. *Am. J. Kidney Dis.* **2014**, *64*, 954–961. [CrossRef] [PubMed]

66. Baracco, R.; Saadeh, S.; Valentini, R.; Kapur, G.; Jain, A.; Mattoo, T.K. Iron deficiency in children with early chronic kidney disease. *Pediatr. Nephrol.* **2011**, *26*, 2077–2080. [CrossRef] [PubMed]

67. Cusick, S.E.; Mei, Z.; Freedman, D.S.; Looker, A.C.; Ogden, C.L.; Gunter, E.; Cogswell, M.E. Unexplained decline in the prevalence of anemia among US children and women between 1988–1994 and 1999–2002. *Am. J. Clin. Nutr.* **2008**, *88*, 1611–1617. [CrossRef] [PubMed]

68. Akbari, M.; Moosazadeh, M.; Tabrizi, R.; Khatibi, S.R.; Khodadost, M.; Heydari, S.T.; Tahami, A.N.; Lankarani, K.B. Estimation of iron deficiency anemia in Iranian children and adolescents: A systematic review and meta-analysis. *Hematology* **2017**, *22*, 231–239. [CrossRef] [PubMed]

69. Fishbane, S.; Pollack, S.; Feldman, H.I.; Joffe, M.M. Iron indices in chronic kidney disease in the National Health and Nutritional Examination Survey 1988–2004. *Clin. J. Am. Soc. Nephrol.* **2009**, *4*, 57–61. [CrossRef] [PubMed]

70. Cappellini, M.D.; Comin-Colet, J.; de Francisco, A.; Dignass, A.; Doehner, W.; Lam, C.S.; Macdougall, I.C.; Rogler, G.; Camaschella, C.; Kadir, R.; et al. Iron deficiency across chronic inflammatory conditions: International expert opinion on definition, diagnosis, and management. *Am. J. Hematol.* **2017**, *92*, 1068–1078. [CrossRef] [PubMed]

71. Centers for Disease Control and Prevention (CDC). Iron deficiency—United States, 1999–2000. *MMWR Morb. Mortal. Wkly. Rep.* **2002**, *51*, 897–899.

72. Haupt, L.; Weyers, R. Determination of functional iron deficiency status in haemodialysis patients in central South Africa. *Int. J. Lab. Hematol.* **2016**, *38*, 352–359. [CrossRef] [PubMed]

73. Knight, T.G.; Ryan, K.; Schaefer, C.P.; D'Sylva, L.; Durden, E.D. Clinical and economic outcomes in Medicare beneficiaries with stage 3 or stage 4 chronic kidney disease and anemia: The role of intravenous iron therapy. *J. Manag. Care Pharm.* **2010**, *16*, 605–615. [CrossRef] [PubMed]

74. Kovesdy, C.P.; Estrada, W.; Ahmadzadeh, S.; Kalantar-Zadeh, K. Association of markers of iron stores with outcomes in patients with nondialysis-dependent chronic kidney disease. *Clin. J. Am. Soc. Nephrol.* **2009**, *4*, 435–441. [CrossRef] [PubMed]

75. Bross, R.; Zitterkoph, J.; Pithia, J.; Benner, D.; Rambod, M.; Kovesdy, C.; Kopple, J.D.; Kalantar-Zadeh, K. Association of serum total iron-binding capacity and its changes over time with nutritional and clinical outcomes in hemodialysis patients. *Am. J. Nephrol.* **2009**, *29*, 571–581. [CrossRef] [PubMed]

76. Cuevas, X.; García, F.; Martín-Malo, A.; Fort, J.; Lladós, F.; Lozano, J.; Pérez-García, R. Risk factors associated with cardiovascular morbidity and mortality in Spanish incident hemodialysis patients: Two-year results from the ANSWER study. *Blood Purif.* **2012**, *33*, 21–29. [CrossRef] [PubMed]

77. Kleine, C.E.; Soohoo, M.; Ranasinghe, O.N.; Park, C.; Marroquin, M.V.; Obi, Y.; Rhee, C.M.; Moradi, H.; Kovesdy, C.P.; Kalantar-Zadeh, K.; et al. Association of pre-end-stage renal disease hemoglobin with early dialysis outcomes. *Am. J. Nephrol.* **2018**, *47*, 333–342. [CrossRef] [PubMed]

78. Roberts, T.L.; Foley, R.N.; Weinhandl, E.D.; Gilbertson, D.T.; Collins, A.J. Anaemia and mortality in haemodialysis patients: Interaction of propensity score for predicted anaemia and actual haemoglobin levels. *Nephrol. Dial. Transplant.* **2006**, *21*, 1652–1662. [CrossRef] [PubMed]

79. Fort, J.; Cuevas, X.; Garcia, F.; Perez-Garcia, R.; Lladós, F.; Lozano, J.; Martín-Malo, A.; ANSWER Study. Mortality in incident haemodialysis patients: Time-dependent haemoglobin levels and erythropoiesis-stimulating agent dose are independent predictive factors in the ANSWER study. *Nephrol. Dial. Transplant.* **2010**, *25*, 2702–2710. [CrossRef] [PubMed]

80. Avram, M.M.; Blaustein, D.; Fein, P.A.; Goel, N.; Chattopadhyay, J.; Mittman, N. Hemoglobin predicts long-term survival in dialysis patients: A 15-year single-center longitudinal study and a correlation trend between prealbumin and hemoglobin. *Kidney Int. Suppl.* **2003**, *87*, S6–S11. [CrossRef]

81. Macdougall, I.C.; Tomson, C.R.; Steenkamp, M.; Ansell, D. Relative risk of death in UK haemodialysis patients in relation to achieved haemoglobin from 1999 to 2005: An observational study using UK Renal Registry data incorporating 30,040 patient-years of follow-up. *Nephrol. Dial. Transplant.* **2010**, *25*, 914–919. [CrossRef] [PubMed]

82. Shi, Z.; Zhen, S.; Zhou, Y.; Taylor, A.W. Hb level, iron intake and mortality in Chinese adults: A 10-year follow-up study. *Br. J. Nutr.* **2017**, *117*, 572–581. [CrossRef] [PubMed]

83. Rheault, M.N.; Molony, J.T.; Nevins, T.; Herzog, C.A.; Chavers, B.M. Hemoglobin of 12 g/dl and above is not associated with increased cardiovascular morbidity in children on hemodialysis. *Kidney Int.* **2017**, *91*, 177–182. [CrossRef] [PubMed]

84. Ishani, A.; Guo, H.; Gilbertson, D.T.; Liu, J.; Dunning, S.; Collins, A.J.; Foley, R.N. Time to target haemoglobin concentration (11 g/dl)—Risk of hospitalization and mortality among incident dialysis patients. *Nephrol. Dial. Transplant.* **2007**, *22*, 2247–2255. [CrossRef] [PubMed]

85. Shoji, T.; Niihata, K.; Fukuma, S.; Fukuhara, S.; Akizawa, T.; Inaba, M. Both low and high serum ferritin levels predict mortality risk in hemodialysis patients without inflammation. *Clin. Exp. Nephrol.* **2017**, *21*, 685–693. [CrossRef] [PubMed]

86. Kalantar-Zadeh, K.; McAllister, C.J.; Lehn, R.S.; Liu, E.; Kopple, J.D. A low serum iron level is a predictor of poor outcome in hemodialysis patients. *Am. J. Kidney Dis.* **2004**, *43*, 671–684. [CrossRef] [PubMed]

87. Koo, H.M.; Kim, C.H.; Doh, F.M.; Lee, M.J.; Kim, E.J.; Han, J.H.; Han, J.S.; Oh, H.J.; Park, J.T.; Han, S.H.; et al. The relationship of initial transferrin saturation to cardiovascular parameters and outcomes in patients initiating dialysis. *PLoS ONE* **2014**, *9*, e87231. [CrossRef] [PubMed]

88. Kalantar-Zadeh, K.; Lee, G.H.; Miller, J.E.; Streja, E.; Jing, J.; Robertson, J.A.; Kovesdy, C.P. Predictors of hyporesponsiveness to erythropoiesis-stimulating agents in hemodialysis patients. *Am. J. Kidney Dis.* **2009**, *53*, 823–834. [CrossRef] [PubMed]

89. Ishigami, J.; Onishi, T.; Shikuma, S.; Akita, W.; Mori, Y.; Asai, T.; Kuwahara, M.; Sasaki, S.; Tsukamoto, Y. The impact of hyporesponsiveness to erythropoietin-stimulating agents on time-dependent mortality risk among CKD stage 5D patients: A single-center cohort study. *Clin. Exp. Nephrol.* **2013**, *17*, 106–114. [CrossRef] [PubMed]

90. Liu, S.; Zhang, D.L.; Guo, W.; Cui, W.Y.; Liu, W.H. Left ventricular mass index and aortic arch calcification score are independent mortality predictors of maintenance hemodialysis patients. *Hemodial. Int.* **2012**, *16*, 504–511. [CrossRef] [PubMed]

91. Ishida, J.H.; Johansen, K.L. Iron and infection in hemodialysis patients. *Semin. Dial.* **2014**, *27*, 26–36. [CrossRef] [PubMed]

92. Jenq, C.C.; Hsu, C.W.; Huang, W.H.; Chen, K.H.; Lin, J.L.; Lin-Tan, D.T. Serum ferritin levels predict all-cause and infection-cause 1-year mortality in diabetic patients on maintenance hemodialysis. *Am. J. Med. Sci.* **2009**, *337*, 188–194. [CrossRef] [PubMed]

93. Kessler, M.; Hoen, B.; Mayeux, D.; Hestin, D.; Fontenaille, C. Bacteremia in patients on chronic hemodialysis. A multicenter prospective survey. *Nephron* **1993**, *64*, 95–100. [CrossRef] [PubMed]

94. Park, K.S.; Ryu, G.W.; Jhee, J.H.; Kim, H.W.; Park, S.; Lee, S.A.; Kwon, Y.E.; Kim, Y.L.; Ryu, H.J.; Lee, M.J.; et al. Serum ferritin predicts mortality regardless of inflammatory and nutritional status in patients starting dialysis: A prospective cohort study. *Blood Purif.* **2015**, *40*, 209–217. [CrossRef] [PubMed]

95. Kim, T.; Streja, E.; Soohoo, M.; Rhee, C.M.; Eriguchi, R.; Kim, T.W.; Chang, T.I.; Obi, Y.; Kovesdy, C.P.; Kalantar-Zadeh, K. Serum ferritin variations and mortality in incident hemodialysis patients. *Am. J. Nephrol.* **2017**, *46*, 120–130. [CrossRef] [PubMed]

96. Brookhart, M.A.; Freburger, J.K.; Ellis, A.R.; Winkelmayer, W.C.; Wang, L.; Kshirsagar, A.V. Comparative short-term safety of sodium ferric gluconate versus iron sucrose in hemodialysis patients. *Am. J. Kidney Dis.* **2016**, *67*, 119–127. [CrossRef] [PubMed]

97. Hoen, B.; Paul-Dauphin, A.; Kessler, M. Intravenous iron administration does not significantly increase the risk of bacteremia in chronic hemodialysis patients. *Clin. Nephrol.* **2002**, *57*, 457–461. [CrossRef] [PubMed]

98. Macdougall, I.C.; Bock, A.H.; Carrera, F.; Eckardt, K.U.; Gaillard, C.; Van Wyck, D.; Roubert, B.; Nolen, J.G.; Roger, S.D.; FIND-CKD Study Investigators. FIND-CKD: A randomized trial of intravenous ferric carboxymaltose versus oral iron in patients with chronic kidney disease and iron deficiency anaemia. *Nephrol. Dial. Transplant.* **2014**, *29*, 2075–2084. [CrossRef] [PubMed]

99. Kalantar-Zadeh, K.; Regidor, D.L.; McAllister, C.J.; Michael, B.; Warnock, D.G. Time-dependent associations between iron and mortality in hemodialysis patients. *J. Am. Soc. Nephrol.* **2005**, *16*, 3070–3080. [CrossRef] [PubMed]

100. Karaboyas, A.; Morgenstern, H.; Pisoni, R.L.; Zee, J.; Vanholder, R.; Jacobson, S.H.; Inaba, M.; Loram, L.C.; Port, F.K.; Robinson, B.M. Association between serum ferritin and mortality: Findings from the USA, Japan and European Dialysis Outcomes and Practice Patterns Study. *Nephrol. Dial. Transplant.* **2018**. [CrossRef] [PubMed]

101. Floege, J.; Gillespie, I.A.; Kronenberg, F.; Anker, S.D.; Gioni, I.; Richards, S.; Pisoni, R.L.; Robinson, B.M.; Marcelli, D.; Froissart, M.; et al. Development and validation of a predictive mortality risk score from a European hemodialysis cohort. *Kidney Int.* **2015**, *87*, 996–1008. [CrossRef] [PubMed]

102. Chauveau, P.; Level, C.; Lasseur, C.; Bonarek, H.; Peuchant, E.; Montaudon, D.; Vendrely, B.; Combe, C. C-reactive protein and procalcitonin as markers of mortality in hemodialysis patients: A 2-year prospective study. *J. Ren. Nutr.* **2003**, *13*, 137–143. [CrossRef] [PubMed]

103. Leonard, M.B.; Donaldson, L.A.; Ho, M.; Geary, D.F. A prospective cohort study of incident maintenance dialysis in children: An NAPRTC study. *Kidney Int.* **2003**, *63*, 744–755. [CrossRef] [PubMed]

104. Chavers, B.M.; Roberts, T.L.; Herzog, C.A.; Collins, A.J.; St Peter, W.L. Prevalence of anemia in erythropoietin-treated pediatric as compared to adult chronic dialysis patients. *Kidney Int.* **2004**, *65*, 266–273. [CrossRef] [PubMed]

105. Van Stralen, K.J.; Krischock, L.; Schaefer, F.; Verrina, E.; Groothoff, J.W.; Evans, J.; Heaf, J.; Ivanov, D.; Kostic, M.; Maringhini, S.; et al. Prevalence and predictors of the sub-target Hb level in children on dialysis. *Nephrol. Dial. Transplant.* **2012**, *27*, 3950–3957. [CrossRef] [PubMed]

106. Dmitrieva, O.; de Lusignan, S.; Macdougall, I.C.; Gallagher, H.; Tomson, C.; Harris, K.; Desombre, T.; Goldsmith, D. Association of anaemia in primary care patients with chronic kidney disease: Cross sectional study of quality improvement in chronic kidney disease (QICKD) trial data. *BMC Nephrol.* **2013**, *14*, 24. [CrossRef] [PubMed]

107. Freburger, J.K.; Ng, L.J.; Bradbury, B.D.; Kshirsagar, A.V.; Brookhart, M.A. Changing patterns of anemia management in US hemodialysis patients. *Am. J. Med.* **2012**, *125*, 906–914. [CrossRef] [PubMed]

108. Miskulin, D.C.; Zhou, J.; Tangri, N.; Bandeen-Roche, K.; Cook, C.; Ephraim, P.L.; Crews, D.C.; Scialla, J.J.; Sozio, S.M.; Shafi, T.; et al. Trends in anemia management in US hemodialysis patients 2004–2010. *BMC Nephrol.* **2013**, *14*, 264. [CrossRef] [PubMed]

109. Charytan, D.M.; Pai, A.B.; Chan, C.T.; Coyne, D.W.; Hung, A.M.; Kovesdy, C.P.; Fishbane, S.; Dialysis Advisory Group of the American Society of Nephrology. Considerations and challenges in defining optimal iron utilization in hemodialysis. *J. Am. Soc. Nephrol.* **2015**, *26*, 1238–1247. [CrossRef] [PubMed]

110. Hassan, R.H.; Kandil, S.M.; Zeid, M.S.; Zaki, M.E.; Fouda, A.E. Kidney injury in infants and children with iron-deficiency anemia before and after iron treatment. *Hematology* **2017**, *22*, 565–570. [CrossRef] [PubMed]

111. Streja, E.; Kovesdy, C.P.; Greenland, S.; Kopple, J.D.; McAllister, C.J.; Nissenson, A.R.; Kalantar-Zadeh, K. Erythropoietin, iron depletion, and relative thrombocytosis: A possible explanation for hemoglobin-survival paradox in hemodialysis. *Am. J. Kidney Dis.* **2008**, *52*, 727–736. [CrossRef] [PubMed]

112. Peyrin-Biroulet, L.; Williet, N.; Cacoub, P. Guidelines on the diagnosis and treatment of iron deficiency across indications: A systematic review. *Am. J. Clin. Nutr.* **2015**, *102*, 1585–1594. [CrossRef] [PubMed]

113. Takasawa, K.; Takaeda, C.; Maeda, T.; Ueda, N. Hepcidin-25, mean corpuscular volume, and ferritin as predictors of response to oral iron supplementation in hemodialysis patients. *Nutrients* **2015**, *7*, 103–118. [CrossRef] [PubMed]

114. Peters, N.O.; Jay, N.; Cridlig, J.; Rostoker, G.; Frimat, L. Targets for adapting intravenous iron dose in hemodialysis: A proof of concept study. *BMC Nephrol.* **2017**, *18*, 97. [CrossRef] [PubMed]

115. Rozen-Zvi, B.; Gafter-Gvili, A.; Paul, M.; Leibovici, L.; Shpilberg, O.; Gafter, U. Intravenous versus oral iron supplementation for the treatment of anemia in CKD: Systematic review and meta-analysis. *Am. J. Kidney Dis.* **2008**, *52*, 897–906. [CrossRef] [PubMed]

116. Albaramki, J.; Hodson, E.M.; Craig, J.C.; Webster, A.C. Parenteral versus oral iron therapy for adults and children with chronic kidney disease. *Cochrane Database Syst. Rev.* **2012**, *1*, CD007857. [CrossRef] [PubMed]

117. Qunibi, W.Y.; Martinez, C.; Smith, M.; Benjamin, J.; Mangione, A.; Roger, S.D. A randomized controlled trial comparing intravenous ferric carboxymaltose with oral iron for treatment of iron deficiency anaemia of non-dialysis-dependent chronic kidney disease patients. *Nephrol. Dial. Transplant.* **2011**, *26*, 1599–1607. [CrossRef] [PubMed]

118. Pisani, A.; Riccio, E.; Sabbatini, M.; Andreucci, M.; Del Rio, A.; Visciano, B. Effect of oral liposomal iron versus intravenous iron for treatment of iron deficiency anaemia in CKD patients: A randomized trial. *Nephrol. Dial. Transplant.* **2015**, *30*, 645–652. [CrossRef] [PubMed]

119. Agarwal, R.; Rizkala, A.R.; Bastani, B.; Kaskas, M.O.; Leehey, D.J.; Besarab, A. A randomized controlled trial of oral versus intravenous iron in chronic kidney disease. *Am. J. Nephrol.* **2006**, *26*, 445–454. [CrossRef] [PubMed]

120. Kalra, P.A.; Bhandari, S.; Saxena, S.; Agarwal, D.; Wirtz, G.; Kletzmayr, J.; Thomsen, L.L.; Coyne, D.W. A randomized trial of iron isomaltoside 1000 versus oral iron in non-dialysis-dependent chronic kidney disease patients with anaemia. *Nephrol. Dial. Transplant.* **2016**, *31*, 646–655. [CrossRef] [PubMed]

121. Macdougall, I.C.; Bock, A.H.; Carrera, F.; Eckardt, K.U.; Gaillard, C.; Wyck, D.V.; Meier, Y.; Larroque, S.; Perrin, A.; Roger, S.D. Erythropoietic response to oral iron in patients with nondialysis-dependent chronic kidney disease in the FIND-CKD trial. *Clin. Nephrol.* **2017**, *88*, 301–310. [CrossRef] [PubMed]

122. Jenq, C.C.; Tian, Y.C.; Wu, H.H.; Hsu, P.Y.; Huang, J.Y.; Chen, Y.C.; Fang, J.T.; Yang, C.W. Effectiveness of oral and intravenous iron therapy in haemodialysis patients. *Int. J. Clin. Pract.* **2008**, *62*, 416–422. [CrossRef] [PubMed]

123. Stoves, J.; Inglis, H.; Newstead, C.G. A randomized study of oral vs intravenous iron supplementation in patients with progressive renal insufficiency treated with erythropoietin. *Nephrol. Dial. Transplant.* **2001**, *16*, 967–974. [CrossRef] [PubMed]

124. Takasawa, K.; Takaeda, C.; Wada, T.; Ueda, N. Optimal serum ferritin levels for iron deficiency anemia during oral iron therapy (OIT) in Japanese hemodialysis patients with minor inflammation and benefit of intravenous iron therapy for OIT-nonresponders. *Nutrients* **2018**, *10*, 428. [CrossRef] [PubMed]

125. Ogawa, C.; Tsuchiya, K.; Tomosugi, N.; Kanda, F.; Maeda, K.; Maeda, T. Low levels of serum ferritin and moderate transferrin saturation lead to adequate hemoglobin levels in hemodialysis patients, retrospective observational study. *PLoS ONE* **2017**, *12*, e0179608. [CrossRef] [PubMed]

126. Sanai, T.; Ono, T.; Fukumitsu, T. Beneficial effects of oral iron in Japanese patients on hemodialysis. *Intern. Med.* **2017**, *56*, 2395–2399. [CrossRef] [PubMed]

127. Kooistra, M.P.; Niemantsverdriet, E.C.; van Es, A.; Mol-Beermann, N.M.; Struyvenberg, A.; Marx, J.J. Iron absorption in erythropoietin-treated haemodialysis patients: Effects of iron availability, inflammation and aluminium. *Nephrol. Dial. Transplant.* **1998**, *13*, 82–88. [CrossRef] [PubMed]

128. Nakanishi, T.; Kuragano, T.; Kaibe, S.; Nagasawa, Y.; Hasuike, Y. Should we reconsider iron administration based on prevailing ferritin and hepcidin concentrations? *Clin. Exp. Nephrol.* **2012**, *16*, 819–826. [CrossRef] [PubMed]

129. Owen, W.F.; Lowrie, E.G. C-reactive protein as an outcome predictor for maintenance hemodialysis patients. *Kidney Int.* **1998**, *54*, 627–636. [CrossRef] [PubMed]

130. Kalender, B.; Mutlu, B.; Ersöz, M.; Kalkan, A.; Yilmaz, A. The effects of acute phase proteins on serum albumin, transferrin and haemoglobin in haemodialysis patients. *Int. J. Clin. Pract.* **2002**, *56*, 505–508. [PubMed]

131. Heidari, B.; Fazli, M.R.; Misaeid, M.A.; Heidari, P.; Hakimi, N.; Zeraati, A.A. A linear relationship between serum high-sensitive C-reactive protein and hemoglobin in hemodialysis patients. *Clin. Exp. Nephrol.* **2015**, *19*, 725–731. [CrossRef] [PubMed]

132. Chan, K.E.; Lafayette, R.A.; Whittemore, A.S.; Hlatky, M.A.; Moran, J. Facility factors dominate the ability to achieve target haemoglobin levels in haemodialysis patients. *Nephrol. Dial. Transplant.* **2008**, *23*, 2948–2956. [CrossRef] [PubMed]

133. Sharain, K.; Hoppensteadt, D.; Bansal, V.; Singh, A.; Fareed, J. Progressive increase of inflammatory biomarkers in chronic kidney disease and end-stage renal disease. *Clin. Appl. Thromb. Hemost.* **2013**, *19*, 303–308. [CrossRef] [PubMed]

134. Aydin, Z.; Gursu, M.; Karadag, S.; Uzun, S.; Sumnu, A.; Doventas, Y.; Ozturk, S.; Kazancioglu, R. The relationship of prohepcidin levels with anemia and inflammatory markers in non-diabetic uremic patients: A controlled study. *Ren. Fail.* **2014**, *36*, 1253–1257. [CrossRef] [PubMed]

135. Goyal, K.K.; Saha, A.; Sahi, P.K.; Kaur, M.; Dubey, N.K.; Goyal, P.; Upadhayay, A.D. Hepcidin and proinflammatory markers in children with chronic kidney disease: A case-control study. *Clin. Nephrol.* **2018**, *89*, 363–370. [CrossRef] [PubMed]

136. Musanovic, A.; Trnacevic, S.; Mekic, M.; Musanovic, A. The influence of inflammatory markers and CRP predictive value in relation to the target hemoglobin level in patients on chronic hemodialysis. *Med. Arch.* **2013**, *67*, 361–364. [CrossRef] [PubMed]

137. Saltissi, D.; Sauvage, D.; Westhuyzen, J. Comparative response to single or divided doses of parenteral iron for functional iron deficiency in hemodialysis patients receiving erythropoietin (EPO). *Clin. Nephrol.* **1998**, *49*, 45–48. [PubMed]

138. Voulgarelis, M.; Kokori, S.I.; Ioannidis, J.P.; Tzioufas, A.G.; Kyriaki, D.; Moutsopoulos, H.M. Anaemia in systemic lupus erythematosus: Aetiological profile and the role of erythropoietin. *Ann. Rheum. Dis.* **2000**, *59*, 217–222. [CrossRef] [PubMed]

139. Van Santen, S.; van Dongen-Lases, E.C.; de Vegt, F.; Laarakkers, C.M.; van Riel, P.L.; van Ede, A.E.; Swinkels, D.W. Hepcidin and hemoglobin content parameters in the diagnosis of iron deficiency in rheumatoid arthritis patients with anemia. *Arthritis Rheum.* **2011**, *63*, 3672–3680. [CrossRef] [PubMed]

140. Seyhan, S.; Pamuk, Ö.N.; Pamuk, G.E.; Çakır, N. The correlation between ferritin level and acute phase parameters in rheumatoid arthritis and systemic lupus erythematosus. *Eur. J. Rheumatol.* **2014**, *1*, 92–95. [CrossRef] [PubMed]

141. Cavallaro, F.; Duca, L.; Pisani, L.F.; Rigolini, R.; Spina, L.; Tontini, G.E.; Munizio, N.; Costa, E.; Cappellini, M.D.; Vecchi, M.; et al. Anti-TNF-mediated modulation of prohepcidin improves iron availability in inflammatory bowel disease, in an IL-6-mediated fashion. *Can. J. Gastroenterol. Hepatol.* **2017**, *2017*, 6843976. [CrossRef] [PubMed]

142. Stein, J.; Haas, J.S.; Ong, S.H.; Borchert, K.; Hardt, T.; Lechat, E.; Nip, K.; Foerster, D.; Braun, S.; Baumgart, D.C. Oral versus intravenous iron therapy in patients with inflammatory bowel disease and iron deficiency with and without anemia in Germany—A real-world evidence analysis. *Clinicoecon. Outcomes Res.* **2018**, *10*, 93–103. [CrossRef] [PubMed]

143. Kronbichler, A.; Mayer, G. Renal involvement in autoimmune connective tissue diseases. *BMC Med.* **2013**, *11*, 95. [CrossRef] [PubMed]

144. Ambruzs, J.M.; Walker, P.D.; Larsen, C.P. The histopathologic spectrum of kidney biopsies in patients with inflammatory bowel disease. *Clin. J. Am. Soc. Nephrol.* **2014**, *9*, 265–270. [CrossRef] [PubMed]

145. Vanarsa, K.; Ye, Y.; Han, J.; Xie, C.; Mohan, C.; Wu, T. Inflammation associated anemia and ferritin as disease markers in SLE. *Arthritis Res. Ther.* **2012**, *14*, R182. [CrossRef] [PubMed]

146. Tripathy, R.; Panda, A.K.; Das, B.K. Serum ferritin level correlates with SLEDAI scores and renal involvement in SLE. *Lupus* **2015**, *24*, 82–89. [CrossRef] [PubMed]

147. Umare, V.; Nadkarni, A.; Nadkar, M.; Rajadhyksha, A.; Khadilkar, P.; Ghosh, K.; Pradhan, V.D. Do high sensitivity C-reactive protein and serum interleukin-6 levels correlate with disease activity in systemic lupus erythematosuspatients? *J. Postgrad. Med.* **2017**, *63*, 92–95. [PubMed]

148. Ripley, B.J.; Goncalves, B.; Isenberg, D.A.; Latchman, D.S.; Rahman, A. Raised levels of interleukin 6 in systemic lupus erythematosus correlate with anaemia. *Ann. Rheum. Dis.* **2005**, *64*, 849–853. [CrossRef] [PubMed]

149. Mohammed, M.F.; Belal, D.; Bakry, S.; Marie, M.A.; Rashed, L.; Eldin, R.E.; El-Hamid, S.A. A study of hepcidin and monocyte chemoattractant protein-1 in Egyptian females with systemic lupus erythematosus. *J. Clin. Lab. Anal.* **2014**, *28*, 306–309. [CrossRef] [PubMed]

150. Zhang, X.; Nagaraja, H.N.; Nadasdy, T.; Song, H.; McKinley, A.; Prosek, J.; Kamadana, S.; Rovin, B.H. A composite urine biomarker reflects interstitial inflammation in lupus nephritis kidney biopsies. *Kidney Int.* **2012**, *81*, 401–406. [CrossRef] [PubMed]

151. Demirag, M.D.; Haznedaroglu, S.; Sancak, B.; Konca, C.; Gulbahar, O.; Ozturk, M.A.; Goker, B. Circulating hepcidin in the crossroads of anemia and inflammation associated with rheumatoid arthritis. *Intern. Med.* **2009**, *48*, 421–426. [CrossRef] [PubMed]

152. Martinelli, M.; Strisciuglio, C.; Alessandrella, A.; Rossi, F.; Auricchio, R.; Campostrini, N.; Girelli, D.; Nobili, B.; Staiano, A.; Perrotta, S.; et al. Serum hepcidin and iron absorption in paediatric inflammatory bowel disease. *J. Crohns Colitis* **2016**, *10*, 566–574. [CrossRef] [PubMed]

153. Iqbal, T.; Stein, J.; Sharma, N.; Kulnigg-Dabsch, S.; Vel, S.; Gasche, C. Clinical significance of C-reactive protein levels in predicting responsiveness to iron therapy in patients with inflammatory bowel disease and iron deficiency anemia. *Dig. Dis. Sci.* **2015**, *60*, 1375–1381. [CrossRef] [PubMed]

154. Ross, D.N. Oral and intravenous iron therapy in the anaemia of rheumatoid arthritis. *Ann. Rheum. Dis.* **1950**, *9*, 358–362. [CrossRef] [PubMed]

155. Anuradha, S.; Singh, N.P.; Agarwal, S.K. Total dose infusion iron dextran therapy in predialysis chronic renal failure patients. *Ren. Fail.* **2002**, *24*, 307–313. [CrossRef] [PubMed]

156. Rambod, M.; Kovesdy, C.P.; Kalantar-Zadeh, K. Combined high serum ferritin and low iron saturation in hemodialysis patients: The role of inflammation. *Clin. J. Am. Soc. Nephrol.* **2008**, *3*, 1691–1701. [CrossRef] [PubMed]

157. Rafiean-Kopaie, M.; Nasri, H. Impact of inflammation on anemia of hemodialysis patients who were under treatment of recombinant human erythropoietin. *J. Ren. Inj. Prev.* **2013**, *2*, 93–95. [PubMed]

158. Tessitore, N.; Girelli, D.; Campostrini, N.; Bedogna, V.; Pietro Solero, G.; Castagna, A.; Melilli, E.; Mantovani, W.; De Matteis, G.; Olivieri, O.; et al. Hepcidin is not useful as a biomarker for iron needs in haemodialysis patients on maintenance erythropoiesis-stimulating agents. *Nephrol. Dial. Transplant.* **2010**, *25*, 3996–4002. [CrossRef] [PubMed]

159. Gaillard, C.A.; Bock, A.H.; Carrera, F.; Eckardt, K.U.; Van Wyck, D.B.; Bansal, S.S.; Cronin, M.; Meier, Y.; Larroque, S.; Roger, S.D.; et al. Hepcidin response to iron therapy in patients with non-dialysis dependent CKD: An analysis of the FIND-CKD trial. *PLoS ONE* **2016**, *11*, e0157063. [CrossRef] [PubMed]

160. Yavuz, A.; Akbaş, S.H.; Tuncer, M.; Kolağasi, O.; Cetinkaya, R.; Gürkan, A.; Demirbaş, A.; Gultekin, M.; Akaydin, M.; Ersoy, F.; et al. Influence of inflammation on the relation between markers of iron deficiency in renal replacement therapy. *Transplant. Proc.* **2004**, *36*, 41–43. [CrossRef] [PubMed]

161. Uehata, T.; Tomosugi, N.; Shoji, T.; Sakaguchi, Y.; Suzuki, A.; Kaneko, T.; Okada, N.; Yamamoto, R.; Nagasawa, Y.; Kato, K.; et al. Serum hepcidin-25 levels and anemia in non-dialysis chronic kidney disease patients: A cross-sectional study. *Nephrol. Dial. Transplant.* **2012**, *27*, 1076–1083. [CrossRef] [PubMed]

162. Chand, S.; Ward, D.G.; Ng, Z.Y.; Hodson, J.; Kirby, H.; Steele, P.; Rooplal, I.; Bantugon, F.; Iqbal, T.; Tselepis, C.; et al. Serum hepcidin-25 and response to intravenous iron in patients with non-dialysis chronic kidney disease. *J. Nephrol.* **2015**, *28*, 81–88. [CrossRef] [PubMed]

163. Drakou, A.; Margeli, A.; Theodorakopoulou, S.; Agrogiannis, I.; Poziopoulos, C.; Papassotiriou, I.; Vlahakos, D.V. Assessment of serum bioactive hepcidin-25, soluble transferrin receptor and their ratio in predialysis patients: Correlation with the response to intravenous ferric carboxymaltose. *Blood Cells Mol. Dis.* **2016**, *59*, 100–105. [CrossRef] [PubMed]

164. Lenga, I.; Lok, C.; Marticorena, R.; Hunter, J.; Dacouris, N.; Goldstein, M. Role of oral iron in the management of long-term hemodialysis patients. *Clin. J. Am. Soc. Nephrol.* **2007**, *2*, 688–693. [CrossRef] [PubMed]

165. Tsuchida, A.; Paudyal, B.; Paudyal, P.; Ishii, Y.; Hiromura, K.; Nojima, Y.; Komai, M. Effectiveness of oral iron to manage anemia in long-term hemodialysis patients with the use of ultrapure dialysate. *Exp. Ther. Med.* **2010**, *1*, 777–781. [CrossRef] [PubMed]

166. Nagaraju, S.P.; Cohn, A.; Akbari, A.; Davis, J.L.; Zimmerman, D.L. Heme iron polypeptide for the treatment of iron deficiency anemia in non-dialysis chronic kidney disease patients: A randomized controlled trial. *BMC Nephrol.* **2013**, *14*, 64. [CrossRef] [PubMed]

167. Bhandari, S.; Kalra, P.A.; Kothari, J.; Ambühl, P.M.; Christensen, J.H.; Essaian, A.M.; Thomsen, L.L.; Macdougall, I.C.; Coyne, D.W. A randomized, open-label trial of iron isomaltoside 1000 (Monofer®) compared with iron sucrose (Venofer®) as maintenance therapy in haemodialysis patients. *Nephrol. Dial. Transplant.* **2015**, *30*, 1577–1589. [CrossRef] [PubMed]

168. Rostoker, G.; Griuncelli, M.; Loridon, C.; Magna, T.; Machado, G.; Drahi, G.; Dahan, H.; Janklewicz, P.; Cohen, Y. Reassessment of iron biomarkers for prediction of dialysis iron overload: An MRI study. *PLoS ONE* **2015**, *10*, e0132006. [CrossRef] [PubMed]

169. Tanaka, A.; Inaguma, D.; Watanabe, Y.; Ito, E.; Kamegai, N.; Shimogushi, H.; Shinjo, H.; Koike, K.; Otsuka, Y.; Takeda, A. Ferrokinetics is associated with the left ventricular mass index in patients with chronic kidney disease. *Acta Cardiol.* **2017**, *72*, 460–466. [CrossRef] [PubMed]

170. Lin, K.C.; Tsai, M.Y.; Chi, C.L.; Yu, L.K.; Huang, L.H.; Chen, C.A. Serum ferritin is associated with arterial stiffness in hemodialysis patients: Results of a 3-year follow-up study. *Int. Urol. Nephrol.* **2015**, *47*, 1847–1853. [CrossRef] [PubMed]

171. Reis, K.A.; Guz, G.; Ozdemir, H.; Erten, Y.; Atalay, V.; Bicik, Z.; Ozkurt, Z.N.; Bali, M.; Sindel, S. Intravenous iron therapy as a possible risk factor for atherosclerosis in end-stage renal disease. *Int. Heart J.* **2005**, *46*, 255–264. [CrossRef] [PubMed]

172. Hsieh, Y.P.; Huang, C.H.; Lee, C.Y.; Chen, H.L.; Lin, C.Y.; Chang, C.C. Hepcidin-25 negatively predicts left ventricular mass index in chronic kidney disease patients. *World J. Nephrol.* **2013**, *2*, 38–43. [CrossRef] [PubMed]

173. Kuragano, T.; Itoh, K.; Shimonaka, Y.; Kida, A.; Furuta, M.; Kitamura, R.; Yahiro, M.; Nanami, M.; Otaki, Y.; Hasuike, Y.; et al. Hepcidin as well as TNF-α are significant predictors of arterial stiffness in patients on maintenance hemodialysis. *Nephrol. Dial. Transplant.* **2011**, *26*, 2663–2667. [CrossRef] [PubMed]

174. Li, H.; Feng, S.J.; Su, L.L.; Wang, W.; Zhang, X.D.; Wang, S.X. Serum hepcidin predicts uremic accelerated atherosclerosis in chronic hemodialysis patients with diabetic nephropathy. *Chin. Med. J. (Engl.)* **2015**, *128*, 1351–1357. [PubMed]

175. Mostovaya, I.M.; Bots, M.L.; van den Dorpel, M.A.; Goldschmeding, R.; den Hoedt, C.H.; Kamp, O.; Levesque, R.; Mazairac, A.H.; Penne, E.L.; Swinkels, D.W.; et al. Left ventricular mass in dialysis patients, determinants and relation with outcome. Results from the COnvective TRansport STudy (CONTRAST). *PLoS ONE* **2014**, *9*, e84587. [CrossRef] [PubMed]

176. Van der Weerd, N.C.; Grooteman, M.P.; Bots, M.L.; van den Dorpel, M.A.; den Hoedt, C.H.; Mazairac, A.H.; Nubé, M.J.; Penne, E.L.; Wetzels, J.F.; Wiegerinck, E.T.; et al. Hepcidin-25 is related to cardiovascular events in chronic haemodialysis patients. *Nephrol. Dial. Transplant.* **2013**, *28*, 3062–3071. [CrossRef] [PubMed]

177. Rostoker, G.; Hummel, A.; Chantrel, F.; Ryckelynck, J.P. Therapy of anemia and iron deficiency in dialysis patients: An update. *Nephrol. Ther.* **2014**, *10*, 221–227. (In French) [CrossRef] [PubMed]

178. Del Vecchio, L.; Locatelli, F. Clinical practice guidelines on iron therapy: A critical evaluation. *Hemodial. Int.* **2017**, *21* (Suppl. 1), S125–S131. [CrossRef] [PubMed]

179. Al-Hawas, F.; Abdalla, A.H.; Popovich, W.; Mousa, D.H.; al-Sulaiman, M.H.; al-Khader, A.A. Use of i.v. iron saccharate in haemodialysis patients not responding to oral iron and erythropoietin. *Nephrol. Dial. Transplant.* **1997**, *12*, 2801–2802. [CrossRef] [PubMed]

180. Canavese, C.; Bergamo, D.; Ciccone, G.; Burdese, M.; Maddalena, E.; Barbieri, S.; Thea, A.; Fop, F. Low-dose continuous iron therapy leads to a positive iron balance and decreased serum transferrin levels in chronic haemodialysis patients. *Nephrol. Dial. Transplant.* **2004**, *19*, 1564–1570. [CrossRef] [PubMed]

181. Rostoker, G.; Griuncelli, M.; Loridon, C.; Magna, T.; Janklewicz, P.; Drahi, G.; Dahan, H.; Cohen, Y. Maximal standard dose of parenteral iron for hemodialysis patients: An MRI-based decision tree learning analysis. *PLoS ONE* **2014**, *9*, e115096. [CrossRef] [PubMed]

182. Vaziri, N.D. Safety issues in iron treatment in CKD. *Semin. Nephrol.* **2016**, *36*, 112–118. [CrossRef] [PubMed]

183. Locatelli, F.; Mazzaferro, S.; Yee, J. Iron therapy challenges for the treatment of nondialysis CKD patients. *Clin. J. Am. Soc. Nephrol.* **2016**, *11*, 1269–1280. [CrossRef] [PubMed]

184. Agarwal, R.; Kusek, J.W.; Pappas, M.K. A randomized trial of intravenous and oral iron in chronic kidney disease. *Kidney Int.* **2015**, *88*, 905–914. [CrossRef] [PubMed]

185. Litton, E.; Xiao, J.; Ho, K.M. Safety and efficacy of intravenous iron therapy in reducing requirement for allogeneic blood transfusion: Systematic review and meta-analysis of randomised clinical trials. *BMJ* **2013**, *347*, f4822. [CrossRef] [PubMed]

186. Bailie, G.R.; Larkina, M.; Goodkin, D.A.; Li, Y.; Pisoni, R.L.; Bieber, B.; Mason, N.; Tong, L.; Locatelli, F.; Marshall, M.R.; et al. Data from the Dialysis Outcomes and Practice Patterns Study validate an association between high intravenous iron doses and mortality. *Kidney Int.* **2015**, *87*, 162–168. [CrossRef] [PubMed]

187. Miskulin, D.C.; Tangri, N.; Bandeen-Roche, K.; Zhou, J.; McDermott, A.; Meyer, K.B.; Ephraim, P.L.; Michels, W.M.; Jaar, B.G.; Crews, D.C.; et al. Developing Evidence to Inform Decisions about Effectiveness (DEcIDE) Network Patient Outcomes in End Stage Renal Disease Study Investigators. Intravenous iron exposure and mortality in patients on hemodialysis. *Clin. J. Am. Soc. Nephrol.* **2014**, *9*, 1930–1939. [CrossRef] [PubMed]

188. Drüeke, T.; Witko-Sarsat, V.; Massy, Z.; Descamps-Latscha, B.; Guerin, A.P.; Marchais, S.J.; Gausson, V.; London, G.M. Iron therapy, advanced oxidation protein products, and carotid artery intima-media thickness in end-stage renal disease. *Circulation* **2002**, *106*, 2212–2217. [CrossRef] [PubMed]

189. Kim, S.M.; Lee, C.H.; Oh, Y.K.; Joo, K.W.; Kim, Y.S.; Kim, S.; Lim, C.S. The effects of oral iron supplementation on the progression of anemia and renal dysfunction in patients with chronic kidney disease. *Clin. Nephrol.* **2011**, *75*, 472–479. [CrossRef] [PubMed]

190. Agarwal, R.; Rizkala, A.R.; Kaskas, M.O.; Minasian, R.; Trout, J.R. Iron sucrose causes greater proteinuria than ferric gluconate in non-dialysis chronic kidney disease. *Kidney Int.* **2007**, *72*, 638–642. [CrossRef] [PubMed]

191. Maruyama, Y.; Nakayama, M.; Yoshimura, K.; Nakano, H.; Yamamoto, H.; Yokoyama, K.; Lindholm, B. Effect of repeated intravenous iron administration in haemodialysis patients on serum 8-hydroxy-2′-deoxyguanosine levels. *Nephrol. Dial. Transplant.* **2007**, *22*, 1407–1412. [CrossRef] [PubMed]

192. Yahiro, M.; Kuragano, T.; Kida, A.; Kitamura, R.; Furuta, M.; Hasuike, Y.; Otaki, Y.; Nonoguchi, H.; Nakanishi, T. The impact of ferritin fluctuations on stable hemoglobin levels in hemodialysis patients. *Clin. Exp. Nephrol.* **2012**, *16*, 448–455. [CrossRef] [PubMed]

193. Wish, J.B. Anemia management under a bundled payment policy for dialysis: A preview for the United States from Japan. *Kidney Int.* **2011**, *79*, 265–267. [CrossRef] [PubMed]

194. Kato, S.; Lindholm, B.; Yuzawa, Y.; Tsuruta, Y.; Nakauchi, K.; Yasuda, K.; Sugiura, S.; Morozumi, K.; Tsuboi, N.; Maruyama, S. High ferritin level and malnutrition predict high risk of infection-related hospitalization in incident dialysis patients: A Japanese prospective cohort study. *Blood Purif.* **2016**, *42*, 56–63. [CrossRef] [PubMed]

195. Ramanathan, G.; Olynyk, J.K.; Ferrari, P. Diagnosing and preventing iron overload. *Hemodial. Int.* **2017**, *21* (Suppl. 1), S58–S67. [CrossRef] [PubMed]

196. Canavese, C.; Bergamo, D.; Ciccone, G.; Longo, F.; Fop, F.; Thea, A.; Martina, G.; Piga, A. Validation of serum ferritin values by magnetic susceptometry in predicting iron overload in dialysis patients. *Kidney Int.* **2004**, *65*, 1091–1098. [CrossRef] [PubMed]

197. Ghoti, H.; Rachmilewitz, E.A.; Simon-Lopez, R.; Gaber, R.; Katzir, Z.; Konen, E.; Kushnir, T.; Girelli, D.; Campostrini, N.; Fibach, E.; et al. Evidence for tissue iron overload in long-term hemodialysis patients and the impact of withdrawing parenteral iron. *Eur. J. Haematol.* **2012**, *89*, 87–93. [CrossRef] [PubMed]

198. Vaziri, N.D. Epidemic of iron overload in dialysis population caused by intravenous iron products: A plea for moderation. *Am. J. Med.* **2012**, *125*, 951–952. [CrossRef] [PubMed]

199. Nissenson, A.R.; Berns, J.S.; Sakiewicz, P.; Ghaddar, S.; Moore, G.M.; Schleicher, R.B.; Seligman, P.A. Clinical evaluation of heme iron polypeptide: Sustaining a response to rHuEPO in hemodialysis patients. *Am. J. Kidney Dis.* **2003**, *42*, 325–330. [CrossRef]

200. Tanemoto, M.; Ishimoto, Y.; Saito, H. Oral low-dose ferric citrate is a useful iron source for hyperphosphatemic hemodialysis patients: A case series. *Blood Purif.* **2017**, *43*, 97–100. [CrossRef] [PubMed]

201. Pandey, R.; Daloul, R.; Coyne, D.W. Iron treatment strategies in dialysis-dependent CKD. *Semin. Nephrol.* **2016**, *36*, 105–111. [CrossRef] [PubMed]

202. Malovrh, M.; Hojs, N.; Premru, V. The influence of need-based, continuous, low-dose iron replacement on hemoglobin levels in hemodialysis patients treated with erythropoiesis-stimulating agents. *Artif. Organs* **2011**, *35*, 63–68. [CrossRef] [PubMed]

203. Deira, J.; González-Sanchidrián, S.; Polanco, S.; Cebrián, C.; Jiménez, M.; Marín, J.; Gómez-Martino, J.R.; Fernández-Pereira, L.; Tabernero, J. Very low doses of direct intravenous iron in each session as maintenance therapy in hemodialysis patients. *Ren. Fail.* **2016**, *38*, 1076–1081. [CrossRef] [PubMed]

204. Schiesser, D.; Binet, I.; Tsinalis, D.; Dickenmann, M.; Keusch, G.; Schmidli, M.; Ambühl, P.M.; Lüthi, L.; Wüthrich, R.P. Weekly low-dose treatment with intravenous iron sucrose maintains iron status and decreases epoetin requirement in iron-replete haemodialysis patients. *Nephrol. Dial. Transplant.* **2006**, *21*, 2841–2845. [CrossRef] [PubMed]

205. Strauss, W.E.; Dahl, N.V.; Li, Z.; Lau, G.; Allen, L.F. Ferumoxytol versus iron sucrose treatment: A post-hoc analysis of randomized controlled trials in patients with varying renal function and iron deficiency anemia. *BMC Hematol.* **2016**, *16*, 20. [CrossRef] [PubMed]

206. Rath, T.; Florschütz, K.; Kalb, K.; Rothenpieler, U.; Schletter, J.; Seeger, W.; Zinn, S. Low-molecular-weight iron dextran in the management of renal anaemia in patients on haemodialysis-the IDIRA Study. *Nephron Clin. Pract.* **2010**, *114*, c81–c88. [CrossRef] [PubMed]

207. Gupta, A.; Lin, V.; Guss, C.; Pratt, R.; Ikizler, T.A.; Besarab, A. Ferric pyrophosphate citrate administered via dialysate reduces erythropoiesis-stimulating agent use and maintains hemoglobin in hemodialysis patients. *Kidney Int.* **2015**, *88*, 1187–1194. [CrossRef] [PubMed]

208. Ferrari, P.; Mallon, D.; Trinder, D.; Olynyk, J.K. Pentoxifylline improves haemoglobin and interleukin-6 levels in chronic kidney disease. *Nephrology (Carlton)* **2010**, *15*, 344–349. [CrossRef] [PubMed]

209. Pergola, P.E.; Spinowitz, B.S.; Hartman, C.S.; Maroni, B.J.; Haase, V.H. Vadadustat, a novel oral HIF stabilizer, provides effective anemia treatment in nondialysis-dependent chronic kidney disease. *Kidney Int.* **2016**, *90*, 1115–1122. [CrossRef] [PubMed]

210. Martin, E.R.; Smith, M.T.; Maroni, B.J.; Zuraw, Q.C.; deGoma, E.M. Clinical trial of vadadustat in patients with anemia secondary to stage 3 or 4 chronic kidney disease. *Am. J. Nephrol.* **2017**, *45*, 380–388. [CrossRef] [PubMed]

211. Besarab, A.; Provenzano, R.; Hertel, J.; Zabaneh, R.; Klaus, S.J.; Lee, T.; Leong, R.; Hemmerich, S.; Yu, K.H.; Neff, T.B. Randomized placebo-controlled dose-ranging and pharmacodynamics study of roxadustat (FG-4592) to treat anemia in nondialysis-dependent chronic kidney disease (NDD-CKD) patients. *Nephrol. Dial. Transplant.* **2015**, *30*, 1665–1673. [CrossRef] [PubMed]

212. Besarab, A.; Chernyavskaya, E.; Motylev, I.; Shutov, E.; Kumbar, L.M.; Gurevich, K.; Chan, D.T.; Leong, R.; Poole, L.; Zhong, M.; et al. Roxadustat (FG-4592): Correction of anemia in incident dialysis patients. *J. Am. Soc. Nephrol.* **2016**, *27*, 1225–1233. [CrossRef] [PubMed]

213. Brigandi, R.A.; Johnson, B.; Oei, C.; Westerman, M.; Olbina, G.; de Zoysa, J.; Roger, S.D.; Sahay, M.; Cross, N.; McMahon, L.; et al. A novel hypoxia-inducible factor-prolyl hydroxylase inhibitor (GSK1278863) for anemia in CKD: A 28-day, phase 2a randomized trial. *Am. J. Kidney Dis.* **2016**, *67*, 861–871. [CrossRef] [PubMed]

214. Kaysen, G.A. Biochemistry and biomarkers of inflamed patients: Why look, what to assess. *Clin. J. Am. Soc. Nephrol.* **2009**, *4* (Suppl. 1), S56–S63. [CrossRef]

215. Hsu, P.Y.; Lin, C.L.; Yu, C.C.; Chien, C.C.; Hsiau, T.G.; Sun, T.H.; Huang, L.M.; Yang, C.W. Ultrapure dialysate improves iron utilization and erythropoietin response in chronic hemodialysis patients—A prospective cross-over study. *J. Nephrol.* **2004**, *17*, 693–700. [PubMed]

216. Sarafidis, P.A.; Rumjon, A.; MacLaughlin, H.L.; Macdougall, I.C. Obesity and iron deficiency in chronic kidney disease: The putative role of hepcidin. *Nephrol. Dial. Transplant.* **2012**, *27*, 50–57. [CrossRef] [PubMed]

217. Sanad, M.; Osman, M.; Gharib, A. Obesity modulate serum hepcidin and treatment outcome of iron deficiency anemia in children: A case control study. *Ital. J. Pediatr.* **2011**, *37*, 34. [CrossRef] [PubMed]

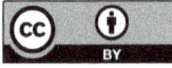

MDPI

St. Alban-Anlage 66

4052 Basel

Switzerland

Tel. +41 61 683 77 34

Fax +41 61 302 89 18

www.mdpi.com

Nutrients Editorial Office

E-mail: nutrients@mdpi.com

www.mdpi.com/journal/nutrients

www.ingramcontent.com/pod-product-compliance
Lightning Source LLC
Chambersburg PA
CBHW051846210326
41597CB00033B/5791